The Home Health Handbook

A Preliminary Guide to Self-Help and Rural Medicine

third edition

THE HOME HEALTH HANDBOOK

Written by

Chris Allen	John Long
Joan Babbott	Ginny Lyman
Elizabeth Baer	Scott Lyman
Michael Beale	James Marmar
Oris Blackwell	Peter Marsh
Consumers Union	James McCarthy
Stuart Copans	Karen McCarthy
Ed Croumey	Barbara McIntosh
Lynne Curtis	Judith Miner
Susan Donnis	Milo Moore
David Giannuzzi	Francis Murray
Steve Goldstein	Sherry Oake
Charles Houston	David Osgood
Jeannie	Charles Phillips
Lleni Jeffrey	Charles Poser
Michael Kupersmith	William Poser
Arie Lindsay	Jim Salander
Owen Lindsay	John Starr
George Little	Janet Young

Edited by Stu Copans and David Osgood

The Stephen Greene Press
Brattleboro, Vermont

Both the first and second editions of this handbook were printed with the support of the following individuals and organizations. These individuals and organizations support the concept of a medical self-help handbook.

All medical information and editorial opinions in the handbook, however, are solely the responsibility of the authors and the editors.

We thank the following for their support and faith:

    Dr. Joan Babbott
    Red Clover Commune
    Dr. Robert Siedman
    Dr. Charles Poser
    Burlington Council of Churches
    Vermont Ecumenical Council
    St. Paul's Cathedral
    Department of Community Medicine, University of Vermont Medical School
    Burlington Ecumenical Action Ministry

Third Edition 1972

Copyright © 1972 by the Burlington Ecumenical Action Ministry
First and second editions copyright © 1971 by Stu Copans

All rights reserved. No part of this book may be reproduced without written permission from the publisher, except by a reviewer who may quote brief passages or reproduce illustrations in a review; nor may any part of this book be reproduced, stored in a retrieval system, or transmitted in any form or by any means electronic, mechanical, photocopying, recording, or other, without written permission from the publisher.

This book has been produced in the United States of America. It was composed by the Stephen Greene Press, printed and bound by The Colonial Press.
It is published by the Stephen Greene Press,
Brattleboro, Vermont 05301.

Library of Congress Catalog Card Number: 72-90930
International Standard Book Number: 0-8289-0175-9

CONTENTS

Foreword ... vii
Preface ... viii
Publisher's Note ... x
Introduction ... xii
THE COMMUNE MEDIC'S GUIDE   *Oris Blackwell, Charles Houston*   1
COMMON EMERGENCIES GUIDE   *James McCarthy, Charles Poser,*
                             William Poser, Susan Donnis   31
IMPORTANT MEDICAL HISTORY EVERYONE SHOULD KNOW ABOUT HIMSELF   50
FIRST AID FOR WOUNDS AND BURNS   *Consumers Union*   51
EXPOSURE AND WIND CHILL EFFECT   *Charles Houston*   55
FIRST AID FOR POISONS   58
POISONS   *Susan Donnis*   59
SANITATION FOR SMALL RURAL GROUPS   *Owen Lindsay*   64
SAFE CANNING (AND FREEZING)   *Arie Lindsay*   82
HEALTH AND NUTRITION   *Linda Fried, Michael Beale*   89
DENTAL HEALTH   *John Long*   119
A PEOPLE'S HERBAL   *Janet Young, Elizabeth Baer*   122
DRUGS   *Lynne Curtis, Ed Croumey, James Marmar,*
          Jim Salander, David Gianuzzi, Francis Murray   136
STRESS   *Barbara McIntosh*   151
MENTAL HEALTH CLINICS IN VERMONT   *Karen McCarthy*   157
PSYCHOLOGICAL PROBLEMS   *Steve Goldstein*   160
WOMEN'S HEALTH: ANATOMY   *Chris Allen, Ginny Lyman*   163
                PHYSIOLOGY   *Ginny Lyman*   170
                A WOMAN'S EXPERIENCE OF
                    PREGNANCY AND CHILDBIRTH   *Ginny Lyman*   173
                PREGNANCY AND CHILDBIRTH   *Stuart Copans*   182
                HOME DELIVERY OF BABIES   *John Starr*   195
                HOME EXPERIENCE OF CHILDBIRTH   *Barbara McIntosh*   201
                RECORDING A BIRTH   203
                BREASTFEEDING   *Judith Miner*   204
BIRTH CONTROL   *Lleni Jeffrey*   209
ABORTION   *Ginny Lyman*   219
A WORD ABOUT ROUTINE PEDIATRIC CARE   *George Little*   223
COMMUNAL DISEASES   *Sherry Oake*   228
VENEREAL DISEASES   *Chris Allen, Barbara McIntosh, Peter Marsh*   231

v

HEPATITIS *Charles Phillips*	236
SAFE USE OF FARM EQUIPMENT *Scott Lyman*	239
HOW TO MINIMIZE FIRE DANGER *Owen Lindsay, Milo Moore*	242
SIMPLE BURIAL *David Osgood*	248
BACK TO THE LAND: POINT *Jeannie—a Farmer's Wife*	252
BACK TO THE LAND: COUNTERPOINT *Joan Babbott*	254
VERMONT LAWS *Michael Kupersmith*	255
SOME HUMAN RESOURCES IN VERMONT	261
APPENDIX I: A FEW THINGS YOU CAN DO AS A BEGINNING	266
APPENDIX II: EMERGENCY CHILDBIRTH	267
APPENDIX III: UNIVERSAL DONOR CONTRACT	279
BIBLIOGRAPHY	280
INDEX	283

FOREWORD

Slowly we are learning not to be dominated by our technology. We are learning once again to fix our own cars, grow our own food, build our own houses, and to create our own culture.

Part of the revolution—the part that is perhaps the slowest in coming—is learning to take care of our own bodies. Some of this is the fault of physicians—who work so hard to become doctors that it's difficult for them to give up some of their prerogatives, even those that others could be taught to exercise—but some of the fault lies with each of us. As individuals committed to the goals of the revolution, if we continue to smoke cigarettes, fail to learn about sewage systems or how to combat venereal disease, and ignore the principles of adequate nutrition, then we destroy both ourselves and the revolution through our ignorance or carelessness.

Compulsive cleanliness is bourgeois. . . .
Sanitation is a revolutionary necessity."
            -Che

PREFACE

The first edition of this Handbook was put together by some people in Vermont for their brothers and sisters in Vermont. We scraped together some money for printing, and we gave away most of the copies we printed. We saved 25 copies to send out in case other people wanted copies of the Handbook, but we soon found ourselves with no copies left, and one or two requests for copies arriving each day.

The second was still printed by mimeograph, and was beautifully printed and bound for us by Chuck Alberts of Burlington. It was financed and distributed by the Burlington Ecumenical Action Ministry (BEAM).

This is the third edition.

We believe very much in this Handbook. It has been revised and improved twice already.

We are still open, however, to any criticism or suggestions.

We know the Handbook will never be finished, complete, or sufficient and we need people's criticisms and comments to help it keep evolving. Please write to us c/o the Stephen Greene Press and tell us what you like, what you disagree with, what seems wrong to you from your experience, and what you think we should include in the next printing. They will forward your letters to us. If you want an answer, send a stamped, self-addressed envelope.

When it became clear that BEAM could not handle the demand for our Handbook, we had to pick a publisher.

We picked the Stephen Greene Press for several reasons:

1. It's a small publishing house.
2. It's located in Vermont, which is our home, and a poor state.
3. Stephen Greene has agreed to let us work with people who are interested in putting out handbooks for their own groups, and to allow others, upon written request, to use reasonable amounts of the Handbook for a reasonable fee (which may turn out to be nothing), provided their purposes generally agree with ours. The Stephen Greene Press will forward the written request to us, we and they will discuss it, and together we'll arrive at what we all consider a reasonable course of action.
4. They have agreed to let us revise articles after each printing, to add to the handbook after each printing (that's why Notes pages appear frequently throughout the book: so we can expand the text where necessary, and so readers can really take notes and make the Handbook even more useful to themselves), and to totally restructure the handbook every two years (if we think it needs it).
5. They seem to understand our vision of the handbook as a model and continuously evolving project rather than as a completed book or a finished product; and we have some understanding of which revisions are easy, and which involve a lot of work for the printers.

PREFACE

Although we have made some changes to make the Handbook appeal to a more general audience, we're still committed to it as a model for small groups interested in developing their own health care systems.

We'd like to see hundreds of small groups of people working with their local physicians and nurses to put together small handbooks in their own language dealing with their own special medical problems.

We'd like to see people do more than just buy our handbook, or even put out their own. We'd like to see them start to learn about their own bodies—how they work, and how to care for them.

We'd like to see physicians teaching medical self-help courses, and we'd like to see communities getting together to develop their own health care systems.

Many of the people in hospitals and most of the people in nursing homes could be cared for in their local communities if the people in the community shared the work and the expense.

Many of the people who wait in physicians' offices or emergency rooms for medical care could be seen by a community medic, and would receive quicker, more relaxed, and probably better medical care.

It is time that people began to explore these possibilities, either by themselves, or together with interested physicians and nurses.

One of the churches connected with BEAM is beginning to develop its own health care system, and people who are interested can write to BEAM at 152 Church St., Burlington, Vt. 05401 for more information about such systems. We've included an appendix with some suggestions for people who want to go beyond the Handbook. Hopefully many of you will.

All profits derived from the sale of the Handbook will be spent in the area of alternative health care delivery. None of the authors or editors will make a personal profit on the book, and each of the contributors will have a say in how the money is used.

Peace, Joy, Good Health

PUBLISHER'S NOTE

Elsewhere the authors of this book have explained why they want to have us publish it. For our part, we do so because we feel that it is a good book, and because we believe that the stated aims of the authors—namely, to help people to keep themselves from getting sick, and, if sick, to help them get well with a minimum of dependence upon the doctor—deserve a wider audience than they have had to date.

Although the authors of *The Home Health Handbook* have chosen not to present their academic and professional qualifications here, the experience of twenty-three of them as doctors, nurses, public health workers, and pharmacists—and of all of the authors as workers in either a lay or professional effort to keep people well—makes them, in our judgment, eminently worth listening to.

INTRODUCTION

Medical care in the United States is rapidly approaching a crossroad. Prior to the early 1900's, when strict licensing of physicians and control over the quality of medical education was instituted, almost everyone in the U.S. had access to medical care, although in many cases treatment obtained was somewhat primitive.

Since that time medicine has gradually become sanctified. It has been moved out of the home, taken away from the country doctor, and locked in its ivory towers. Medical empires have been built, and they send unusual patients and young physicians back and forth like feudal emissaries, only rarely letting a physician escape to return to the country and practice medicine.

An ideology has been created and spread which states that we are all in imminent danger of disease or death, and only the physician or the specialist can sense the unseen danger and protect us. The invisible worm is present everywhere, but he can only be seen with the aid of magical devices, x-rays, sigmoidoscopes, blood tests, etc.

Most proposals to improve medical care in the United States start with this ideology as a basic premise, and then propose to provide more super-specialists, more miraculous machines, and more accessibility to these.

The war companies, fearing an impending end to the arms race, have already begun tooling up to make cardiac monitors, telemeters, and a large variety of other magical medical machines which are expensive, rapidly become obsolete, and are as easily justified to the American public as ICBM's and antimissile missiles. (It is no longer "stop the Chinese communists before they get to San Francisco" but instead "a cure for cancer before your grandchildren are born.")

Both these companies and the medical empires, seeing a chance to expand their areas of control as well as their profits, are working to get a government program set up that will increase their power.

None of the proposed national health care plans talks about nutrition, sanitation, decent housing, pollution or education. Prevention is not a concern of the politicians, and is positively anathema to the medical empires. They all talk about yearly testing and ignore the fact that several studies suggest that these yearly screening tests are of little or no benefit and of great expense. They do not talk about school lunch programs, day care centers, improved housing, or the overuse of insecticides. None of the present proposals even mentions the education of people to understand their bodies, and to start to take care of themselves.

The present proposals for a national health plan would do little more than centralize control of all medical resources in the hands of a few large medical empires, which would be under the direct financial domination of the federal government. Although they ostensibly are designed to improve health care of the poor, they would simply serve to strengthen the medical empires, which we already know are insensitive to the health needs of the poor.

There is no question that medical specialists, fancy machines, and medical centers are occasionally necessary; they should not, however, be in control of medical care, but should simply be one of the available resources to be called upon when needed.

Instead of strengthening the medical empires, instead of putting the federal government in control of all medical resources, instead of creating a federal monopoly on health care, a program could be set up to give more people access to medical resources, to educate people so they could begin to take care of themselves, and to begin looking at the nutritionally deficient foods, the environmental pollution, and the societal stresses responsible for much of the poor health in America today.

In an experimental program in the Midwest, 500 telephone numbers were created which a physician can call for information about 500 different problems related to care of cancer patients. At each number is a 4 to 5 minute lecture dealing with the specific topic assigned to that number. Each physician in the area has a list of the 500 problems and their assigned telephone numbers as well as the name and number of a resource person to call for further information.

There is no reason why this approach could not be used to make medical information available to the general public, both as a means of education, and as a means of providing people with basic resources but giving them control over the decisions affecting their lives.

Previously, when medicine was exclusively diagnosis-oriented, such an approach would have been unthinkable; for it was felt that unless you knew all the possible diagnoses that could cause a problem, you couldn't hope to take care of it.

As a result of the pioneering work of Weed with the problem-oriented medical record, it is becoming clear that you can deal with a medical problem on any level of sophistication as long as you have resources which deal with the problem at that level, and have someone available who can work on a more sophisticated level if necessary. The article on child care by George Little is probably the best example of this problem-oriented approach, and hopefully this approach will be applied to more problems by the next edition of this handbook.

Hopefully in the near future there will be an increasing number of courses and publications, formal or informal, designed to teach people about their bodies, and about taking care of themselves.

Physicians are now faced with a choice between forming an unholy alliance with the federal government and big business, or beginning to teach people how to avoid illness and how to take care of themselves.

Hopefully, with the help of the people, they will make the right choice.

The organization of this handbook reflects both its history and its commitment to preventive medicine and to educating people so they can become medically self-reliant. The original idea for this handbook grew out of a meeting in San Francisco of people interested in medical problems associated with communal living. Several of the articles grew out of a series of small meetings in which people from several Vermont communes came together to discuss common health problems and ways of dealing with them.

A number of the articles were written as part of a course set up to train people from

INTRODUCTION

communes to deal with many of their own health problems. Two of the most important articles in the handbook ("Stress" and "Communal Diseases") were written by students in the course.

A lot of great people helped in the production of this handbook. Among them were:

Chuck Alberts	Debbie Ordahl
Peggy Davis	Ellie Schufter
Ann Ellis	Sarah Stahl
Patt Hennessy	Jack Mayer
Jerri Lamell	Adrienne
Cindy Lane	Judy Ingalls

Hopefully, this handbook will serve as a small step towards the day when the people will think like physicians, and physicians act like people.

It is dedicated to three who already do:

Allen Barbour
Mary Wertheim
Michael Moynihan

THE COMMUNE MEDICS GUIDE

The Constitution of this Republic should make special provision for Medical Freedom as well as Religious Freedom . . . To restrict the art of healing to one class of men and deny equal privileges to others will constitute the Bastille of medical science. All such laws are un-American and despotic. They are fragments of monarchy and have no place in a Republic.

—Benjamin Rush, M.D., Surgeon General of the Continental Army of the United States; Signer of the Declaration of Independence

The best way to deal with sickness is to prevent it. To do this, especially in communes, requires a consciousness of what causes sickness and of basic sanitary requirements. Prevention is a continuing task and can be dealt with in two ways. The simplest way is to appoint a member interested in health to act as a medic, and assume responsibilities for sanitation, preventive medicine, and education of the other commune members. Another alternative for communes opposed to any specialization would be to have weekly preventive medicine meetings to discuss any sanitary problems or sickness which occurred during the previous week.

The following guide was written for communes, but it would be a simple matter for a family or a small town without a physician to appoint someone as medic. Although medics could not prescribe certain medicines, and although they could not legally perform certain procedures, they can still do a great deal. This is particularly true in the areas so often ignored by physicians, who are forced by their workloads to practice symptomatic medicine and who cannot inspect homes for unsanitary conditions, visit people to talk about their diets or drinking water, talk with people about the stresses of their present life-style, and alternative ways of living.

If you want to, you can start to take care of your own health. Do it!

I. PREVENTIVE MEDICINE, PUBLIC AND ENVIRONMENTAL HEALTH

   A. Role of Commune Medic. The overall responsibility for the general health in the community rests with the community. The community also is responsible to refrain from any practices that would cause health hazard or discomfort to neighboring communities. Both of these community responsibilities rest more directly with the commune medic. The medic must aid the commune in protecting the health of its members and in maintaining a healthful environment. The medic must plan and recommend health measures and programs that preserve and promote the well-being of commune members and surrounding communities.

B. The extent of involvement of the medic in the prevention of illness and the promotion of good health will depend on many factors.

   1. The background, understanding, and experience of the medic in preventive programs. With or without such background the medic should seek consultation and cooperation of local health specialists (physicians, nurses, sanitarians, etc. —check the "resources" list).

   2. Prevailing conditions of commune (i.e. location, climate, housing, feeding patterns, number of people, surrounding area, etc.).

   3. As a minimum the commune medic should teach all members about individual and community actions that prevent disease and promote well-being. The medic should also plan, supervise, and, in some cases, personally carry out preventive measures.

C. Prevention of illness and promotion of health falls into two general categories: (a) Those involving individual health status such as specific immunizations, routine physical check-ups, and the prompt, proper diagnosis and treatment if illness occurs; and (b) Those having to do with environmental factors as they effect health.

   1. Individual health status must, to a large extent, involve the physician and the nurse. This in no way relieves the individual and the community of responsibility here. Nutrition, for example, which is of great importance to health status, can usually be well managed by the individuals (with care). Much of this book deals with concerns in this category. When problems arise, or preferably before, contact local health agency resources for help (see "See Human Resources in Vermont").

   2. Environmental factors that effect health are quite rightfully receiving increased attention. A number of the articles in this book deal with environmental problems. At this point a list will perhaps serve as a guide to thinking of whole problems. The largest group of environmental concerns may be seen as part of the physical environment—e.g.:

      a) air pollution (including smoking)
      b) water pollution—water supplies
      c) sewage and garbage disposal
      d) houses and living places
      e) accident prevention
      f) noise pollution

      Other concerns relate more to the biological aspect of the environment—e.g.:

      a) rodent and insect control
      b) communicable disease control
      c) food hygiene and food protection

Still other concerns are more related to the social aspects of the environment—e.g.:

- a) motivation of individuals and groups to deal with the environment in a way that preserves and promotes good health
- b) appropriate support for research, education, and legislation re: the environmental concerns
- c) the inter-relationship of environment and mental health and well-being

3. Obviously, the aspects of the total environment—physical, biological, and social—as listed above, can not be sharply separated. They are *closely* interrelated. It sometimes helps to see the whole if we can for analysis sake visualize the parts.

II. FOOD HYGIENE AND THE COMMUNE MEDIC

Care in the selection, use, and preparation of foods and liquids can make the difference between an effective brother or sister and a medical casualty.

- A. Milk and dairy products: Milk and dairy products from sick cows should not be used for human consumption. All milk and dairy products should be stored under refrigeration.

- B. Meats
   1. Beef: Beef should be fresh, come from healthy animals which are inspected at the time of slaughter, should be handled to protect it against contamination from insects and filth, and should be transported and stored in the most sanitary manner possible. Following the slaughtering and dressing of the animal, the meat should be consumed on the same day unless refrigeration facilities are available or the meat is to be cured. Only thoroughly cooked meat should be eaten. If meat remains red in the center, it has not been thoroughly cooked.
   2. Pork: The rules for freshness, health, and cleanliness are the same as for beef. The cardinal rule for pork is "cook thoroughly and eat no pink pork." Only thorough cooking prevents trichinosis.
   3. Poultry and eggs: Should also be thoroughly cooked. The general rules provided for beef and pork should be followed.
   4. Fish, sea foods, and fresh water life: Fish should be thoroughly cooked before eating.
      - a) Indications of early spoilage of fish:
         - (1) Sunken eyes
         - (2) Flesh pits with pressure
         - (3) Sticky surfaces
         - (4) Scales removed with ease
         - (5) Off odor at the gills and inside the body cavity

b) A fresh fish has:
   (1) Prominent eyes and firm flesh
   (2) Surface will be slimy and scales are not easily removed
   (3) Gills are bright red in color
   (4) No off-odor at the gills or inside the body cavity

C. Food Sanitation Checklist

1. All food should be wholesome and safe (i.e., from sources known to be disease and toxin free).
2. All persons involved in food transport storage, preparation, and serving to be free from communicable disease, to have clean clothes and well-washed hands. They should also be aware of the basics of food hygiene.
3. Adequate provision for storing readily perishable food (milk, eggs, cheese, butter, fish, and meat) at or below 45 deg. F.
4. No rodents or insects should be in the storage, preparation, or serving areas.
5. All surfaces of tables, equipment, and utensils that come in contact with food, either cooked or raw, must be kept clean.
6. All solids (garbage) and liquid (dishwater) should be disposed of properly (underground is usually best).
7. Adequate and safe water supply.
8. No toxic or harmful substances should be allowed in food storage or preparation area.

III. HEALTH OF ANIMALS IN COMMUNE

The Commune Medic should assume an important role in maintaining the health of farm animals and pets in the community. The general practices that tend to keep animals well include:

1. proper, clean food in adequate quantity
2. clean, fresh water in adequate quantity
3. clean living quarters with protection from severe weather
4. careful handling to avoid injury
5. if any animal shows evidence of illness (listness, lame, feverish) a qualified person (usually a veternarian) should be consulted
6. specific immunization programs are recommended for Bang's Disease (undulant fever, infectious abortion) in cows, distemper in dogs and cats, rabies in dogs, cats, pet skunks, etc. The local veterinarian should be consulted.

Poor health in animals is of real concern for many reasons. The Humane Society's contention that animals in our care should be well treated is valid. There are good economic reasons such

THE COMMUNE MEDIC'S GUIDE

as loss of food source. Perhaps of more critical importance, however, is the fact that many diseases of animals are transmissible to man with serious results. Some of the more common of these that might be seen in the New England area are listed below.

COWS

Bang's Disease: (undulant fever, infectious abortion, brucellosis): organisms responsible shed into milk—if infected raw (unpasturized) milk is used, person acquires the disease.

Prevention: "Bangs free" cows (the Vet can test) and/or pasturization of all milk (145 deg. F. for 30 minutes or 165 deg. F. for 12 seconds—both with quick cooling to below 50 deg. F.).

Tuberculosis (Bovine or Human type): organisms shed into milk if ingested many lead to intestinal or osteo tuberculosis.

Prevention: "T.B. free" cows (the Vet can test) and/or pasturization of all milk.

Mastitis: an infection of one or more quarters of the udder with any of several bacteria. Usually staphylococcus or streptococcus. Either of these can cause serious disease in man. Organisms are shed with milk.

Prevention: this infection is usually "given" to the cow by man during the milking—from infected persons (sore throat, bad "cold", pimples, boils, infected cuts); from unwashed dirty hands; from dirty equipment, especially milking machines, and each of these sources are a greater hazard to the cow if there is rough handling of teats and udder and/or "over milking". Mastitis can also be acquired from dirty quarters, pens, and even pasture. Prior to milking (either by hand or machine) the udders should be washed with clean warm water and a mild soap and rinsed with clean water. The "fore milk" from each quarter should be milked out into a "strip cup" (any cup covered with a fine wire mesh). Abnormal mastitis milk will show up as "flaky"; i.e., it will leave clumps of cellular material—white flakes—on the wire mesh. When a cow is found to have mastitis it should be treated (preferably by a vet) with an appropriate antibiotic. Milk from cows with mastitis should not be used.

CHICKENS—poultry in general

Salmonellosis: Young chickens usually die from the disease. Some survive to be old, sick chickens and spread the disease to other chicks and man through infection on eggs and through improper handling of chickens used for food. Up to 20 percent of raw chicken meat in the retail market has been found to contain salmonella organisms. In man the disease may vary from a mild gastro-enteritis (diarrhea and vomiting) lasting a few hours to a severe debilitating disease leading to death. The latter course is more common in the very young and the old.

Prevention: Get chicks or chickens from reliable disease-free sources; don't crowd in pens; feed whole grains or salmonella-free mixes. Cook all eggs—do not allow raw chicken meat to contact (directly or indirectly) food that is not going to be cooked—salad vegetables, for example, or cooked food that will not be further cooked.

PIGS

Swine diseases that can effect man include erysipelas, leptospirosis, brucellosis, and tuberculosis, but these diseases are quite rare in the New England area. Trichinosis is caused by eating meat containing live trichina worms. Many animals from horny-tail lizards to bear and man, may contract trichinosis, but swine are the most implicated in transmission of the disease to man.

Prevention: Do not feed uncooked garbage to hogs. Thoroughly cook all pork (to at least 137 deg. F. in all parts) or by freezing (to 0 deg. F.) for several weeks. Salting and curing meat may kill the larva but thorough cooking is still indicated.

DOGS AND CATS

These pets may harbor disease that can infect man; most of these are intestinal worms that are eaten or inhaled by man. The animal feces may be eaten directly by children (a two-year old baby died recently in New Jersey of a massive intestinal worm infestation which followed the eating of a dog turd from in front of her house!) It may be advisable to de-worm these pets on a regular basis—consult the local vet. In any event the feces should be considered infectious and disposed of accordingly.

Rabies is a serious disease that all warm blooded animals seem to be susceptible to. Dog bites are the major source of rabies for man, but cats, skunks, bats may also transmit rabies. Pets should receive anti-rabies shots regularly. The vaccination lasts 2½ years, with annual boosters recommended in areas where the disease is especially prevalent.

IV. LICE AND OTHER INSECT PESTS:

Insects have profoundly affected history. Locusts cause famine, flies spread epidemics of cholera and other diseases, lice spread typhus, fleas spread plague, and mosquitoes carry malaria to hundreds of millions of people. We're blessed in our country with relative freedom from insect-borne disease, but there's enough about to make it necessary to be careful.

Besides, being lousy is uncomfortable.

Lice are common where sanitation is poor and human contact great. Lice are classified as head, body, and public lice depending on their preferred homes. Lice are small—about the size of a pinhead; they cause itching and scratching and they transmit certain virus diseases. Lice can't survive for more than a day without human blood, but as long as they are on you they'll get blood and lay tiny white eggs which hatch and spread on you as their planet. Lice in long hair are most unpleasant and hard to get rid of; ditto for beards. Pubic lice (crabs) are a specially irritating variety; shaving pubic and axillary hair is easier than shaving the head, but is pretty uncomfortable—and won't cure the condition. You need to get rid of the nits and lice on clothes—by washing and sunning and keeping away from human contact for a couple of days (to destroy the nits). You need to get rid of your own nits by a pesticide

(DDT powder is best but of course ecologically bad), by kerosene (ouch), or by Lindane or Chlordane ointments. You have to shave the head to really get rid of a bad case. Remember, the nits can be in your bedding—and usually are—so stay away from that bedding till it has been thoroughly sunned, brushed, aired, and inspected.

Fleas from dogs and cats bite people, too, but not often or badly, and are usually not a human parasite. They can infect your furniture and bedding and make life miserable. Get them off the dog and they'll stop bothering you.

Ticks are not much of a problem in New England, but can infect animals, get into woodwork, and they do transmit disease (Rocky Mountain Spotted Fever is not rare in southern Massachusetts), so keep an eye on your dogs and cats, and on yourself. Pull off the tick, or better, bring a cigarette (lighted) near him and he'll drop off complete with head. Main consideration here is inspection and early management.

Bedbugs can be a terrible problem in old substandard housing. They get into the woodwork, under plaster covered with paper, and especially into bedding. Though bedbugs don't carry disease, they leave a characteristic row of bites—three to six little itching red bumps an inch or two apart in a curving line on arms, legs, body, or face. Bedbugs characteristically bite, fill up with blood, and leave in a few minutes, so the sleeper may never see the biter, only the bite. Fumigation of bedding and house is essential if there's much infestation: burning sulfur for a few hours with all openings sealed will work; HCN Discoids produce very deadly hydrocyanic gas and *should be used only under professional supervision;* it's the most effective. Bedbugs have gotten used to DDT, so this is no longer fully effective. Bedding may have to be burned. Bedbugs sleep over in the day time, in bedding and woodwork—and are seldom found on people.

Mites belong to a large family, some of whose members transmit disease (mouse mites carried an epidemic of fever in Kew Gardens some years ago), but most of which are merely annoying. The worst diseases are Tsutsugamushi disease (not in the USA) and Scrub Typhus, also not here. But the itching from the female who has burrowed into the skin between the fingers, in the elbows and armpits can be intolerable. It's hard to make the diagnosis, except by suspicion, but often a rash appears—around the waist, in the armpits and groin, which is a secondary reaction to *scabies,* because it does not occur where the burrows are most common. This should help settle the diagnosis, but best of all is to explore the red itching bump between the fingers with a sterile needle and dig out the ugly little beast. Sulfur ointment (10% sulfur in Vaseline) or an emulsion of Benzyl Benzoate rubbed into all the possible infected areas usually cures after one application—but a second treatment is wise. The main thing is to get cleaned up—another argument for frequent soap and water and clean clothes. The itch of scabies is almost as bad as from chiggers.

Chiggers are little red mites that also burrow into the skin and cause a reddish bump, usually on the legs or buttocks since the bugs get on from the ground and don't migrate much. Camphorated oil rubbed into the affected area will help. Chiggers don't cause much disease in this part of the world, but they can and do result in secondary infection from scratching.

Cockroaches are a nuisance, spoiling food, cluttering up the house, scaring the babies. They give off a foul odor and have been shown to carry filth diseases, such as Salmonella food poisoning, from place to place. Get rid of them by cleaning up. Cockroaches are a sign of bad kitchen habits and it's these that lead to diseases from spoiled food, dirt, and from other insects.

Flies don't cause diseases either, but they certainly do carry bacteria and viruses—like from a fresh stool alive with cholera onto your dinner, or from the urine of a patient with hepatitis onto your drinking glass. Fly control depends on getting rid of natural breeding and feeding places—by covering the manure, liming a pit privy or covering with dirt, by keeping food undercover, refrigerated, and dishes clean—and above all by proper garbage and waste disposal. Most of the insecticides that kill flies (and house flies are almost immune to DDT and other insecticides) are harmful to our environment. The Vapona strips are just ways of dispensing continuous small amounts of insecticide vapor. They are poisonous and should not be used. Sticky flypaper is a nice old-fashioned way of getting rid of flies—safe and neat; you can make your own with honey or molasses. Swatting is what the Chinese did so effectively that the house fly is said to be almost unknown in China, if you can believe that.

Spiders bite. The *black widow* causes terrible abdominal pains and cramps and, rarely, death; you need to get a doctor; the spider is black and has an orange hourglass on her underside. She is usually found in piles of wood or lumber or other rummaging around places. The *brown recluse* spider's bite is an unhealing wound in some people. The spider is brown with a fiddle head pattern on its back. It stays in closets, cellars, and other places where it isn't disturbed. Several harmless spiders look a lot like this one. But most spiders are really helpful —killing and enjoying lots of more bothersome insects—so in general encourage them, especially the large wolf spider.

TREATMENT FOR LICE

Choose any of these medications (available at a drug store) and follow the directions; some are much easier than others.

    A-200 "Pyrinate" liquid

    Kwell Shampoo, Cream or Lotion

    Xylol 15 to 20% in Petrolatum or Aquaphor

    Topocide (Benzyl Benzoate Compound)

Bathe and shampoo often. Comb hair with a fine-toothed comb.

Lice and nits get on clothing and bedding and then reattack you.

Hang clothes and bedding outdoors for 24—48 hours. Lice cannot live for more than 24 hours without blood to feed on.

Wear different clothes each day for a while.

Toilet seats and other washable articles should be scrubbed. Medicated shampoo or regular soap can be used.

Medically Important Arthropods	Approximate Duration of Life Cycles at 75 deg. C.			Where Found
Flies i.e., housefly	Egg Larva Pupa Adult	10 5 5 30	hours days days days	Animals or human waste, garbage, grass, decomposing animals, and mud contaminated with organic material.
Mosquitoes i.e., yellow fever mosquito	Egg Larva Pupa Adult	4 10 2 14	days days days days	Standing water which may be found in ponds, tin cans, old tires and tree holes. (A large variety of places and conditions of breeding have been noted.)
Fleas i.e., oriental rat flea	Egg Larva Pupa Adult	7 15 8 365	days days days days	Nests or beds of animals.
Lice i.e., human body lice	Egg Nymph Adult	7 16 30	days days days	Head hair and clothing of humans. Lice cannot exist on a clean human.
Cockroaches i.e., German cockroach	Egg Nymph Adult	30 60 200	days days days	Cracks and crevices which provide warmth, moisture and food such as around water, garbage, and food facilities.
Ticks and Mites	Life cycle completed: 6 weeks to 2 years.			Tall grass, underbrush, animal watering places, and shady rest areas of animals.

V. REVISED SCHEDULE FOR ACTIVE IMMUNIZATION AND TUBERCULIN TESTING OF NORMAL INFANTS AND CHILDREN IN THE UNITED STATES

2 months	DTP[1]	TOPV[2]
4 months	DTP	TOPV
6 months	DTP	TOPV
12 months	(Measles, rubella, and mumps)[3] Tuberculin Test[4]	
18 months	DTP booster	TOPV booster
4–6 years	DTP booster	TOPV booster
10–12 years	DTP booster	

(DTP booster should be repeated at 10-year intervals or as injury demands.)

---

1. DTP: Diphtheria and Tetanus toxoids combined with Pertussis vaccine.
2. TOPV: Trivalent Oral Polio Virus vaccine. The above recommendation is suitable for breast-fed as well as bottle-fed infants.
3. These are available singly, or as double or triple combined vaccines. They should be given as soon after one year as possible. Most health departments will administer without charge.
4. Frequency of repeated TB tests depends on risk of exposure of child and the prevalence of tuberculosis in the population group.

Tetanus toxoid at time of injury: For clean, minor wounds, no booster dose is needed by a fully immunized child unless more than 10 years have elapsed since the last dose.

For contaminated wounds, a booster dose should be given if more than 5 years have elapsed since the last dose.

Other vaccines and biologicals available for special circumstances (travel, exposure, etc.):

Cholera Vaccine (travel to endemic area)
Tetanus Toxoid (after open wounds)
Immune Serum Globulin (intimate household contacts of infectious hepatitis and measles)

Influenza Vaccine (for persons over 65 or persons with chronic illness)
Mumps Vaccine (special circumstances)
Plague Vaccine (special circumstances)
Rabies antiserum—rabies vaccine (exposure)
Smallpox Vaccine (travel to endemic area)
Typhoid Vaccine (travel or special circumstances)
Yellow Fever Vaccine (travel or special circumstances)

The U.S. Public Health Service no longer recommends routine Smallpox vaccination in the United States.

VI. FEATURES OF SOME INFECTIOUS DISEASES

DISEASE	AGENT V=Virus B=Bacteria R=Rickettsia H=Helminth P=Protozoa	TRANSMISSION	INCUBATION PERIOD	ISOLATION	CONTROL	TREATMENT When there is a choice of drug it is indicated by (1)
ADENOVIRUS INFECTION	V	Droplets, contact	2–10 days	None	Immunization	Symptomatic
AMEBIC DYSENTERY	P	Feces, water, food, flies	days–months	None	Carrier control food, sanitation, water	Prescribed antibiotic
ANCYLOSTOMIASIS (hookworm disease)	H	Soil, skin contact	2–10 weeks	None	Sanitary disposal of feces, wearing of shoes	(1)
ANTHRAX	B	Contact, inhalation, ingestion of contaminated animal tissue	1–4 days	of lesions	Sterilization of animal tissue, hides, bristles, etc.	Prescribed antibiotic
ASCARIASIS	H	Feces to mouth	2 months	None	Sanitation, disposal of feces	(1)
BRUCELLOSIS	B	Contact with an infected animal, ingestion of milk, etc.	6–60 days	None	Eradication of disease in animals. Pasteurization	Prescribed antibiotic
CHANCROID	B	Sexual contact	1–10 days	Modified	Prevention of exposure	Prescribed antibiotic
CHICKEN POX	V	Respiratory droplets	2–3 weeks	10 days after exposure until 1 wk. after vesicles appear.	Isolation	Symptomatic
DIPTHERIA	B	Respiratory droplets from cases and corners	2–5 days	Strict until culture negative	Active immunization	Prescribed antibiotic

Features of Some Infectious Diseases - continued

DISEASE	AGENT	TRANSMISSION	INCUBATION	ISOLATION	CONTROL	TREATMENT
DYSENTERY AMEBIC	See "Amebic Dysentery"					
DYSENTERY BACILLARY	B	Infected feces, water, food, flies	1–7 days	Strict until culture negative	Breaking transmission, chain chemotherapy	Prescribed antibiotic
GERMAN MEASLES (Rubella)	V	Respiratory droplets	14–21 days	exclude from school 10 days after exposure	Exposure of girls before childbearing age	Symptomatic. Gamma Globulin immediately after exposure if patient is pregnant
GONORRHEA	B	Contact of mucus membrane with infected pus	1–8 days	Modified	Sex hygiene, treatment of cases	Prescribed antibiotic
GRANULOMA INGUINALE	B	Sexual contact	8–12 weeks	Modified	Sex Hygiene	Prescribed antibiotic
HEPATITIS, INFECTIOUS	V	Fecal contamination. Contact? Water? Shellfish?	15–35 days	Stool isolation	Stool isolation	Symptomatic, high protein diet. Rest
HEPATITIS SERUM	V	Blood or blood product transfusion, contaminated syringes, needles	2–6 months or longer	None	Disposable syringes & needles. Careful selection of blood donors	Symptomatic. High protein diet. Rest
INFLUENZA	V	Respiratory contact	1–4 days	During acute illness	Isolation vaccine	Symptomatic

13

Features of Some Infectious Diseases - continued

DISEASE	AGENT	TRANSMISSION	INCUBATION	ISOLATION	CONTROL	TREATMENT
LYMPHOGRAN-ULOMA VENEREUM	V	Venereal contact	1–6 weeks	Modified	Treatment of cases	Prescribed antibiotic
MALARIA	P	Bite of female Anopheles mosquito	Variable	Screens	Mosquito control personal protection measures. Chemoprophylaxis	Complex treatment regime
MEASLES (Rubeola)	V	Respiratory droplet or contact	10–15 days	From 7 days after exposure to 5 days after rash starts	Vaccination, isolation	Symptomatic
MENINGITIS MENINGOCOCCIC	B	Respiratory droplet or contact	2–10 days	Strict	Avoidance of overcrowding fatigue	Prescribed antibiotic
MUMPS	V	Respiratory droplet or contact	18–21 days	Modified	Isolation, Vaccination	Symptomatic
PARATYPHOID FEVERS	B	Water, food, flies' excrement	1–14 days	Strict	Sanitation, immunization	Prescribed antibiotic
PERTUSSIS (Whooping Cough)	B	Respiratory contact, droplets	5–10 days	Modified	Immunization only in early life	Prescribed antibiotic
STREPTOCOCCAL INFECTIONS	B	Respiratory droplets	1–5 days	None	Treatment of cases	Prescribed antibiotic
SYPHILIS	B	Venereal, transfusion, trans-placentae	1–6 weeks (usually 2 weeks)	Modified	Case finding, treatment of cases	Prescribed antibiotic

Features of Some Infectious Diseases - continued

DISEASE	AGENT	TRANSMISSION	INCUBATION	ISOLATION	CONTROL	TREATMENT
TUBERCULOSIS	B	Discharge from lesions, infected cow's milk. Respiratory droplets	Variable	Strict	Case finding, treatment	Prescribed antibiotic
TYPHOID	B	Water, food, contaminated with excreta of infected man	10–14 days	Strict until 2 successive neg. stool cultures	Sanitation, immunization	Prescribed antibiotic

(1) If concomitant roundworm infestation (ascariasis) exists or is strongly suspected, the patient should be treated with piperazine for roundworms *before* regular hookworm therapy is begun.

Oris Blackwell
Charles Houston

VII. DESCRIPTION AND OPERATION OF THE COMPOST PRIVY*

A reasonably safe way for a villager to prepare excreta for use as fertilizer is for him to compost it in a privy pit. After the required period of composting, the pit can be emptied, thus eliminating the handling of the raw excreta.

The method is a modification of the Bangalore composting process and is based on anaerobic decomposition of organic wastes which are left undisturbed during a period of at least six months to ensure destruction of pathogens and ova of helminths. The procedure would be as follows:

1. Dig a pit of required size, the bottom of which should always be above ground-water level.
2. Before the slab is placed, cover the bottom 50 cm (20 in.) of the pit with grass cuttings, fine leaves, garbage, paper, etc.; but allow no rubbish such as metal cans, glass bottles, or similar materials to be deposited therein.
3. Place slab, and complete superstructure, keeping in mind that they will both be moved periodically to another site.
4. In addition to depositing human excrement, throw the daily garbage into the pit, along with cow, horse, sheep, chicken and pig manure, as well as urine-soaked earth or straw. The latter materials are important, as urine is rich in nitrogen, an essential plant nutrient.
5. About once a week throw a few kilograms of grass clippings and fine-texture leaves into the pit. After some experimentation, one can arrive at a pit mixture which will provide a good fertilizer.
6. When the pit's contents reach a level 50 cm (20 in.) below ground, a new pit is dug 1.50-2m (5-6.5 ft.) away (more if desired), and the superstructure and slab are moved over it. The first pit is levelled, finally with 15 cm (6 in.) of grass clippings and leaves, and the top 35 cm (14 in.) with well-tamped earth.
7. When the second pit is filled as indicated above, the first pit is uncovered and the compost removed. It should be stable, and will provide a good fertilizer which can be applied immediately to the fields or stored.

The volume of the pit depends on the needs for fertilizer and the number of people using the privy. The proportion of night-soil that can be added to refuse for satisfactory composting should be about 1 to 5 by volume. From the data given above, it will be noted that a family of five will produce, on the average, one cubic metre (35 cu. ft.) of partly digested excreta in about four years. On this basis, one-fifth of a pit of one cubic metre (35

---

* This section on compost privys and the diagrams that appear at the end of this section are from the following W. H.O. Publications:
W.H.O. Publication No. 39, 1958, E. G. Wagner and J. N. Lanoix, *Excreta Disposal for Rural Areas and Small Communities.*
W.H.O. Publication No. 42, 1959, E. G. Wagner and J. N. Lanoix, *Water Supply for Rural Areas and Small Communities.*
Used by permission.

cu. ft.) capacity would be filled with excreta in approximately 9–10 months, which would be a good composting cycle for such a pit. (The other four-fifths of the contents would consist of refuse and other wastes thrown in as explained above.)

Before applying or recommending this method in a rural area where it is not familiar, it is desirable to try it first on a pilot scale under adequate control in order to determine the proper operating schedule and materials suitable and available in the area under consideration.

To obviate moving the superstructure and slab back and forth over two separate pits, the system may be amended by building what may be called a "double-vault" latrine (see fig. 59). This latrine consists of a large vault divided into two compartments, each of which is topped by a slab and a hole. The superstructure is likewise partitioned into two houses with separate entrances. In practice, the vaults are filled and emptied alternately in the same manner as described above for the compost privy. They should be large enough to allow sufficient time for the materials to compost thoroughly before their removal. The vaults need not be water-tight but should be built well above the ground-water table. The difficulty with the double-vault privy is that often both compartments are used simultaneously, thus defeating their purpose.

NOTES

FIG. 2. TRANSMISSION OF DISEASE FROM EXCRETA

CHANNELS OF TRANSMISSION OF DISEASE FROM EXCRETA

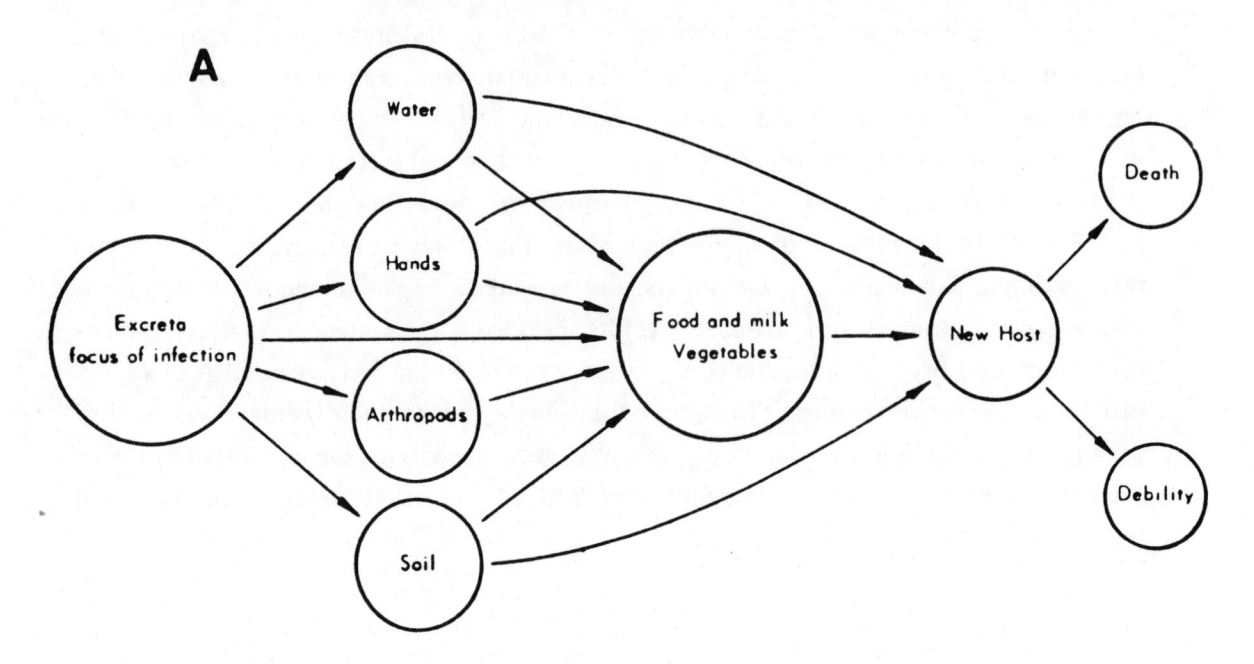

STOPPING THE TRANSMISSION OF FAECAL-BORNE DISEASES BY MEANS OF SANITATION

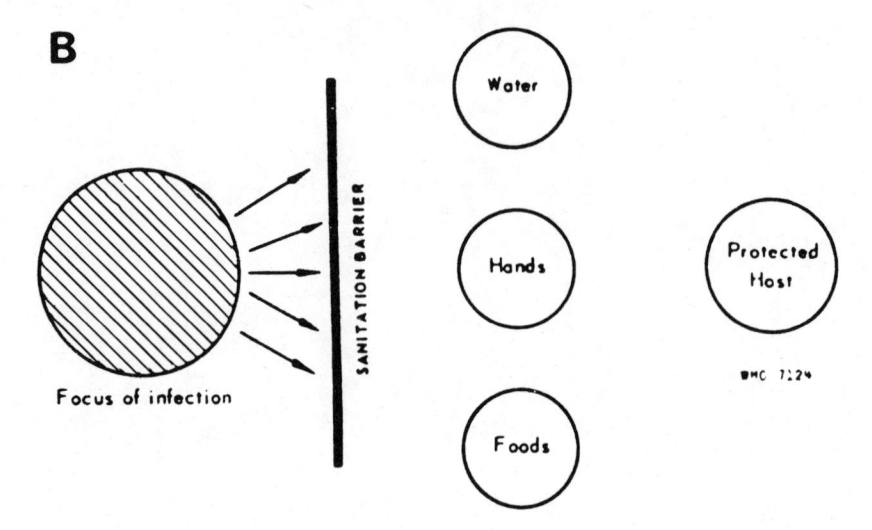

THE COMMUNE MEDIC'S GUIDE

FIG. 26. SQUARE CONCRETE SLAB FOR PIT AND BORED-HOLE LATRINE

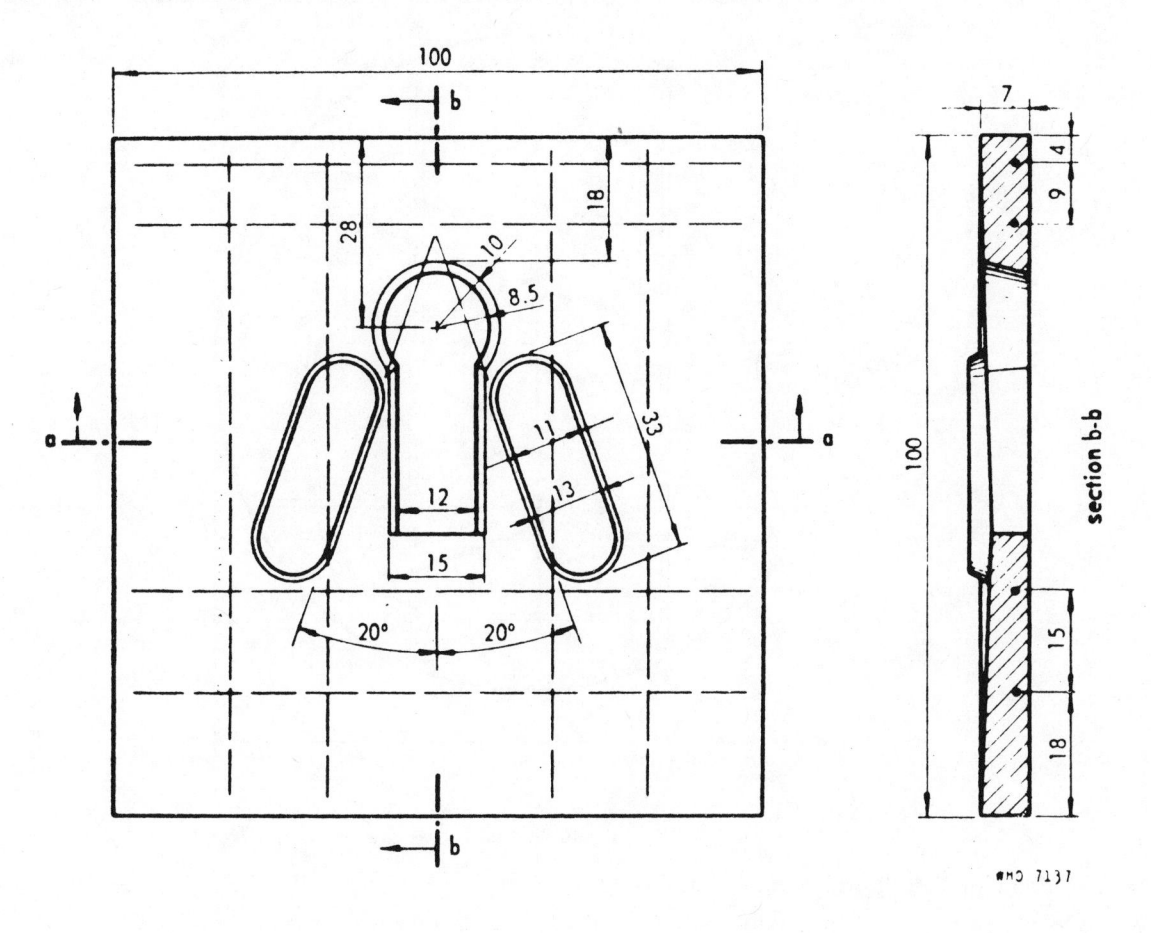

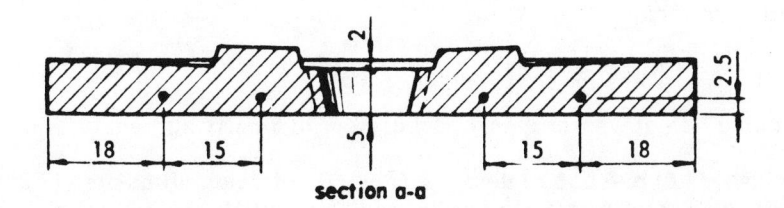

Measurements shown are in centimetres.

20   *THE HOME HEALTH HANDBOOK*

FIG. 27. CIRCULAR SLAB FOR BORED-HOLE LATRINE*

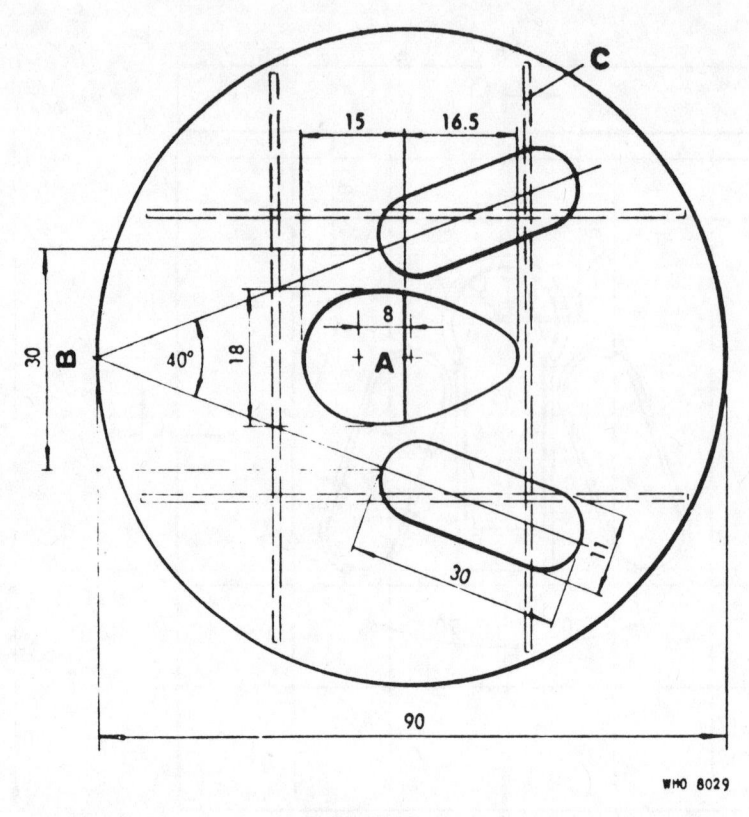

Measurements shown are in centimetres.

* Built in East Pakistan. See also Fig. 52.

A = Centre open hole 2.5 cm (1 in.) back of centre if slab is 80 cm (31 in.) in diameter; centre open hole 8.0 cm (3 in.) back of centre if slab is 90 cm (35 in.) in diameter
B = Between back centre foot-rests
C = Reinforcement

Notes on construction of slab

Concrete for slabs should be not weaker than 1 part cement to 6 parts aggregate, with a minimum of water.

Slab is reinforced with strips of bamboo of timber quality. Reinforcing strips are about 2.5 cm (1 in.) wide, have had inner, weaker fibres stripped away, and have been soaked in water overnight before use.

Slabs are cast upside down in one operation. Base of form is of wood with indentations for foot-rests. Base of form is encircled by sheet metal strip which makes outer wall of form. Side walls of hole form and foot-rests are made with slight slope so as to come out easily. Form for open hole is removed when concrete has taken initial set. Slabs are removed from form in about 40 hours and stored under water, preferably for 10 days or more. Since these slabs are round, they may be rolled some distance when conveyance is difficult.

THE COMMUNE MEDIC'S GUIDE

FIG. 59. DOUBLE-VAULT LATRINE

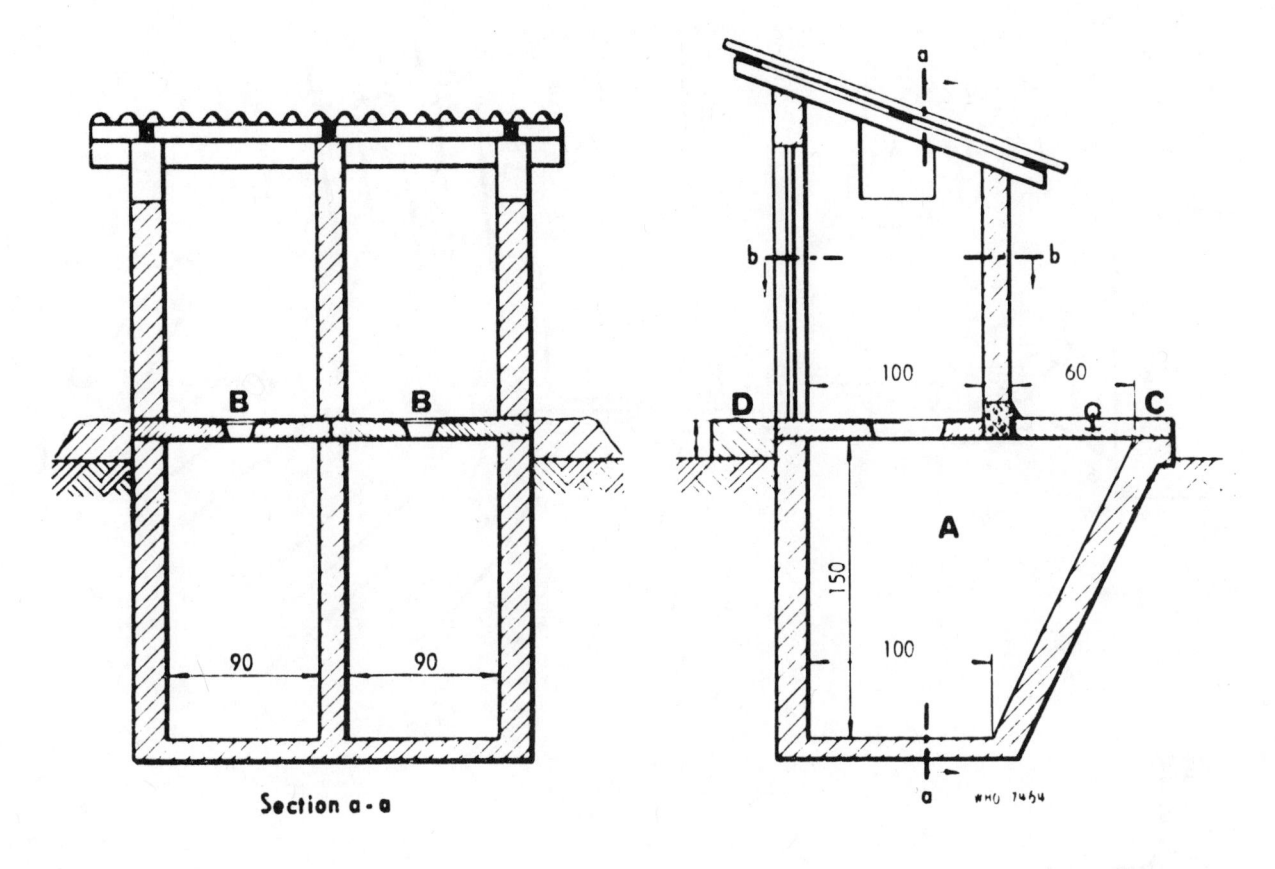

Section a-a

Section b-b

Measurements shown are in centimetres.

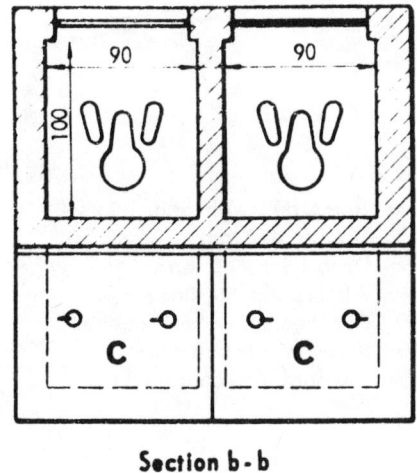

A = Two vaults
B = Squatting slabs
C = Removable covers
D = Step and earth mound

FIG. 63. TYPICAL LAYOUT OF SEPTIC-TANK SYSTEM

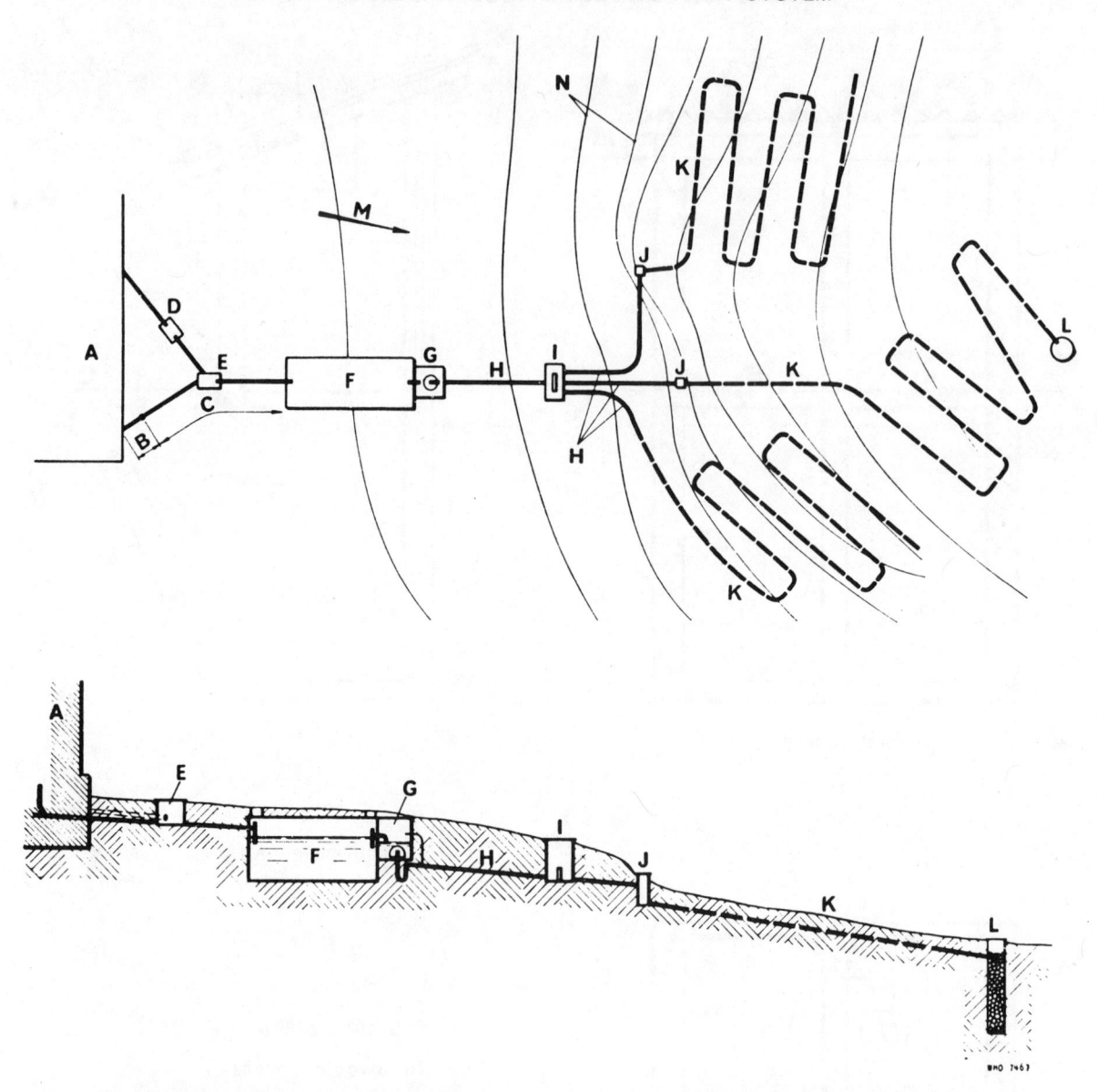

A = Private house or public institution
B = House sewer
C = Building sewer
D = Grease interceptor on pipe line from kitchen
E = Manhole
F = Septic tank
G = Dosing chamber and siphon
H = Pipes laid with tight joints
I = Distribution box
J = Drop-boxes or terracotta L's
K = Absorption tile lines
L = Seepage pit, when required
M = Slope of ground surface
N = Topographic contour lines

FIG. 64. TYPICAL HOUSEHOLD SEPTIC TANK

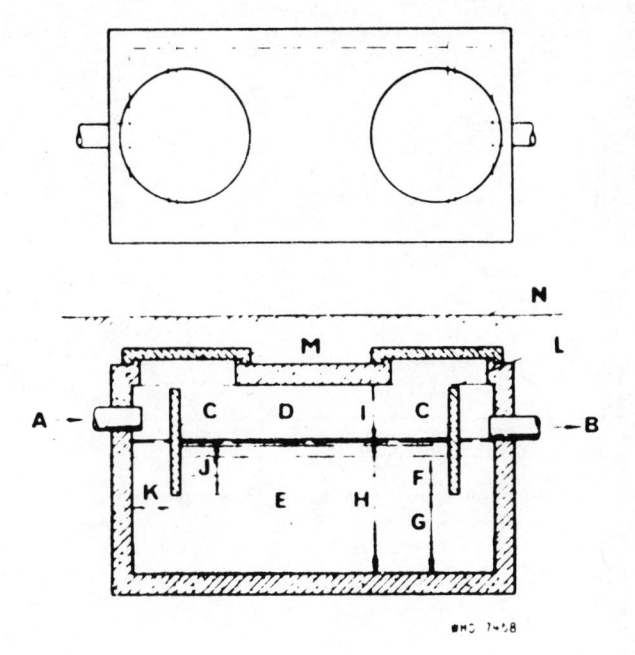

A = Inlet
B = Outlet
C = Baffle
D = Floating scum
E = Sludge
F = Scum-clear space
G = Sludge-clear space
H = Depth of water in tank
I = Clearance
J = Depth of penetration of baffle
K = Distance of baffle to wall, 20-30 cm (8-12 in.)
L = Top of baffle 2.5 cm (1 in.) below roof for ventilation purposes
M = Tank covers, preferably round
N = Ground level, less than 30 cm (12 in.) above tank (if less, raise tank covers to ground surface)

Fig. 20. DRIVEN WELL WITH DROP-PIPE AND CYLINDER AND PROTECTIVE PLATFORM

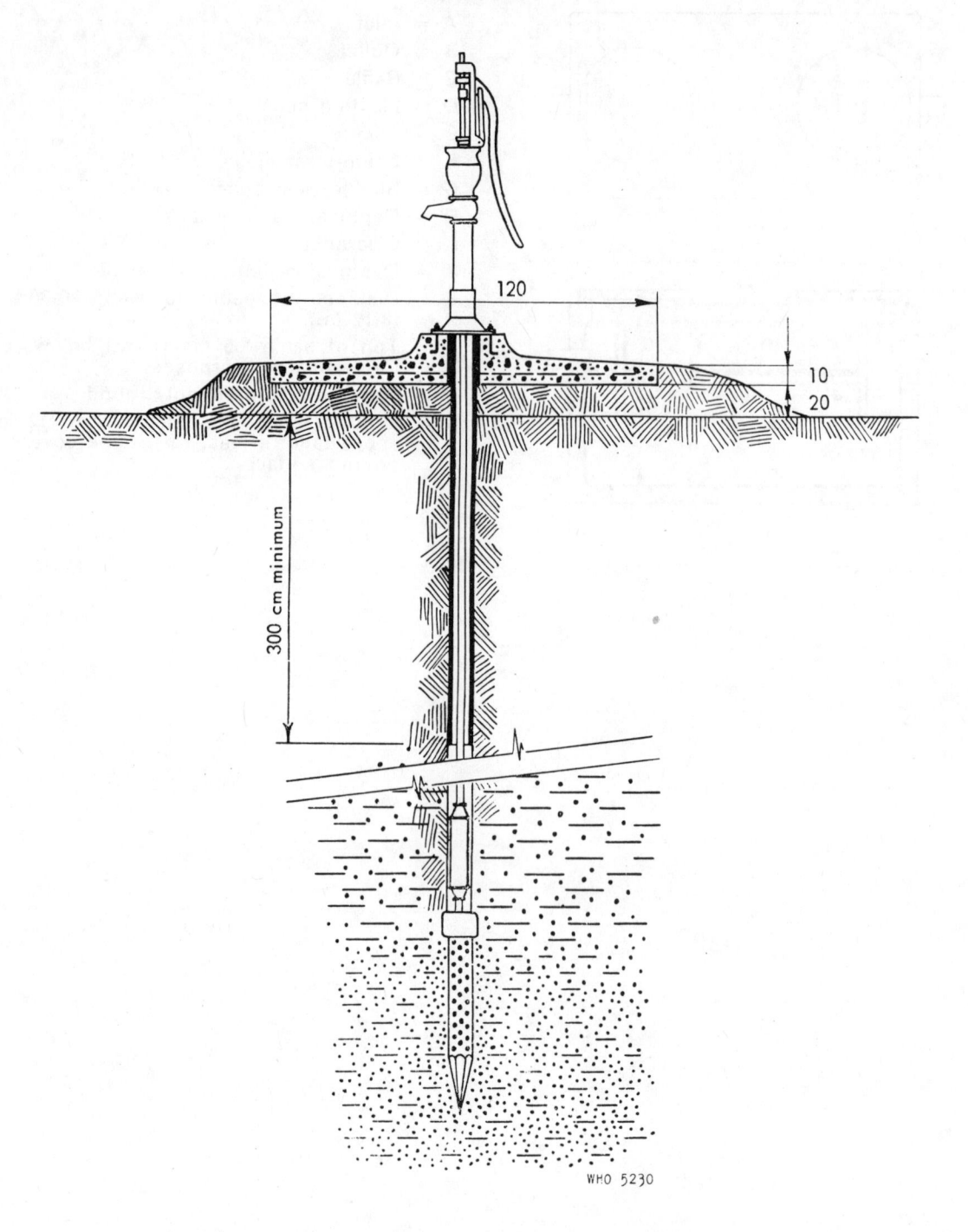

In areas with relatively coarse sand, driven wells can be an excellent and very cheap means of obtaining water. They can be driven rapidly and put into operation quickly. With proper technique, this well can be developed to increase its capacity. Note the water-tight casing which extends down to a minimum of 3 m (10 ft) below ground surface.

THE COMMUNE MEDIC'S GUIDE

Fig. 14. DUG WELL LINED WITH CONCRETE OR CLAY TILE

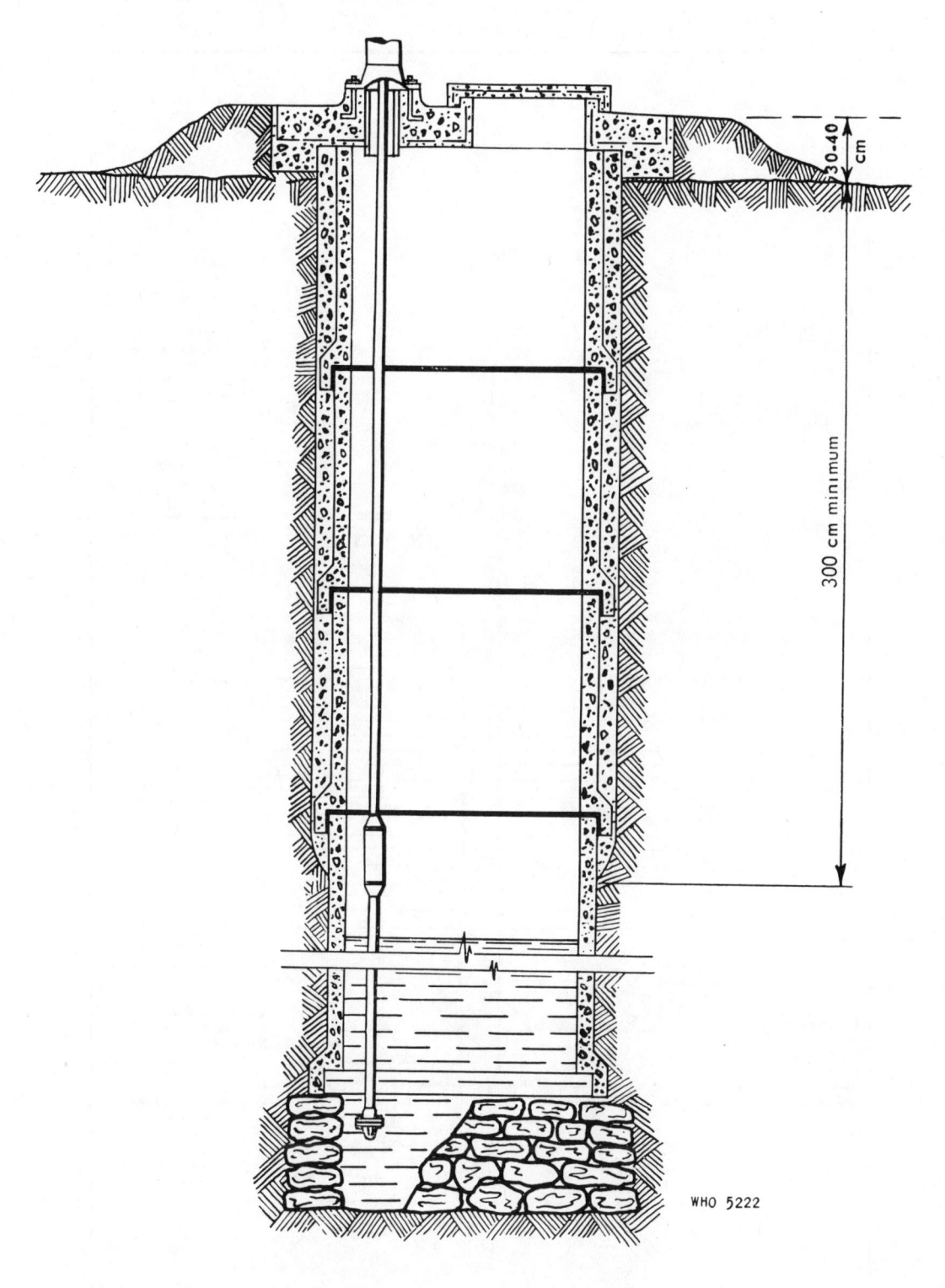

Concrete or clay tiles make excellent well casing and can be placed quickly and easily into the well by the use of a simple A-frame or other temporary structure for lowering tile into a well. Note the outside, protective layer of concrete which extends down to 3 m (10 ft) minimum to ensure water-tightness of the upper walls.

Fig. 15. RECONSTRUCTED DUG WELL WITH BURIED SLAB

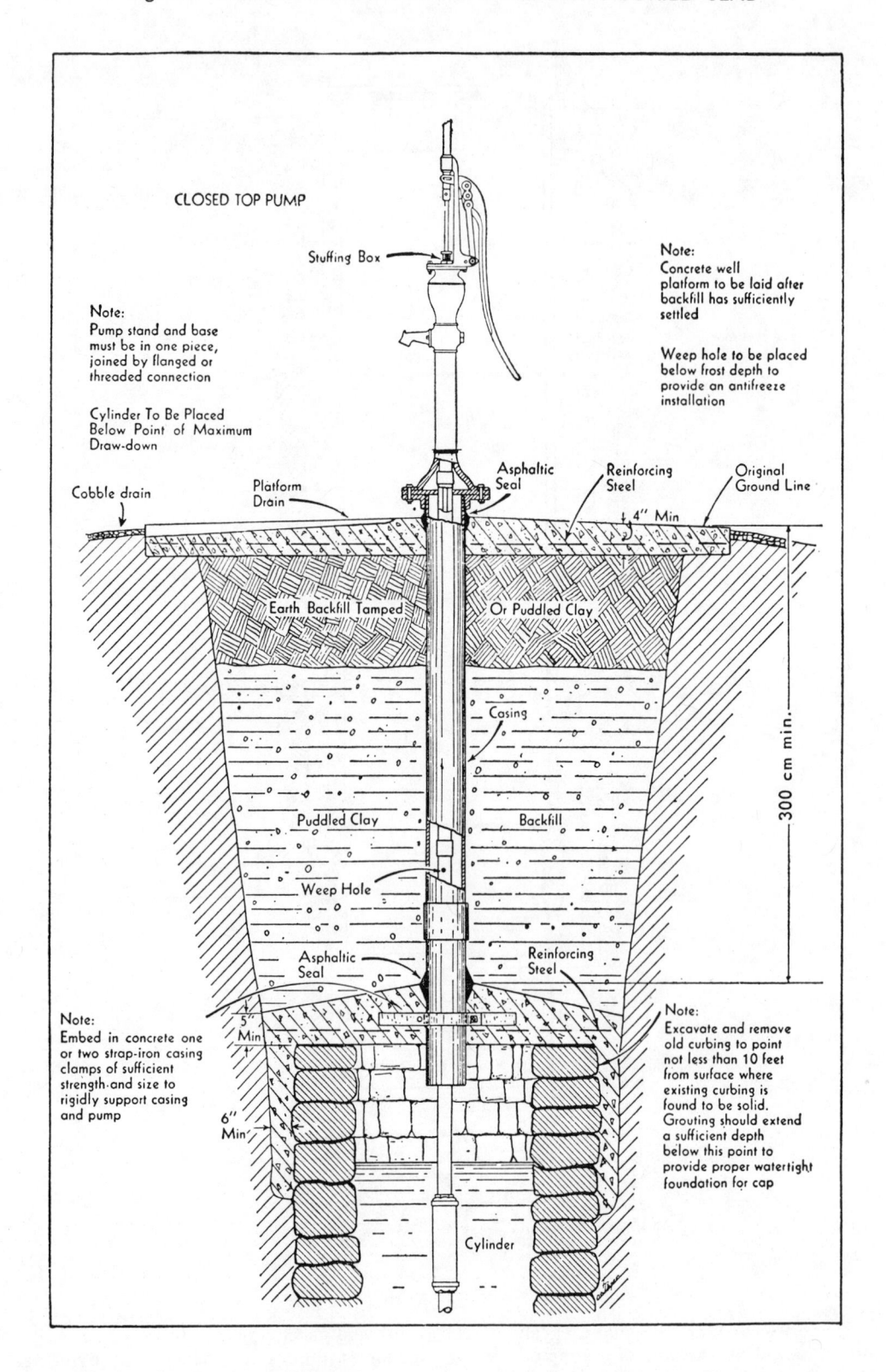

Reproduced from US Public Health Service, Joint Committee on Rural Sanitation (1950) *Individual water supply systems*, Washington, p. 25

THE COMMUNE MEDIC'S GUIDE 27

Fig. 32. IMPROVEMENT OF EXISTING WELLS (I)

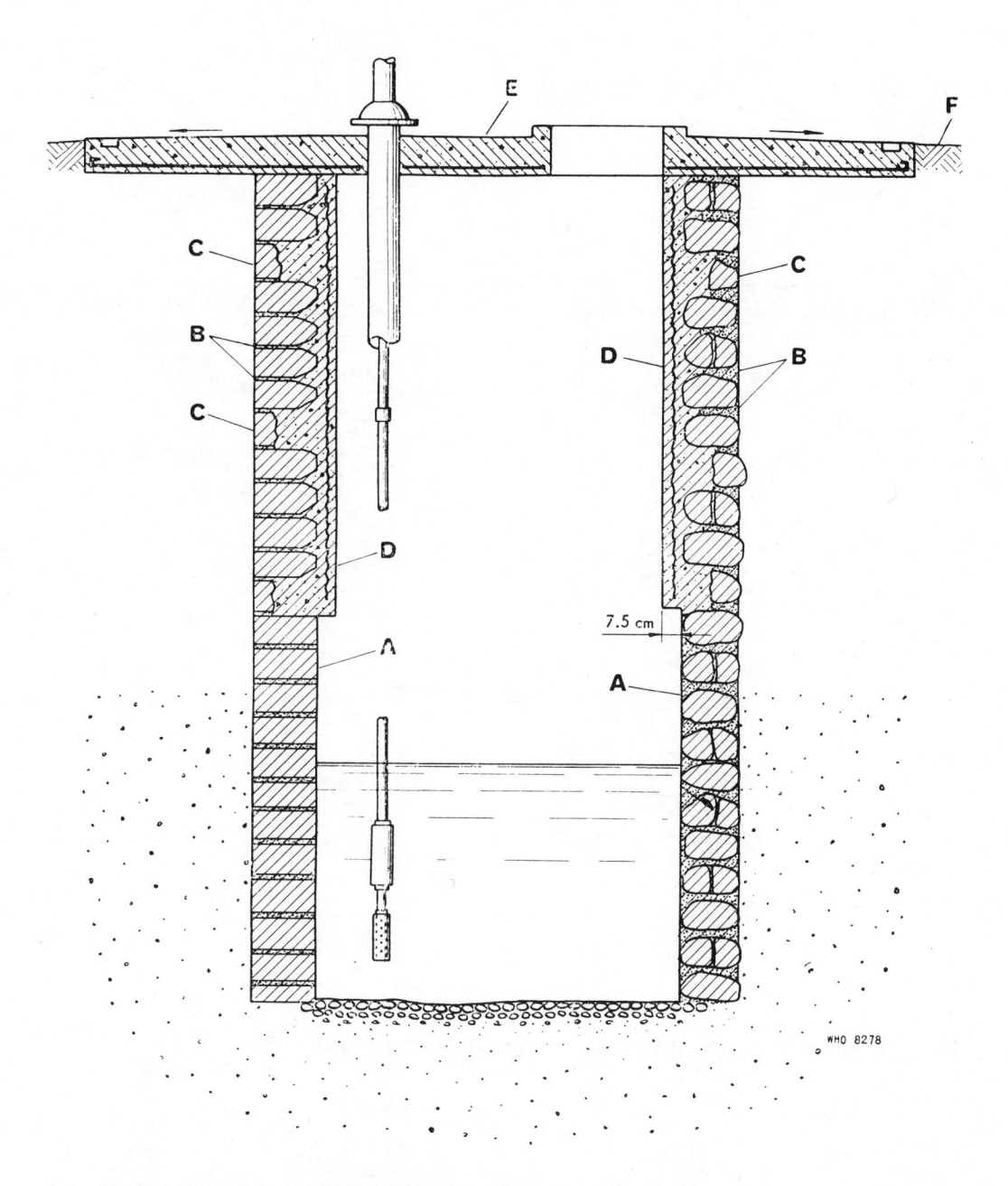

A = Existing masonry or brick walls with cracke mortar joints
B = Old mortar removed with chisel as far back as possible
C = Stone or bricks ug out to provide key for new concrete lining
D = New concrete lining, built to a depth of at least 3 m (10 ft) below outside ground level, or to low water level in well. For concrete, use pea-sized gravel and wire-mesh for temperature reinforcement.
E = New concrete well top, incorporating sanitary features (manhole with raised edges, slope for proper drainage, proper pump installation, etc.).
F = Outside ground level (adequate drainage being provided for excess water or surface run-off)

28 THE HOME HEALTH HANDBOOK

Fig. 32 (continued). IMPROVEMENT OF EXISTING WELLS (II)

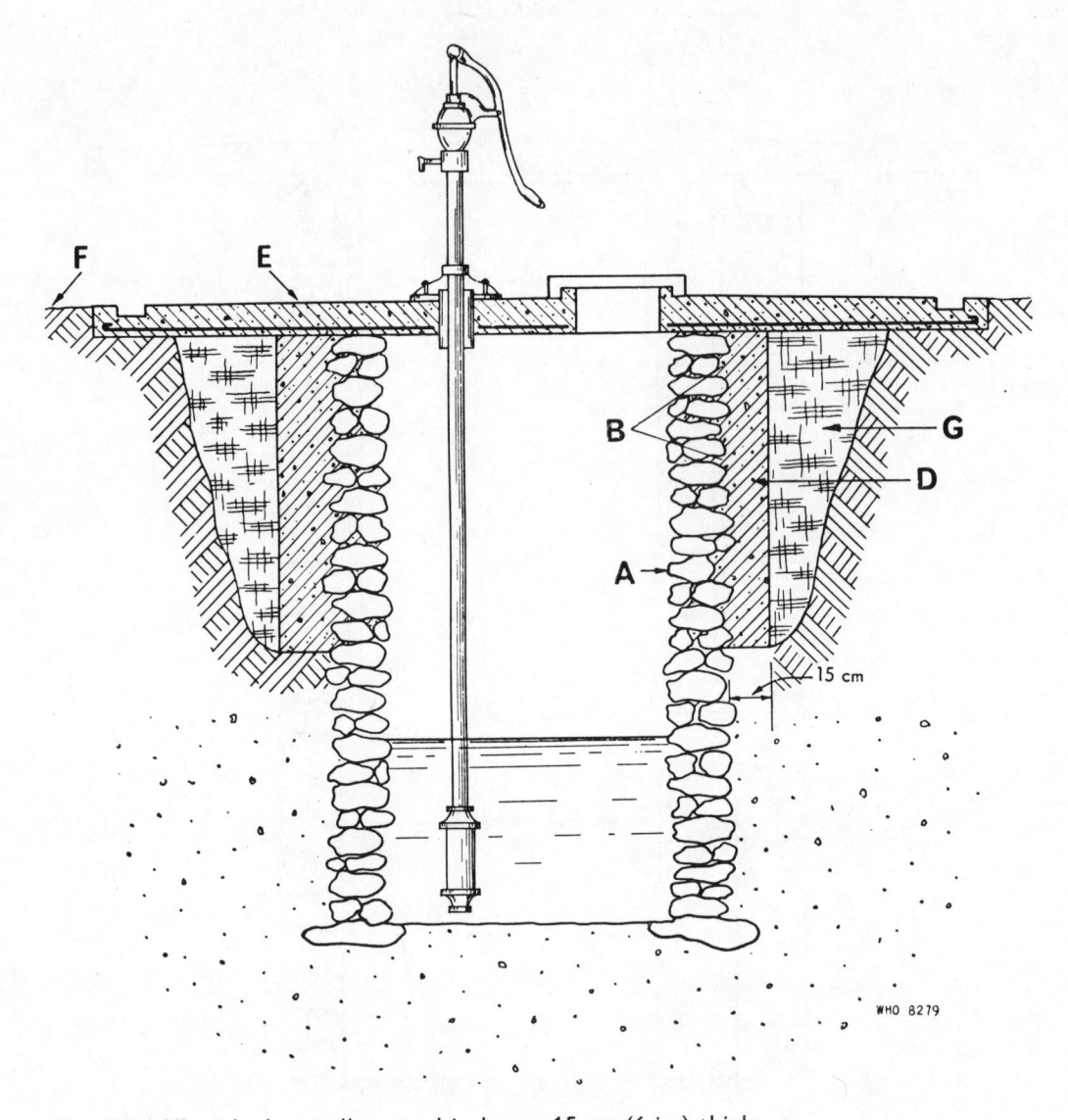

G = Backfill with clay, well tamped in layers 15 cm (6 in.) thick

Fig. 33. PROPERLY PROTECTED SPRING (I)

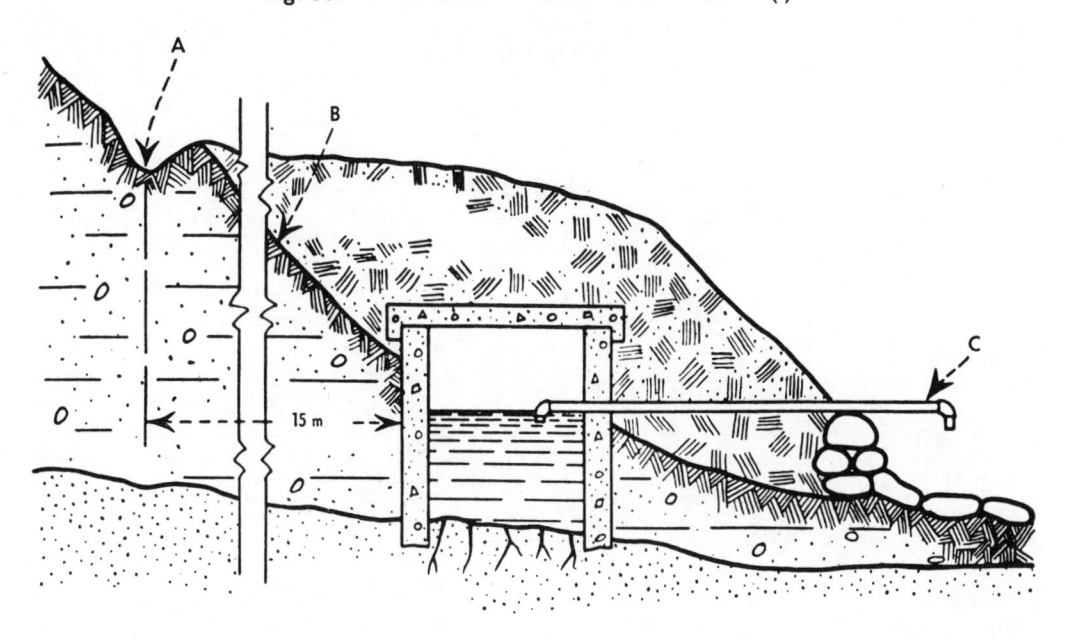

A = Protective drainage ditch to keep drainage water a safe distance from spring
B = Original slope and ground line
C = Screened outlet pipe : can discharge freely or be piped to village or residence

Springs can offer an economical and safe source of water. A thorough search should be made for signs of ground-water outcropping. Springs that can be piped to the user by gravity offer an excellent solution. Rainfall variation may influence the yield, so dry-weather flow should be checked.

Fig. 34. PROPERLY PROTECTED SPRING (II)

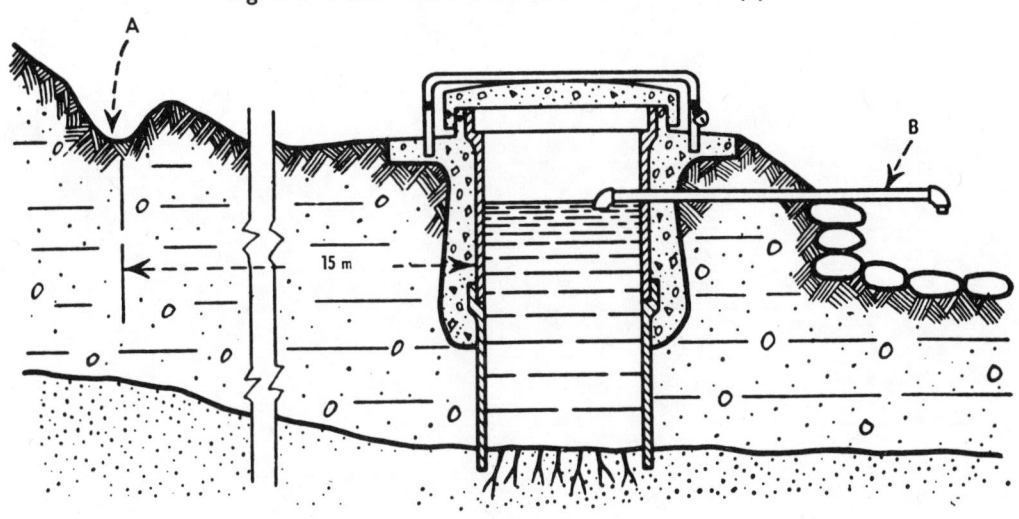

A = Protective drainage ditch to keep drainage water a safe distance from spring
B = Screened outlet pipe : to discharge freely or be piped to village or residence

NOTES

COMMON EMERGENCIES GUIDE

Introduction: This chapter is based on a government pamphlet entitled *Family Guide Emergency Health Care.* The pamphlet was written to advise citizens as to what to do for the period following a nuclear attack when outside assistance might not be available. Since this unavailability of professional help has happened already (without the intervening nuclear holocaust) we feel this review is appropriate. Some sections have been deleted as irrelevant, other sections shortened because they have been covered elsewhere in the Handbook.

I. MANAGEMENT OF COMMON EMERGENCIES

When confronted with an emergency one should remember two extremely (albeit self-evident) principles: (1) If the person is not breathing . . . breath for him and (2) If the heart is not beating—replace the action of the heart by compressing the chest. After you have first taken care of these two things, then you have time to consider what else should be done, i.e., bandaging, treating burns, etc. This section of the Handbook is thus divided into three sections: (A) Artificial Maintenance of Life, (B) Major Emergencies, and (C) Minor Emergencies.

A. Artificial Maintenance of Life. (Breathing, Heart Beat)

1. Breathing

The best method to substitute for the person's own breathing is the mouth-to-mouth method (See Fig. 1). Since most people die if breathing has stopped for more than six minutes, artificial breathing should be started as soon as possible. One should breathe about 12 times per minute for the person and should continue until either the person begins to breathe spontaneously or you are positive he is dead.

2. Heart Beat

If you can't feel a heart beat or pulse you should press with the heel of the hand (other hand on top of this one) with enough force to compress the breast bone about one-half to one inch. This should be done approximately three times more frequently than you breathe for the person. If you are fortunate enough to have someone helping you, be synchronous! i.e., don't be blowing air in while he is pushing down on the chest (wait until he lets up).

B. Major But Not Immediately Life-Threatening Emergencies

The most important rule to remember in the care of these problems is don't make things worse than they already are by moving a fractured limb, putting a tourniquet on too tight, etc. If you are not sure what you are doing . . . do the minimal life saving maneuvers and get help.

1. Bleeding and Bandaging.

The first step in controlling bleeding is to cover bleeding area and exert pressure.

MOUTH-TO-MOUTH AND MOUTH-TO-NOSE METHOD FIG. 1

A. Before starting any type of artificial respiration be sure that the mouth and throat are completely clear of mucus and foreign objects. Use your fingers to clean the mouth. You may cover fingers with a piece of cloth to help remove mucus and slippery objects.

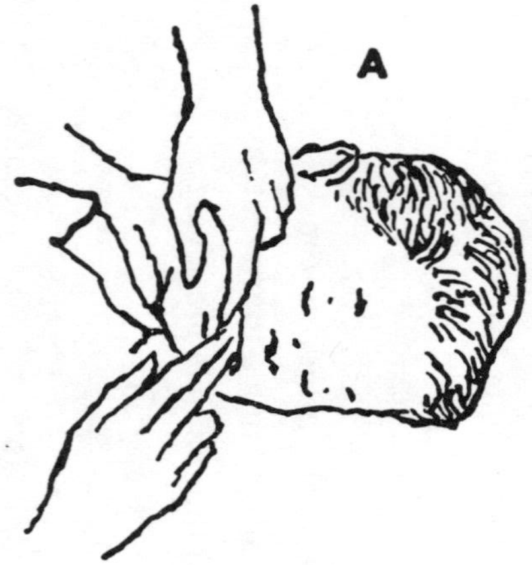

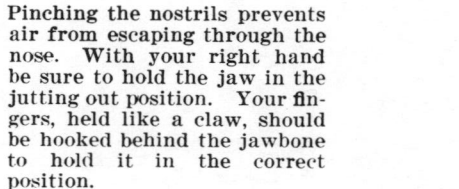

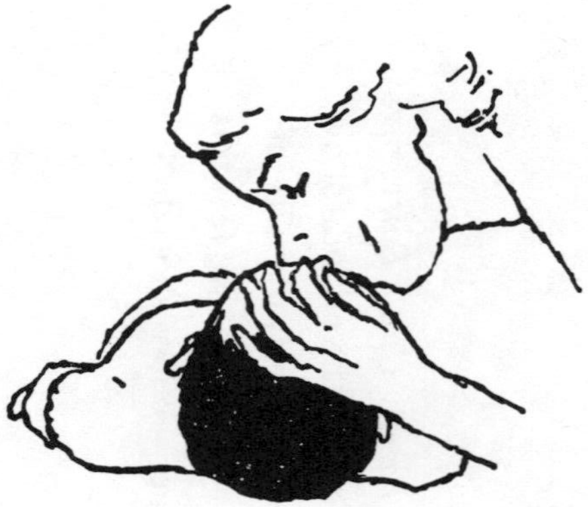

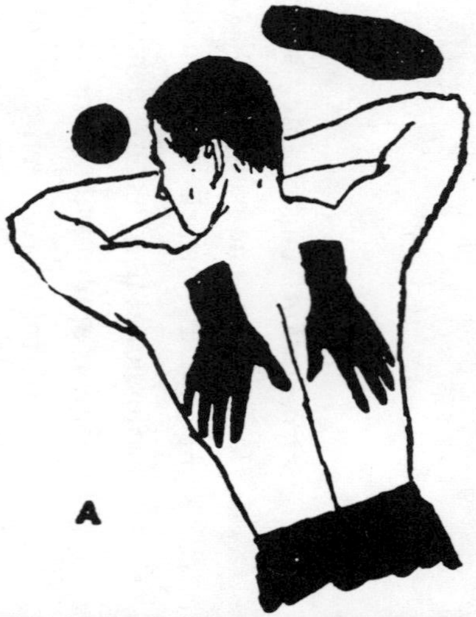

B. The head must be tipped back to allow a free air passage with the jaw held in a jutting out position. The more you can achieve the "sword swallower" position the better.

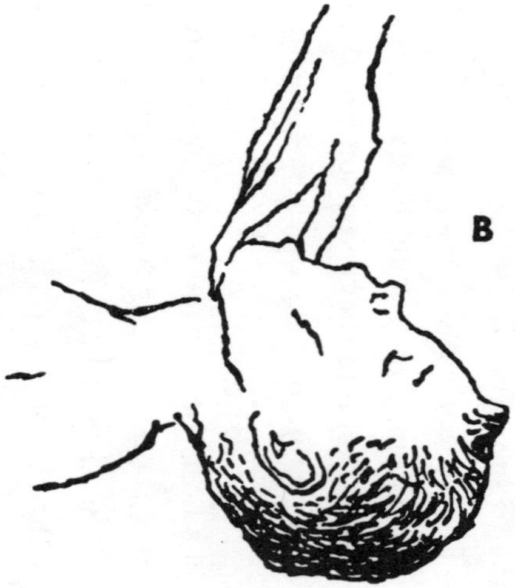

C. Remember—Don't blow too hard. Your mouth and the mouth of the person receiving treatment should be wide open with a complete seal between them. Inhale more than usual before exhaling into person's mouth. In this way he will get more oxygen.

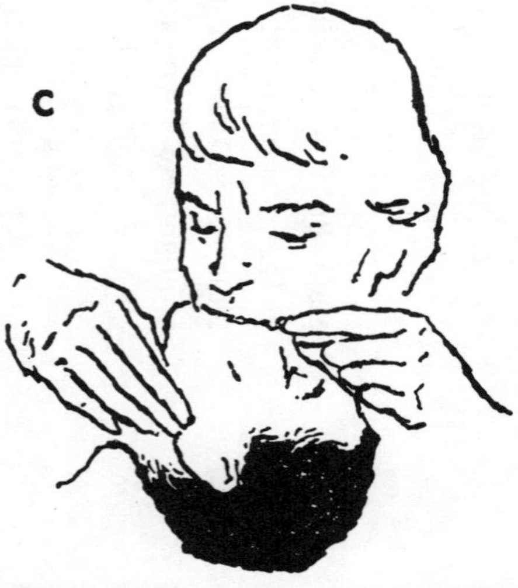

D. Pinching the nostrils prevents air from escaping through the nose. With your right hand be sure to hold the jaw in the jutting out position. Your fingers, held like a claw, should be hooked behind the jawbone to hold it in the correct position.

E. This is the mouth-to-nose type of respiration with the lips being sealed by the two fingers of the right hand. This would be used when an obstruction is in the mouth that cannot be removed, or a severe mouth injury prevents proper contact.

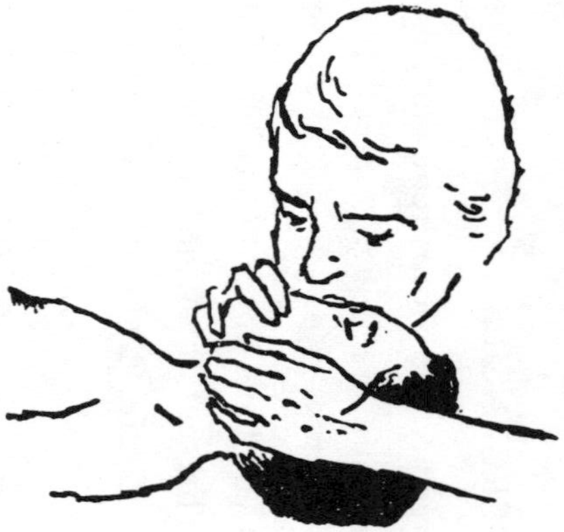

BACK PRESSURE ARMLIFT METHOD

A. This picture shows the correct position of the knee, foot, and hands in the first step of back pressure armlift method. The knee and foot may be alternated to make it less tiring for the person administering this type of artificial respiration.

The cleaner the cloth used to cover the less the chance of infection, but if nothing is available you may temporarily have to use your hand while someone looks for a cloth. The pressure works by squeezing shut the open blood vessel, and allowing clotting to take place.

After the bleeding has been controlled, then the second step takes place, i.e., application of the bandage. The material put directly over the cut should be as sterile as possible, it doesn't really matter for the rest of the bandage. Make sure the bandage is not too tight because you may do more harm than good (bandage should be just tight enough to stop bleeding).

2. Sucking Wounds in the Chest.

"Sucking wounds" are chest wounds in which an opening is created from the lungs to the outside air. The air enters the chest causing frothing and a hissing sound. As the person breaths out immediately cover the hole with a sterile bandage making it as airtight as possible with tape.

3. Caring for Wounds Including Infection. (see "First Aid for Wounds and Burns," p.

4. Fractures and Splinting.

(a) Broken bones—If ends are not through the skin the fracture is called simple; if broken bone breaks through the skin it is called compound (can be serious because of infection). The usual findings in a fracture include; tenderness over area, swelling, irregular feel to bone (or even gross distortion of the shape of the bone).

(b) Treatment—If you even remotely consider the possibility of a fracture, treat as one until you are sure. The important first thing to do is to prevent motion of the site of the break (i.e., splint until a cast can be put on). Occasionally one has to straighten the limb before the splint is applied. (See Fig. 2) If the fracture is compound, first clean the area around the wounds by pouring sterile water over it, then allow the end of the bone to ease itself back (don't push it in), and finally cover with sterile bandage. Almost any rigid material (stick, folded newspaper, etc., will act as an adequate splint. Do not make splint too tight (check color of limb, as person if limb feels numb).

FIG. 2

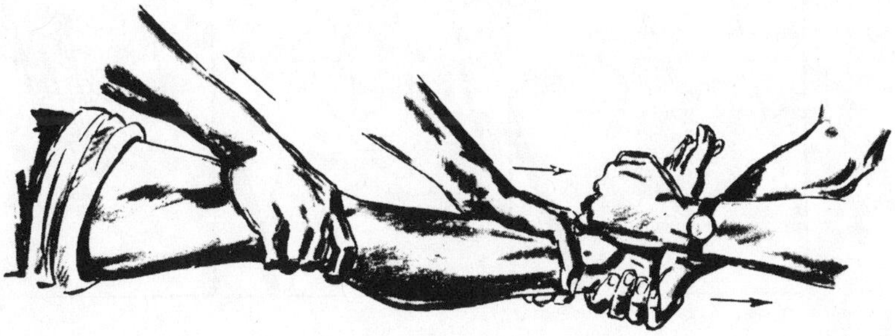

Fractured collar bone—is treated with a sling and then binding arm to body.

Fractured rib—may be taped but these are probably best left alone and treated with analgesics.

Fracture of the back—is very serious because of potential damage to the spinal cord; when the patient is moved he should be held as rigidly as possible and put on a stiff board or door.

Fractured neck—is extremely serious because of the danger to the spinal cord. It is important that the head, neck, and shoulders be maintained in the relative positions in which they are found. The head should be immobilized by placing soft but firm material such as sandbags on either side of the head.

All fractures should be treated for shock. (see item 7 below)

Never force traction.

5. Sprains.

Sprains are caused by abnormal stretching (and occasionally tearing) of the ligaments of the joints. Severe sprains shall be treated as fractures. To retard swelling the area should be covered with ice, the limb elevated on a pillow.

6. Burns.

These are usually classified in degrees of severity: (see Fig. 3)

A first-degree burn only reddens the skin and if it does not cover more than 25 percent of the body, usually is not serious.

In second-degree burns blisters develop and there is now the very real danger of infection. Extensive second-degree burns will require giving additional fluids to the burned person. Do not apply grease or salve. Cover with sterile or clean dressing.

Third-degree burns even in a relatively small area are serious. The injury is deep and the underlying tissue has been destroyed. Keep this type of burn clean to avoid infection.

FIG. 3

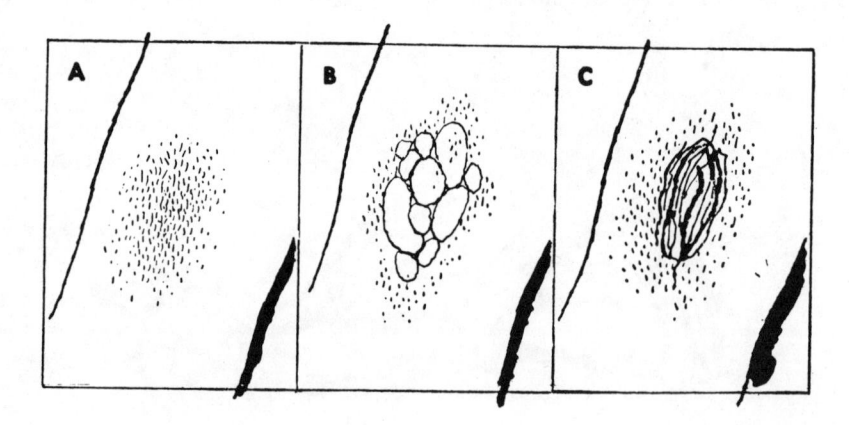

What to do: Treat for shock (see item 7 below).
  Relieve pain.
  Prevent infection, cover area with a sterile cloth.
  Encourage fluids to replace fluid loss from body.

What *not* to do: Do *not* pull clothes over burned area;
  Do *not* remove pieces of cloth stuck to burn;
  Do *not* clean burn;
  Do *not* break blister;
  Do *not* use grease-ointment-petroleum jelly;
  Do *not* use iodine or antiseptics;
  Do *not* change dressing unless absolutely necessary.

7. Shock.

Refers to a condition that frequently comes with serious injury such as severe wounds, burns, bleeding, and broken bones. It is thought to be due to shortage of blood in various parts of the body. This causes the heart to beat faster. Shock may cause death if not treated promptly. Shock is usually easy to recognize. (see Fig. 4)

Treatment of shock:
  Have injured person lie down.
  Elevate feet and legs 12 inches or more (unless chest or head injury).
  Keep person warm.
  Give him liquid, about a glassful of solution (made up of one quart of water and
    ½ teaspoon baking soda and 1 teaspoon of salt) every 15 minutes. Don't give if
    the patient is unconscious or vomiting.
  Keep person quiet.

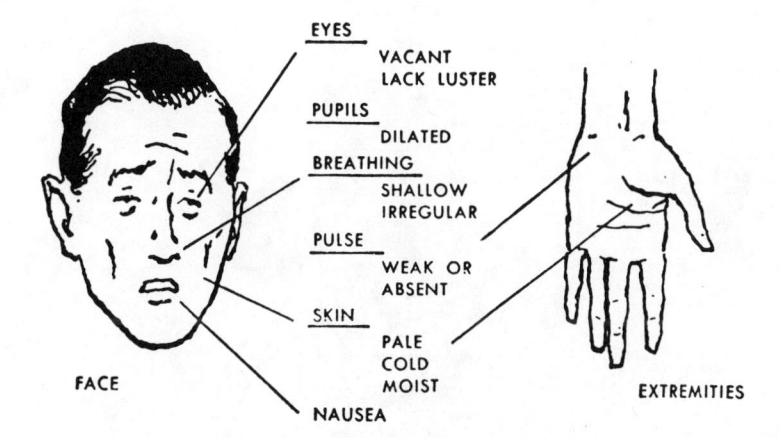

FIG. 4

8. Transport of the Patient.

This should only take place after all emergency measures have been carried out. The following pictures are self explanatory. (Fig. 5)

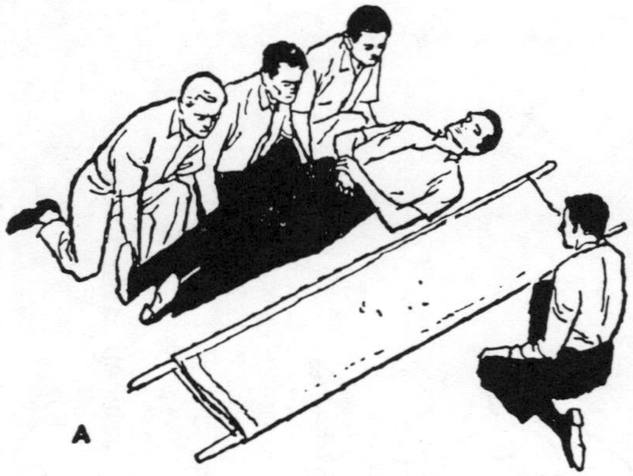

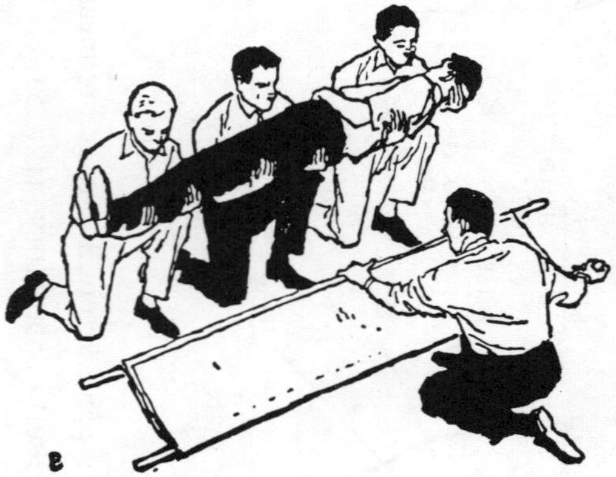

This saddle-back carry is simple and effective for moving an injured person a short distance, when his injuries are not serious.

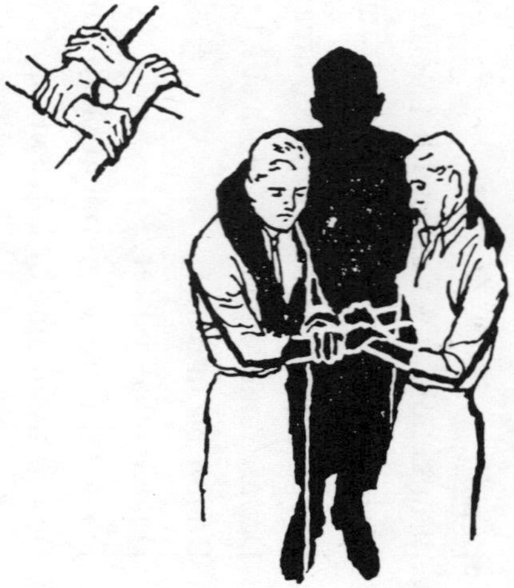

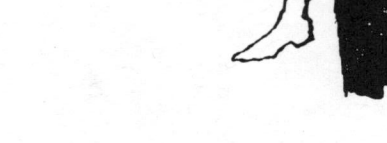

The four-hand seat carry shown above is an excellent method for carrying conscious, not too seriously injured persons a short distance.

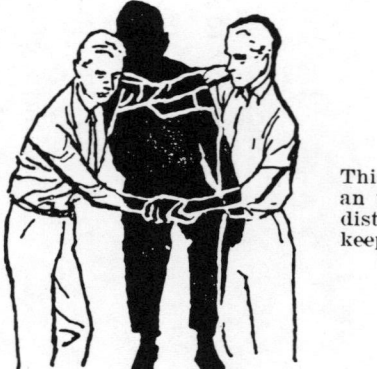

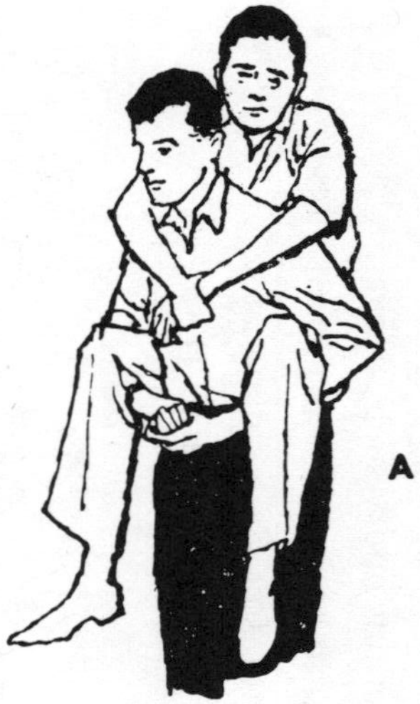

This is an effective method of carrying an unconscious injured person a short distance provided it is not necessary to keep him flat.

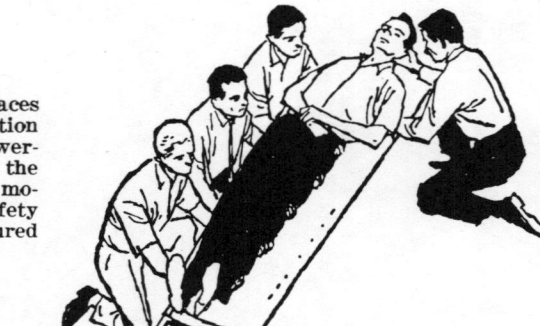

This is the first step in the correct method of using four people to load a seriously injured person on a stretcher. In this first step the fourth man does not touch the injured person.

The three persons now lift slowly and all together and roll the injured person gently toward them on injured side.

The fourth man now places the stretcher into position and then assists in lowering the person into the stretcher. Even, slow motion assures greatest safety and comfort of the injured person.

FIG. 5

COMMON EMERGENCIES GUIDE

C. Common Problems Which are Usually Not Life-Threatening. (In alphabetical order.)

1. Abscess and boils (skin infections).

   What to do: Leave it alone if it is closed.

   Wait for it to open by itself.

   Cover with a sterile or clean dressing if draining.

   Apply hot packs.

   Give aspirin for pain.

   When possible keep clothing away from area.

   What *not* to do: Do not squeeze pimple, boil or carbuncle.

   Do not pick it with a pin or needle.

2. Animal bites.

   What to do: Wash the wound thoroughly with soap and water.

   Catch the animal and confine for 14 days (if practical).

3. Asthma attack.

   What to do: Place victim in comfortable sitting position.

   Reassure the victim.

   Determine if he has his own medication.

   Administer his medication only after checking with victim as to exact dosage and proper administration.

4. Blisters.

   What to do: Wash blister area clean.

   Sterilize a needle.

   Open blister from edge.

   Gently squeeze out fluid and cover with dressing.

   Keep it clean.

5. Chills.

   What to do: Put person to bed.

   Keep person warm.

   A chill or sudden cold feeling will usually be associated with fever. This may be an indication of a severe illness and should be investigated by a physician.

6. Choking.

   (see Fig. 6)

7. Common cold

   What to do: For adults, 2 aspirin every 4 hours. (1 aspirin every 4 hours for children.

   Drink ample amounts of fluids.

   Rest.

   Use nose drops from medical kit.

CHOKING

What To Do

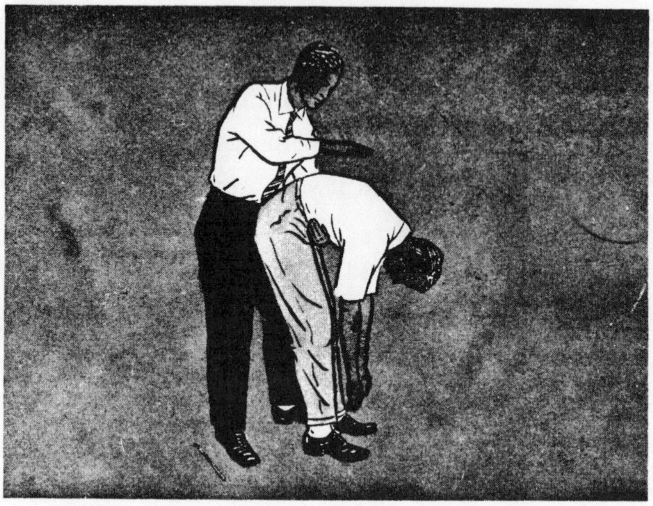

Hold as shown above—a vigorous slap on the back will help dislodge obstruction in throat.

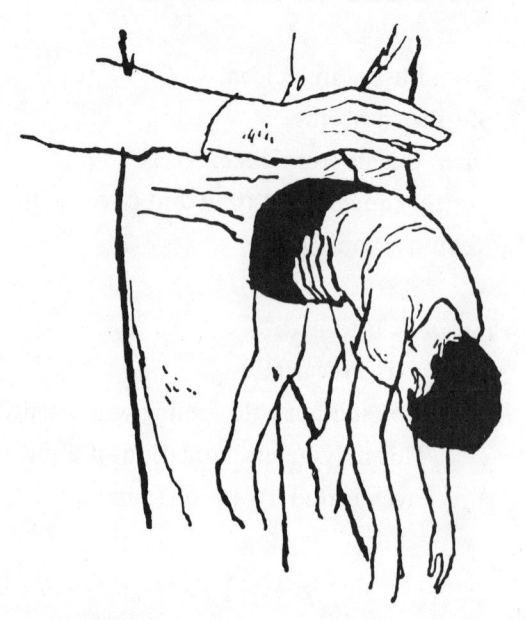

When objects are caught in the throats of children and cannot be reached with the fingers, they may be dislodged as shown above. If breathing stops quickly try above methods of removing obstruction and start artificial respiration immediately.

FIG. 6

Sore Throat.
> What to do: Gargle with hot water and salt (1 teaspoon to a pint).
>
> Cold compresses over throat.
>
> Aspirin every four hours.

8. Convulsions.

Epileptic convulsions may occur at any time, including during sleep, and affect people of all ages. While the popular picture of a convulsion—that of a person suddenly losing consciousness, shaking, foaming at the mouth, and losing control of his bladder or bowel—is frequent, other types of seizures also occur which are much less dramatic, less easy to recognize but equally as important.

Convulsions occuring in babies and young children frequently indicate the presence of a serious illness and medical attention should be sought as soon as possible. In the older child, the adolescent or the adult the urgency is not as great, but certainly consultation with a physician is always indicated as early as possible.

Convulsions are caused by an abnormal activity of the brain and can result from many different causes which include infections such as meningitis, injuries to the head, etc. Recurrent episodes of fainting may in actuality be what are called fragments of convulsions and need to be recognized and treated as such.

With modern medical therapy three-fourths of individuals with a convulsive disorder can be treated and lead a completely normal life.

There is very little that can or should be done for the individual who is having a convulsion except to move him or her, if possible, to a bed or on the floor and remove objects or furniture from the vicinity so that he or she will not get hurt. A pillow should be placed under the head, collar, belt and tight clothing should be loosened. No attempt should be made to insert any object between the clenched teeth. Since many individuals will be very confused and sleepy after a convulsion, it is best to have them rest quietly for several hours afterwards.

If a baby or young child has a seizure during the course of a febrile illness, attempts should be made to reduce the fever by using sponging with cool water and by using aspirin.

Once a person with convulsions has been started on anticonvulsant medication, it is imperative that the medication be taken exactly as prescribed. Even missing a single dose may result in a seizure. As a rule, such medication must be taken every single day and may have to be continued for many years. Many people think that medication can be stopped because seizures no longer occur, while in reality the seizures do not occur *because* of the medication.

Unfortunately in the minds of many, there is still a stigma attached to convulsions or to the term epilepsy. This is totally unwarranted since the overwhelming majority of epileptics are perfectly normal in every other respect and should be treated as such. There are very few things that epileptics should not do, such as drive a car (unless they have been seizure-free and under good medical control for a least two years), work near potentially dangerous machinery, or engage in dangerous sports such as mountain climbing. In regard to swimming, the buddy system should always be used in such instances.

With appropriate medical care, the future of the epileptic child or adult in the great majority of cases can be considered to be quite excellent.

9. Croup.

Usually begins suddenly at night when the child wakens with a hoarse cough, and has difficulty in breathing.

    What to do: Inhalation of steam from boiling water or hot shower provides the best means of relief.

10. Diabetic Emergencies.

There are two types of diabetic emergencies. One results from lack of insulin (flushed face, drowsiness, rapid gasping breaths, sweet odor to breath) and the other from too much insulin (white face, moist clammy skin, confused state).

    What to do: Put victim to bed.

        Prop him in a partial sitting up position.

        Keep him warm.

        If lack of insulin (see above), give person his regular dosage.

        If too much insulin, give a teaspoon of sugar.

11. Diarrhea.

    What to do: If child, see "A Word About Routine Pediatric Care" (p. 223).

        If adult, withhold food for 24 hours.

        Give water if person does not have nausea or vomiting.

        If diarrhea persists for 2 to 3 days give person sugar-salt solution (1 level teaspoon of salt and 1½ tablespoons of sugar in a quart of water).

12. Earache.

    What to do: Apply ice bag or water bottle to affected ear (try ice bag first).

        Apply 2 to 3 drops of ear drops from the medical kit (unless ear is draining).

        Give aspirin for pain.

13. Eye irritations

    What to do: Use corner of a clean handkerchief to gently remove foreign object.

        Remove chemicals and very fine dust by flushing with water. Turn head to one side. Use plenty of water.

    What *not* to do: Do not rub the eye.

14. Fever.

    What to do: Determine the amount of fever.

                      Put person to bed.

                      Give 2 aspirin every four hours.

                      If temperature severe, i.e., greater than 101 deg. F., consult physician.

                (See item 22, Meningitis, below)

15. Frostbite.

Frostbite occurs when flesh is exposed to extreme cold. The flesh first becomes pink, then numbs and becomes white as it freezes. There is usually no pain, as the freezing deadens the nerves. If the freezing is stopped while the flesh is still pink, before it is completely frozen, the condition is called chillblains, which, though extremely painful on warming, require no special treatment. Frostbite is most likely to occur in the hands, feet and face. Improper clothing, exhaustion, and high altitude contribute to frostbite.

If the freezing is noticed early enough it may be checked by rubbing the flesh gently to restore circulation.

The treatment of frostbite consists mainly of rapid rewarming of the frostbitten part. The best way to do this is to soak the frostbitten part in water at a temperature of 112 deg. F. (44.5 deg. C) until it thaws. If this is not possible hold the injured part against a warm part of the body. If you cannot measure the temperature, use water that feels warmer than your own (normal) hand. DO NOT use a light bulb or hot water bottle unless you are certain that the temperature will not be higher than 110 deg.; many frostbitten persons have received bad burns from excess zeal in warming. Insulating the part is not much good as a way of thawing it, because the frozen part cannot generate much heat. As it thaws, the frostbitten part will become red, swollen, and painful. The flesh will be sensitive for quite a while, so if it is a hand or foot that is injured, it may be necessary to put padding between the fingers or toes. Warm drinks will add to the injured's comfort. Alcohol should not be given.

In all cases of frostbite the patient should be warmed thoroughly, in a sleeping bag, hot room or hot bath, to enable warmed blood to reach the frozen part. Do not give alcohol, but hot drinks speed up the re-warming process effectively.

In severe cases of frostbite, large blisters form; these must not be broken if possible, but covered gently with large sterile dressings, loosely bound. If the blisters break, dead skin can be clipped away with sterile scissors and scrubbed hands, and dry sterile dressings applied. Within a few days badly frostbitten parts turn purple, then black—gangrene has set in and this is a medical problem. In some cases the gangrene is dry, a demarcation line forms over a period of several weeks and part of the member (usually less than expected) falls off. Wet gangrene is usually infected and may poison the rest of the body.

In any case of bad frostbite, anti-biotics should be started at once and kept up until the victim is hospitalized—which he must be.

Under no circumstances rub with snow. Rub with the hands. Do not rub vigorously or hard, but softly and for a long time. Warming against the belly or groin or armpits of a warm person is effective if out in the field.

If the person has frozen feet—white, hard without feeling—do not warm or try to thaw until it is no longer necessary for him to walk or stand. He will do better to walk on the frozen foot than to walk after it has thawed.

Remember: warming the whole body, and protecting the frozen part from tissue damage and infection are the crucial parts of treatment. (See also Exposure article, p. 55).

16. Headache.

Headaches constitute the single most common complaint of mankind! As a general rule, the overwhelming majority of headaches are not serious (although they may be quite painful and disabling to the patient). The number of individuals with severe headaches who actually have a brain tumor is infinitesimal in spite of the widely held popular belief to that effect.

There are basically two different types of headaches, the muscle-tension type and the vascular or migraine type.

Headaches are actually relatively easy to treat. If they are not as a rule relieved by a couple of aspirins, they probably require treatment by a physician. Many people put off obtaining medical advice for headaches in the belief that they will get used to it, or that they will go away, that they are not dangerous or that is simply a condition of life that one has to bear! This is far from true and in the proper hands, even the most severe and disabling headache can be prevented and the individual may be almost completely headache free. Self-medication for chronic, recurring, long-duration headache is usually self-defeating. The earlier the headache is brought under control, the better the results.

17. Heart Emergencies.

What to do: Administer medication person usually takes.

Place person in a comfortable position (usually sitting up).

Reassure person.

When able to eat, give salt-free, soft diet.

If chest pain, get medical help immediately.

18. Heat Illness (headache, nausea, vomiting, muscle cramps, heavy perspiration).

What to do: Put person to bed or lay him down in a cool place.

Give him cool salted water to drink (1 teaspoon of salt to 1 quart of water).

19. Heat stroke (high fever, no evident perspiration, headache, dizziness, sometimes coma).

What to do: Undress the person and put him to bed.

Sponge body freely with tepid water to reduce temperature to

102 deg. F. or less.

Administer salt solution (½ teaspoon of salt in a glassful of water every 15 minutes).

This is an emergency and person should be seen by a doctor.

What *not* to do: Do not give stimulants such as coffee or tea.

20. Hernia (section of bowel has found its way out of abdominal cavity into scrotum or thru abdominal wall).

What to do: Have person lie flat on his back with knees drawn up.

Apply cold compresses to the site of the hernia.

If the first two procedures fail, have person kneel with his buttocks raised.

What *not* to do: Don't attempt to push back the hernia with finger.

Don't give laxative or cathartic.

21. Insect bites.
    (a) Bees, wasps, hornets—remove stinger

    Apply paste of baking soda.

    (b) Scorpions—Apply tourniquet above the sting. (Remove after 5 minutes).

    Apply ice pack.

    Keep person warm.

    Keep affected limb lower than the rest of the body.

    (c) Spiders (black widow)— Keep person quiet.

    Elevate hips and legs in shock position.

    Apply hot packs if abdominal cramps develop.

22. Meningitis.

Meningitis means that the coverings of the brain, inside the skull, are infected, usually by some type of bacteria.

The patient with acute meningitis usually complains of headache, very often has a stiff neck (he has difficulty, discomfort, and occasionally pain in trying to touch his chin to his chest) and has a fever. The disease is particularly dangerous in infants and young children, and may be recognized only by the fact that the child is fussy, refuses to eat, and may have a fever. The baby may appear flushed, be restless and be sleepier than usual. Infection of the nervous system is an extremely serious condition and requires immediate medical attention. Convulsions may occur, especially in young children. The appearance of a rash, especially one that looks like many small pinpoints of blood immediately under the skin, is a very dangerous sign. Some types of meningitis are extremely contagious and it may be necessary for all those who have had contact with the patient to be examined by a physician and possibly also receive medication to protect them against the infections.

23. Nausea and vomiting.

What to do: Determine cause if possible.

Put person to bed.

If cause can be determined, refer to appropriate section of Handbook.

Give warm, clear liquids only when tolerated.

Start soft foods after liquids have been retained for 24 hours.

24. Nosebleed.

    What to do: Place person in sitting position, head back slightly.

                Gently grasp lower end of nose between thumb and index finger, firmly press the sides of the nose against the center for 5 minutes.

                Release pressure gradually.

                Apply cold cloths or ice.

                If bleeding persists, plug the nostrils with small strip of gauze.

25. Pain.

    What to do: Locate, determine severity and type of pain.

                Determine cause if possible.

                If cause can be determined, refer to appropriate section of Handbook.

                Give aspirin 2 tablets every four hours.

  (a) Pain in chest accompanied by arm pain and difficulty breathing indicates heart disease; person should see a doctor.

  (b) Pain in stomach may be due only to minor upset, but it may be more serious; person should see a doctor if there is tenderness in the belly, if the belly is rigid, or if a fever is present. Do not give a laxative, since it may make the trouble worse.

26. Poisoning. (See also Susan Donnis's "Poisons," p. 59, and Elizabeth Baer's and Janet Young's "A People's Herbal," p. 122.)

    What to do: For *general poisoning:* Dilute with large amount of luke warm water and salt.

                For *acid* (e.g. phenol, hydrochloric) and *alkali* (e.g. lye, ammonia, drano) dilute and neutralize (for acid—milk of magnesia or baking soda; for alkali—vinegar or lemon juice; then give milk). *Don't induce vomiting in acid or alkali poisoning.*

                For *kerosene*—give ½ cup of mineral oil. *Do not* cause vomiting, keep person warm.

                For carbon monoxide (starts as headache, nausea, dizziness or sleepiness)—get person fresh air as soon as possible.

27. Skin rash.

    What to do: To relieve itching, apply compress soaked in cool soda solution (3 teaspoons of baking soda and a glass of cool water).

                For rashes with small pimples or eruptions cover generously with paste of bicarbonate of soda.

                Caution person not to scratch or rub area.

28. Snakebite.

a) GENERAL. Poisonous snakes of one type or another are found in most parts of the world. Different species live in different geographical areas. The medic should familiarize himself with the kinds found in the area where he is working. One of the first concerns in treating snakebite is to properly identify the kind of snake. Treatment with antivenin involves a certain amount of risk and should not be given if the bite was from a non-poisonous snake. About one-third of the time a poisonous snake strikes it does not inject venom. Treatment is not necessary in these cases. The presence of fang marks and the development of pain, redness, and edema (accumulation of fluid) are indications that venom has been injected.

b) TREATMENT

(1) Immobilize the bitten area and keep the patient as quiet as possible. Do not let him walk or run. Do not give stimulants such as alcohol.

(2) A loose constricting band should be placed between the bite and the heart until definitive therapy can be started. One should be able to easily slip a finger under the band; it should impede lymphatic flow, but must not be so tight that it stops blood flow. It should *not* be loosened and tightened as this pumps the venom into the system faster. Once other therapy has been started, the constricting band should be removed and left off.

(3) If the bite is seen within the first 30 minutes, a single longitudinal incision about one-quarter inch deep and one-quarter to one-half inch long should be made over each fang mark, and suction applied by cup, bulb, or mouth (safe unless you have open sores). Crossed incisions or multiple incisions should not be used. If more than 30 minutes have passed since the bite, incision and suction are of no value and should not be used. Sterile technique should be observed as much as possible.

(4) Antivenin is the most important therapy in the treatment of snakebite. In North America the polyvalent antivenin made by Wyeth can be used for all but the coral snake. In many other areas of the world, specific antivenins are available for the snakes in the area. If the snake is a pit viper of any kind, the polyvalent antivenin will probably be of benefit. Antivenins are all made from horse serum. Since some people are highly allergic to horse serum, a skin test should be done before administering the antivenin. Children, in general, require more antivenin than adults. The antivenin is normally given intramuscularly, but particularly in severe cases may be diluted in 250 cc normal saline and given intravenously. Local infiltration of antivenin in the area of the bite should not be done.

(5) Antibiotics should be given because the puncture wounds from the fangs are often highly contaminated by bacteria from the snake's mouth. Broad spectrum antibiotics are preferred (tetracycline, ampicillin, etc.).

(6) Persons being treated for snakebite should be given a booster dose of of tetanus toxoid. If they are previously unimmunized for tetanus, it will be necessary to use tetanus antitoxin.

(7) The bite of a poisonous snake is very painful and requires the judicious use of analgesics. Intravenous administration of whole blood, destran, or saline solution may be required to combat shock. Vasopressors such as aramine may be necessary to maintain blood pressure.

29. Stroke (paralysis, unconsciousness).

    What to do: Put person to bed, propped up on pillows if he is more comfortable.

        When breathing is difficult, turn face to one side so fluid may drain from his mouth.

        Remove any loose dental bridges.

30. Tetanus.

Tetanus is a serious disease of the nervous system. Tetanus bacteria are commonly introduced and grow in an infected wound. The reservoir of infection is in infected domestic animals, especially horses, and in man. Immediate source of infection is soil, street dust, and animal and human feces.

Puncture wounds (a small, often insignificant wound, whose opening is covered by a skin flap; an example of a puncture is a wound that is caused by stepping on a nail) are especially prone to tetanus infection. The risk of tetanus also occurs with second- and third-degree burns. Prompt treatment should be given.

Symptoms of infection appear in two to seven days or later. If the wound area becomes tender, red, warm, and swollen, see a physician. A tetanus antitoxin or booster and penicillin will be given. If red streaks extend from the wound up to the arm or leg, see a doctor immediately. This means the infection has progressed and needs immediate treatment.

Home care: To relieve tenderness, soak wound in warm (as warm as can be tolerated) water. Keep clean and keep protected.

IMPORTANT: The tetanus bacteria can enter and grow in small, insignificant wounds. Never dismiss the possibility of infection, especially if the object involved in the accident was rusted, old, or otherwise unclean. Tetanus can be easily prevented by keeping immunizations up to date.

31. Toothache.

    What to do: If available, apply oil of cloves or toothache drops (from medical kit) on a small piece of cotton and gently pack into the tooth cavity.

        Repeat 2 or 3 times daily.

    Ice packs or hot packs may provide relief.

    Aspirin may be used to relieve the pain. (2 tablets every four hours).

32. Unconsciousness.

It would be literally impossible, as well as quite useless, to list all the conditions that may result in loss of consciousness. Except for unconsciousness of very short duration, which is seen with simple fainting or with some types of convulsions, prolonged unconsciousness always requires immediate medical attention.

Among the more common causes are the unconsciousness following head injury, that associated with sugar diabetes, and that of certain infections of the nervous system.

In general, while awaiting medical attention, collars, belts, and clothing in general should be loosened. It is important to try to prevent the person from "swallowing" his tongue. To accomplish this, be sure that the patient is turned on his or her side, or even better put him face down with the head turned to the side. Never attempt to give an unconscious person any food or liquids by mouth. It is better to keep the head at the same level or even slightly lower than the rest of the body. If the unconsciousness is the result of a head injury, handle the head and neck as little as possible. If the person must be moved from the scene of the accident, he or she should be transported on a hard surface such as a door or a wide plank, taking care to move the head and neck as little as possible.

James A. McCarthy
Charles M. Poser
William Poser

BASIC MEDICAL SUPPLIES

MINOR MEDICAL TREATMENT: Let wound bleed a little; wash thoroughly but gently with soap and water. Apply alcohol for more protection *around* the wound, but not in it. Cover with dry, clean gauze and adhesive tape.

BASIC SUPPLIES

Alcohol (70% isopropyl): The only essential antiseptic needed for first aid treatment. Rubbing alcohol differs from 70% isopropyl alcohol in that it contains glycerin to prevent skin dryness.

Aspirin: Buy the cheapest brand you can find that meets U.S.P. standards, evidenced by 'U.S.P.' printed on the label of the bottle. Avoid using flavored aspirin for children—small children may identify this as tempting candy.

Calamine Lotion: For relief of skin itching (mosquito bites, poison ivy).

Adhesive tape: 1"–2" wide.

Flashlight

First Aid Manual

Sterile needle: For extracting slivers, splinters.

Safety Pins

Sterile gauze pads: 4" wide.

Elastic bandage (Ace bandage): To support sprained joints. Be careful not to wrap tightly.

Tweezers

Hot Water Bottle: For relief of cramps. Avoid burning the skin by covering with a towel-thickness of cloth. With persistent cramps of the abdomen, see physician.

Ice Bag: A hot water bottle can double as an ice bag if ice is crushed small enough. Use cold to relieve pain and minimize swelling or bleeding. Apply immediately after injury, for three to four hours. *Never use heat.* Cold constricts; heat dilates.

ITEMS NOT RECOMMENDED

1. Any first aid antiseptics or ointments except alcohol.
2. Cough syrups—any cough not relieved by a heavily steamed bathroom or shower, hot fluids, or hard candies should be treated by a physician.
3. Ready-made first aid kits—commercial kits are expensive. A good collect-it-yourself first aid kit is cheap and just as convenient.

Susan Donnis

NOTES

IMPORTANT MEDICAL HISTORY EVERYONE SHOULD KNOW ABOUT HIMSELF

MAJOR MEDICAL ILLNESSES (such as required hospitalization or prolonged doctor's care)

    Date   Illness   Type of continuing problem
                                                               from this illness.

MAJOR OPERATIONS OR INJURY

    Date   Type of Operations or Injury

CURRENT MEDICAL PROBLEMS (diabetes, for example) or medications

MAJOR ALLERGIES (to foods or medications, for example)

    IMMUNIZATIONS   Date of last shot

      Tetanus—
      Diphtheria—
      Smallpox—
      Polio—
      Measles—

Person(s) to notify in case of emergency: _____
_____

Such information may be extremely useful to you in case you become ill while you are traveling. It would be a good idea to keep a copy of this information with you at all times.

FIRST AID FOR WOUNDS AND BURNS

Scratches, cuts, and other small wounds can best be treated by cleansing with soap and water and covering with a small bandage for protection from bumps and additional contamination. Anyone who feels he must use an antiseptic should shun the highly promoted brand-name products, choosing instead isopropyl (rubbing) alcohol. It (and any other antiseptic) should be applied, if at all, *around* the wound, never on the wound or in it.

The makers of branded antiseptic products do not share these views; indeed, in their advertising they often imply dire consequences if their products are not used. Consumers are the targets, for example, of a sharp promotional contest between purveyors of the many liquid antiseptics of one type or another; of attempts by sellers of the newer or less familiar types of antiseptic and antibiotic products (aerosols, sprays, creams) to carve a deeper niche in the market; and of an ever-renewed barrage of claims that "new" products are safer and more effective than the familiar standbys of the first-aid kit.

But whatever the advertisements and labels may say, the truth is that first-aid antiseptics used as commonly directed (that is, applied directly to the wound) probably do less good than harm. The amount of either will vary to some extent with the type and amount of active ingredients in the preparation's formula. The agents most commonly used in first-aid antiseptic products fall into several categories:

Alcohols, most frequently isopropyl and ethyl. The former is much cheaper and just as effective. In concentrations ranging from fifty per cent to ninety-five per cent, alcohols are probably as effective in killing most skin bacteria as any other type of germicide in common use. For first-aid use, alcohol is considered the most effective and least irritating of all antiseptics and is devoid of allergic effects.

Halogens, principally iodine and most often in alcoholic solution; that is, as a tincture. Recently, aqueous (water) solutions of iodine compounds (Isodine, Betadine) have been marketed. They cause less straining of the skin and less pain and they are possibly as effective as the tinctures for first-aid use; but they are more expensive.

Heavy-Metal Compounds (mercurial compounds such as ammoniated mercury, phenyl mercuric compounds, Merthiolate, Mercurochrome, or Metaphen and silver compounds such as silver nitrate or Argyrol). Many are available both as tinctures and in aqueous solution. Recently it has been shown that these compounds do not consistently kill the bacteria with which they come in contact, though they may prevent these bacteria from actively multiplying. *Allergic skin reactions are fairly common.*

Phenol (carbolic acid, cresol). To be effective, phenol and substituted phenols must be used in such high concentrations that they irritate the skin. Phenol itself is thought to penetrate the

---

Reprinted, with permission, from *The Medicine Show,* by the editors of Consumer Reports, published by Consumers Union. Copyright 1971 by Consumers Union of United States, Inc., Mount Vernon, New York—a nonprofit organization.

skin; if it does penetrate in sufficient quantity, systemic reactions may occur. This chemical still shows up in some proprietary remedies. And a number of branded antiseptic products, including Listerine Antiseptic and S.T. 37 Antiseptic, contain substituted phenols.

Quaternary Ammonium compounds. These substances are effective against one of the two broad classes of bacteria—gram-positive organisms, including staphylococci, commonly the cause of skin infections. But they have poor effectiveness against many gram-negative bacteria, which can also cause infection. Also, they are less effective against the gram-positive organisms on the skin than in a test tube. Proprietary products containing this class of antiseptics include Bactine, Phemerol Chloride, and Sephiran Chloride.

Bis-Phenols (hexachlorophene, bithionol). The bis-phenols are effective in preventing the multiplication of bacteria on the skin surface, but they do not kill the bacteria as quickly or as completely as alcohol. Among first-aid products containing hexachlorophene are Medi-Quick, Solarcaine, and Pepsodent Antiseptic. Bithionol is one ingredient in Johnson & Johnson First Aid Cream.

Antibiotics. Antibiotic preparations intended for use on the skin are available without a doctor's prescription. Neomycin and bacitracin are the antibiotics most commonly used, but not the only ones; Tyroderm, for example, contains tyrothricin. The wisdom of using antibiotics without medical supervision is to be questioned. When used repeatedly, they may encourage the development of resistant strains of bacteria; they would then be useless if these strains later caused a serious infection. The use of antibiotics can also lead to super-infections by resistant micro-organisms. And allergic reactions are reported frequently.

One other product often found in home medicine chests, hydrogen peroxide, is also sometimes used on small wounds. But it is not an effective first-aid antiseptic.

Tinctures are generally more effective than aqueous solutions of a given germicide. But alcohol alone is as effective as an equal amount of many tinctures. Consumers Union's consultants do not recommend any antiseptics packaged as sprays or aerosols, because it is almost impossible to use them without getting the medication into the wound. Also, the sprays and aerosols are needlessly expensive products.

Of late, ointments have been actively promoted as "first-aid creams." Very few data are available to show how effective they are. Claims that they aid in healing wounds should not be taken to mean that they speed healing.

The widespread belief that every break in the skin should be dosed with an antiseptic is founded mainly on the fact that large numbers of bacteria normally are present on the skin surface at all times. Most, however, are harmless. Indeed, one school of thought maintains that such micro-organisms aid in maintaining a healthy skin. Most disease bacteria do not find conditions on the skin surface suitable for growth. And the large majority of organisms that do enter a wound probably are killed most effectively not by an applied germicide, but by the body's own natural defenses.

These defenses, which are not fully understood, nearly always seem able to cope with the bacteria in a small wound. Certainly, one of the defenses is the physical barrier offered by the

FIRST AID FOR WOUNDS AND BURNS

skin itself. At the immediate point of a wound, the body must rely on other defenses—including white blood cells, serum, and fixed phagocytic cells which mobilize in a wound. These defenses probably are most effective when the skin is damaged as little as possible, and when conditions in and around the wound are as little favorable to bacterial growth as possible. Dead tissue in the wound provides an excellent medium for bacteria to grow on—a strong reason against the use of antiseptics directly on the delicate cells inside a fresh wound.

With this background, it is not difficult to outline a rational program for the treatment of minor wounds—comparatively small scratches, cuts, or abrasions. Deep puncture wounds (because of the difficulty of cleansing them through the small break in the skin) and large cuts or badly lacerated wounds (because of the great danger of massive bacterial invasion combined with the larger healing task confronting the body) should not be treated at home. Such wounds should be protected with a sterile dressing while the patient is taken promptly to a physician. Excessive bleeding from such wounds can usually be controlled by firm hand pressure on the sterile dressing. Never use a tourniquet unless absolutely necessary.

In treating a minor wound, three points need attention: cleansing the area gently; permitting the body's defenses to work; protecting the area from further damage by contamination.

The cleansing process should be gentle to avoid further injury, but foreign bodies must be removed even though removal may cause further injury. Water running from a faucet usually will do a good job of cleansing the wound itself. Bits of foreign matter not removed this way should be lifted out as gently as possible with tweezers sterilized by boiling in water. Bleeding also helps to cleanse the wound.

Ordinary soap and water are adequate for the removal of bacteria from the surface of normal skin. Such soaps are poor germicides, but they help wash away most of the bacteria. Soaps containing antibacterial agents, such as hexachlorophene, are little if any better than plain soap for this purpose because their antibacterial agents are not very effective germicides. *They are able to produce a significant reduction in the bacterial population of the skin only after they are used regularly for two to four days.*

Most of the organisms which remain after the washing can be killed by moistening the skin around the wound with alcohol for two minutes. It is difficult to apply antiseptics without getting them into the wound. And very few infections will result if this step is omitted.

When the cleansing is completed, allow a scab to form. It is not as effective a physical barrier as intact skin, but it helps protect the new cells during healing.

Because the scab is more easily damaged than skin, external protection is often advisable. A covering of sterile gauze and adhesive tape ordinarily suffices. The bandage should not be medicated. Nor should it be airtight. Moisture given off by the skin may be trapped and encourage the growth of bacteria. Plastic adhesive tape is bad in this respect. Adhesive bandages with plastic-coated gauze will not stick to a wound.

If the wound should bleed after the bandage is applied, and the gauze becomes stuck, it is best to leave it on as long as the wound is healing normally. Pulling the scab loose to change the dressing can only retard healing and increase the chances of infection. If a stuck bandage must be removed, hydrogen peroxide used to help soften the scab can reduce the damage.

Burns are classified according to the depth of damage. In a first-degree burn there is reddening of the skin, caused by the swelling of small blood vessels. In a second-degree burn, serum or fluid escapes from the swollen vessels into the skin, causing blisters. In a third-degree burn, the entire depth of the skin and some subcutaneous tissues are destroyed. Only first-degree and small second-degree burns can be safely treated at home.

The pain of such burns can be relieved by immediate immersion of the affected part in ice water or in cold, running water. Cold, wet compresses may also be useful for as long as there is pain. Sterile gauze impregnated with petroleum jelly, which can be bought specially packaged in most drugstores, is good for covering the burn. If a blister forms, a firmly applied dressing of this gauze helps prevent rupture and guards against secondary infection.

Leading authorities on first aid and the treatment of burns recommend that proprietary burn ointments never be used. Most of these remedies contain one or more of the following: analgesic drugs (Nupercaine, Butesin Picrate, Benzocaine), antiseptics, tannic acid, antihistamine drugs, cod-liver oil, vitamins, and chlorophyll. None of these materials has been shown to have any special pain-relieving value beyond that provided by the petroleum jelly or similar vehicles in which they are contained. Nor has it been established that burn ointments are of value in preventing infection or in assisting healing; in some instances, ointments may interfere with healing. The analgesic and antiseptic ingredients in many proprietary burn ointments have been known to cause many allergic reactions.

Extensive burns, irrespective of their depth, should be considered as emergencies and treated by a physician as soon as possible. It is hazardous to apply any ointment, oil, salve, or solution to a third-degree burn, because the drugs in the preparation can be absorbed and cause toxic reactions. Also, burn preparations can seriously interfere with later professional care.

Sunburn resembles an ordinary burn. If it is mild, without blistering, the pain may be relieved by compresses of cold water or cool baths. Extensive sunburn or deep, blistered sunburn calls for medical treatment.

EXPOSURE AND WIND CHILL EFFECT

Exposure to low temperatures results in hypothermia, or lowered body temperature which can be fatal. In most cases the individual has been chilled by being motionless and inadequately clothed in temperatures below zero. (Note the additional chilling from wind shown in the attached wind-chill table.)

Most commonly the person has passed out from drinking too much or has been knocked unconscious by an assault or fall. Frostbite and freezing generally occur under these conditions.

Exposure to cold tends to diminish judgement, decrease will, weaken strength and thus the person travelling in cold weather often wishes to rest; many persons have frozen to death from exposure in the wintry north because of falling asleep while resting. Activity is protective.

Symptoms of exposure include:

    Unreasonable behavior and violent language.

    Complaints of fatigue, cold, and sleepiness.

    Weak, slurred speech and poor vision and dulled hearing.

    Decreased mental ability and physical lethargy.

    Loss of judgment and perseverance.

    Loss of consciousness and, later, death.

Persons caught out in the cold without adequate protection must keep moving, stay awake, and strive for shelter. The will to go on often permits survival under fantastically bad conditions.

If the exposure victim is conscious when found, wrap him warmly in blankets or clothing, give hot sweet drinks (but not alcohol) and rewarm slowly. A warm tub (115 deg. F. or 46 deg. C) is helpful. Protect from wind. Examine for frostbite or freezing as soon as possible, and treat accordingly (see "Common Emergencies Guide," item IC15).

If the exposure victim is unconscious, look with special care for frozen areas (buttocks, fingers, toes, face), since these must be handled with special care. Watch pulse and breathing—both tend to be slow and either may stop suddenly. Rewarming must be slow and under constant supervision—if possible with a rectal thermometer in place (axillary is less satisfactory and oral temperature should not be taken on the unconscious person).

If the pulse stops, start closed-chest cardiac massage at once, along with mouth-to-mouth breathing. If respiration stops, do mouth-to-mouth breathing at once (see "Common Emergencies Guide," items IA1 and IA2). Keep up both procedures for a long time, since it is difficult to tell when an unconscious exposure victim is really dead. Medical help is essential.

                                                                        Charles Houston

WIND-CHILL EFFECT: EQUIVALENT EFFECTIVE TEMPERATURE

Actual air temperature (degrees F.)

Windspeed (mph)	50	40	30	20	10	0	−10	−20	−30	−40	−50	−60
5	48	36	27	17	−5	−5	−15	−25	−35	−46	−56	−66
10	40	29	18	5	−8	−20	−30	−43	−55	−68	−80	−93
15	35	23	10	−5	−18	−29	−42	−55	−70	−83	−97	−112
20	32	18	4	−10	−23	−34	−50	−64	−79	−94	−108	−121
25	30	15	−1	−15	−28	−38	−55	−72	−88	−105	−118	−130
30	28	13	−5	−18	−33	−44	−60	−76	−92	−109	−124	−134
35	27	11	−6	−20	−35	−48	−65	−80	−96	−113	−130	−137
40	26	10	−7	−21	−37	−52	−68	−83	−100	−117	−135	−140
45	25	9	−8	−22	−39	−54	−70	−86	−103	−120	−139	−143
50	25	8	−9	−23	−40	−55	−72	−88	−105	−123	−142	−145

Note: This table gives the effective temperature which, due to the wind-chill effect, is equivalent to the actual temperature in still air. The zero wind condition is taken as the rate of chilling when one is walking through still air (an apparent wind of 4 mph).

The above table is reproduced by permission of the Museum of Science, Boston, U.S.A.

NOTES

FIRST AID FOR POISONING

A. In *all* cases of poisoning it is important to get out *or* to dilute the poison.

B. Remember—If anyone swallows a poison it is an emergency. Any non-food substance is a potential poison. Always call for help *PROMPTLY*.

C. In cases of swallowed poison, HERE'S WHAT TO DO:
 1. Call Doctor, Hospital, or Poison Center *PROMPTLY*.
 2. Dilute the poison whenever possible. Give glass of water.
 3. Make patient vomit, if so directed, *BUT DO NOT IF*:

 —Patient is unconscious or is having fits.
 —Swallowed poison was a strong corrosive.
 —Swallowed poison contained kerosene, gasoline or other petroleum distillates (unless it contains dangerous insecticide as well, which must be removed).

 4. Directions for making patient vomit:

 Give one tablespoonful (one-half ounce) of Syrup of Ipecac for child one (1) year of age, plus at least one cup of water. If no vomiting occurs after 20 minutes this dose may be repeated one time only.
 If no Ipecac Syrup is available, try to make patient vomit by tickling back of throat with spoon or similar blunt object after giving water.
 Do not waste time waiting for vomiting, but transport patient, if indicated, to a medical facility. *Bring package or container with intact label.*

CALL FOR HELP PROMPTLY

IN VERMONT—THE MEDICAL AND HEALTH CARE

INFORMATION CENTER

1-802-864-0454

BE SURE TO HAVE 1 OZ. SYRUP OF IPECAC ON HAND

D. Keep the following important phone numbers handy, near telephone, in case of emergency:

Doctor's Office Phone _____ Police _____
Doctor's Home Phone _____ Poison Control Center _____
Local Hospital (Emergency Room) _____
Rescue Squad _____

Adapted from literature provided by American Association of Poison Control Centers.

POISONS

ACCIDENTAL CHILD POISONING. One child 5 years of age or under dies every day from accidental poisoning at home. This age group is the largest segment of our population being poisoned each year. The incidence of such poisoning is increasing. This is mainly due to a lack of awareness of the dangerous potential of many substances common to every home—medicines, cosmetics, household cleaners, pesticides—and carelessness in storing these products.

Experts list three major factors that contribute to accidental poisoning:
- (1) an inexperienced person
- (2) a potentially toxic material
- (3) an unsafe environment

Children aged 5 years or younger will always be inexperienced. It's up to you to recognize and prevent the other two factors.

Sue Donnis

TOXICITY OF SOME COMMON HOUSEHOLD ITEMS NOT GENERALLY REVIEWED AS POISONS*

There are numerous common household items that children tend to ingest. The following list contains products that are less frequently discussed either because they are generally assumed to be common knowledge or considered unimportant in a toxicologic review. This is obviously a partial list, there being many other such products. Our attempt here is to stimulate an awareness of the potential danger of household products.

(1) Aerosol Sprays: The most common propellants are the freons. In ordinary exposure they are harmless, but in deliberate, concentrated inhalations they have caused rapid death, possibly due to sensitization of the myocardium.

(2) After Shave Lotions: Contain alcohol, water and perfume. Observe for alcohol intoxication. In a few cases, in children, ethyl alcohol has been reported to cause hypoglycemia (abnormal decrease in blood sugar).

(3) Airplane Glue: These adhesive products are resins with a solvent to keep them fluid. The solvent is usually largely composed of toluene and not harmful unless deliberately inhaled in high concentrations, as in "glue-sniffing."

(4) Alcohol Drinks: The ethyl alcohol present may cause the common signs of intoxication. •In a few cases, in children, it has been reported to cause hypoglycemia.

*Adapted from Bulletin of National Clearinghouse for Poison Control Center, March - April, 1969.

(5) Ball Pen Inks: In the amounts available in ball-point pen cartridges the ink is not a hazard.

(6) Barbecue Fluid: The petroleum hydrocarbons may produce chemical pneumonia if aspirated into the lungs. This is very likely because of the low viscosity of the fluid.

(7) Bath Tub Floating Toys: Water, water-glycerin combinations and sometimes mineral oil are found inside of these toys. Occasionally an oil with a strong kerosene odor has been reported. The latter should be suspect for producing chemical pneumonia.

(8) Battery (Dry Cell): Flashlight and pen-type batteries are not swallowed but may be bitten into by children. A conventional flashlight battery (size D) contains only 1/5 of a minimum lethal dose (MLD) of mercuric chloride for a child. Other ingredients would not be expected to cause harm in amounts present.

(9) Beer: The ethyl alcohol present may cause the common signs of intoxication.

(10) Bleach: Mixed with bowl cleaners or ammonia, bleach forms chlorine or chloramine gas. Both are irritating if inhaled but the latter has more transient symptoms.

(11) Body Conditioners: Contain alcohol, water and perfume. Observe for alcohol intoxication. In a few cases, in children, ethyl alcohol has been reported to cause hypoglycemia.

(12) Bubble Bath Soaps: These are composed of detergents. If a child drinks it from bath water the most toxic effect would be vomiting.

(13) Candles: Neither beeswax nor paraffin, with or without scent or color, is likely to cause symptoms.

(14) Caps for toy pistols: The toxic ingredient is potassium chlorate present at approximately 4 mg/cap. The estimated MLD for a child is 4 to 5 grams of potassium chlorate, which would make a roll of caps nontoxic.

(15) Cigarettes: One cigarette or cigar contains a large amount of nicotine. However, the absorption of nicotine from tobacco apparently is delayed. The initially absorbed fraction causes vomiting, removing much of the tobacco from the stomach. Since nicotine is a liquid volatile alkaloid, it would not be expected to be present in cigarette ash in significant amounts.

(16) Cigarette Lighter Fluid: The petroleum hydrocarbons may produce chemical pneumonia if aspirated into the lungs. This is very likely because of the low viscosity of the fluid.

(17) Cocktails: The ethyl alcohol present may cause the common signs of intoxication. In a few cases, in children, ethyl alcohol has been reported to cause hypoglycemia.

(18) Colognes: Contain alcohol, water and perfume. Observe for alcohol intoxication. In a few cases, in children, ethyl alcohol has been reported to cause bypoglycemia.

(19) Crayons: Those bearing the C.P. or A.P. designation are nontoxic. Do not confuse children's crayons with industrial crayons.

(20) Dehumidifying Packets: Medicine bottles frequently contain small packets of moisture-absorbent materials—most often dried silica gel or charcoal—that are nontoxic.

(21) Deodorizer Cakes: Blocks are usually p-dichlorobenzine and less commonly naphthalene. The latter is more toxic to those with a glucose-6-phosphate dehydrogenase

POISONS

deficiency. Both these products should be removed from the stomach if child has eaten as much as a teaspoonful.

(22) Fish Bowl Additives: These products contain chemicals used to control the amount of chlorine or to kill fungus. Since small fish tolerate these chemicals they would not be expected to be harmful to children. At the most these products might cause G. I. symptoms (diarrhea).

(23) Golf Balls: The child who peels the ball down to its fluid core might experience an explosion of its liquid contents due to pressure. The most serious effect reported has been a mechanical injury to the eyes.

(24) House Plants: There is very little information on the toxicity of most house plants [But see pp. 127-129 —Ed.]. When no information can be found, we may assume that they are nontoxic in small amounts, since they are frequently ingested without reported symptoms.

(25) Kerosene: The petroleum hydrocarbons may produce chemical pneumonia if aspirated into the lungs. This is very likely because of the low viscosity of the fluid.

(26) Marking, indelible and special-purpose inks: These must be held suspect because of the possibility that they include analine dyes or toxic solvents.

(27) Matches: Less than twenty wooden matches or two books of paper matches do not contain enough potassium chlorate to be harmful to a child.

(28) Model Cement: These adhesive products are resins with a solvent to keep them fluid. The solvent is usually largely composed of toluene and not harmful unless deliberately inhaled in high concentrations as in "glue-sniffing."

(29) Paint: Most new indoor paints do not contain lead, and so are nontoxic if just a few flakes are ingested. However, repeated ingestion of leaded outdoor paint chips (or any other paint chips containing lead) may result in serious lead poisoning.

(30) Pencils: Lead and coloring pencils may be considered nontoxic. Even if they contain toxic pigments, coloring pencils ordinarily would not be ingested in toxic amounts.

(31) Plastic Cement: These adhesive products are resins with a solvent to keep them fluid. The solvent is usually largely composed of toluene and not harmful unless deliberately inhaled in large concentrations as in "glue-sniffing."

(32) Play-doh: This is composed of edible, digestable ingredients.

(33) Polaroid Pictures: The pod that breaks to develop the picture contains a small amount (1 cc) of highly alkaline material (pH 13-14). The fluid used to coat the photograph is not harmful.

(34) Porous-tip ink-marking devices (felt-tip markers): The Federal Hazardous Substances Act exempts these devices providing they meet certain requirements.

(35) Putty: Unless more than 2 or 3 ounces are ingested at one time there is no cause for alarm. If larger amounts are ingested there probably should be more concern for mechanical obstruction than for chemical toxicity.

(36) Roach Tablets: May contain a number of chemicals including arsenic and boric acid.

However, the child in most cases eats only 1 or 2 and has no significant symptoms. All legal insecticides must be labeled as to ingredients.

(37) Sachets: Used in drawers or closets, they usually contain an inert of edible powder that has absorbed essential oils. There is probably more danger from a massive inhalation of the powder than from ingestion. Those containing crushed petals have not been reported to cause problems.

(38) Shaving Creams: Aerosol shaving creams usually contain a soap. Most have a perfume and some have menthol and antiseptics in small amounts. The most serious symptom resulting from ingestion would be vomiting. The new "Thermal" shave creams contain 8% to 10% of sodium or potassium sulfite in the soap base with a 9% hydrogen peroxide solution in a separate compartment. These are mixed as dispensed from the container, producing a controlled exothermic reaction (heat). The resultant soap base contains about 10% of the sulfate salt and a small remainder of unreacted sulfite, but would have little toxicity.

(39) Silly Putty: Is made of silicones and 1% boric acid. No problems anticipated, although there are warnings of possible obstruction if large amounts are ingested.

(40) Smoke Pellets for Train Sets: These are usually supplied as capsules containing mineral oil or deodorized kerosene. If the kerosene-containing pellet is chewed before swallowing, there is danger of aspiration and chemical pneumonia.

(41) Soaps: Ordinary bar soaps may cause vomiting if ingested, but no other toxic effects are expected. Those bar soaps which contain antibacterial substances like hexachlorophene do not present additional hazards because of the small amounts present and the small quantities which are usually ingested.

(42) Teething Rings: These usually contain water (sterility questionable) or a glycerin-water combination.

(43) Thermometers: Broken glass may cut the mouth of children. The amount of mercury present is not harmful.

(44) Toilet Water: Contains alcohol, water and perfume. Observe for alcohol intoxication. In a few cases, in children, ethyl alcohol has been reported to cause hypoglycemia.

(45) Tooth Paste: Considered nontoxic—but those containing stannous fluoride have caused vomiting.

(46) Vitamins: Liquid and chewable vitamins are not harmful in the usual size bottles. However, if they contain iron, gastrointestinal symptoms might be expected.

(47) Dangerous Plants: For a list of dangerous plants with indication of the parts considered dangerous, see "A People's Herbal."

NOTES

SANITATION FOR SMALL RURAL GROUPS

PREFACE

Most of us think of sanitation in terms of public health regulations—too fussy, irrelevant. When you consider 10 or 20 people living together it becomes a matter of collective hygene—you are watching out for the health of your sisters and brothers. Good sanitary practice seems good for other things . . . keeping compost covered is good for the garden as well as the water; keeping infected fingers out of the dishpan is good for the infection as well as the dishes; keeping food covered, cooked, and cooled properly reduces vitamin-killing enzymes as well as people-killing diseases.

The importance of sanitary consciousness increases with the number of people involved. I have written here with groups of 10 to 20 in mind; you will have to stick to these suggested measures more stringently if your group is larger. Even if yours is a small group that occasionally has a crowd, you are better off to develop good sanitary habits now to cope with the wild bugs those people will bring.

There are a couple of topics here that I have not thoroughly researched and therefore mention only for their relevance to other things:

1. The matter of using human shit in the garden involves a lot of variables, like how long it sits before use, how well it decomposes, and what viruses it had to start with. There are people around who use it, and there are books (see Appendix 9 to this article; also see pp. 19-21, 78). Find them before you dig in. A good way to disperse potential hepatitis virus is to separate human shit from other animal and vegetable waste. Use the human manure to fertilize hay fields, the other on the garden. By the time that the hep virus gets into the food that the animals who eat the hay produce, or the shit they produce, it will be so diffused that it should be harmless.

2. Whether or not to pasteurize is a question harder to research. All public health types say emphatically "yes," most health food types say emphatically "no," old time country farmers don't give a shit. I do know that pasteurizing reduces the chance of someone getting sick from the milk of a cow or goat that happens to contain disease-producing organisms. See my Appendix 12 if you are interested.

I apologize for resorting to lengthy appendices, charts, and other toys of academia, as well as for numerous redundancies. I wanted to keep issues of limited interest out of the main test. The various topics are hard to separate, which means that I repeat myself often.

GENERAL PRINCIPLES OF SANITATION

In New England, public health types worry mostly about communicable diseases carried by people into isolated communities—things like hepatitis, typhus (from lice), flus, and a bag of organisms that cause infectious diarrhea. There is another article covering the treatment of various degrees of diarrhea. Yet some of the animals that are part of our families (dogs, cats, cows, pigs, etc.) bring us diseases, like screw worms, tape worms, trichinosis, dysentery, and some strange infections. We get all of these things generally two ways: by eating something infected; by getting infection into our bloodstream through an open cut. Fleas, crabs, and lice are transmitted through body contact (more on that later). Since the art of dressing open cuts is someone else's article, I'll leave that with only this advice: keep open cuts clean and covered, away from animals and manure, and out of the dishpan.

One of the things we accept when we live collectively is that if one person has a bug, everybody has it. There are two general ways to eliminate epidemics; if either one worked completely, there would not be any epidemics:

1. Eliminate the sources, which means screening everybody who visits you even just for a meal. This is difficult as well as unhospitable.
2. Practice maniac sanitation, which means separate washing, eating, and living facilities for everyone, and sterilization of food, utensiles, and people. Somehow this violates the spirit of a collective.

A lot of us have reacted to the mores of grade-school sanitation with all of its germ-phobia and compulsive cleanliness. That is as much of a head disease as hypochondria. But if you have so little as a sore throat, you would do your brothers and sisters a favor to isolate yourself, eat from paper plates for a few days (or keep your own plate and wash it after the other dishes), use a separate towel and clothes, and stay out of the kitchen. Unfortunately many diseases, like hep, are in you before you know it; you could go to Siberia, and the others would still get it. Most of my advice concerns isolating bugs already around you.

WATER

There are some myths we better clear up first:

1. "Running water (in a brook) purifies itself in 25 feet." Bull! Filtering through 25 feet of sand is one thing, flowing over open rocks is another. No matter how uninhabited the land is above you, some squirrel or deer will still dump his load (or his dead cousin) in the stream. Rotting leaves and branches in the brook add to the unpalatability of the water.
2. "Deep wells are always safe." Varying subsoils and the increasing sophistication of the chemicals used in cleaning, on farms, and in factories mean that a lot is not filtered out

even at depths of 250 feet. Often return water from a jet pump infects deep streams. People living in a rural part of New Jersey poured dye down their toilets and found it in their drinking water in a few days.

3. "Just pour in some Clorox." You should NEVER use chlorine (whether bleach or chlorinated lime) to disinfect a well, spring, settling basin, or storage tank unless it is ventilated and you are prepared to go without water for at least a week. Chlorine is a good disinfectant, but it is more poisonous than what you are trying to kill if used improperly. More on that later.

4. "Shallow wells are OK if 100 feet from the barn, drywell, or shithouse." That's a misquoted magic number from public health handouts that doesn't consider where wells, barns, outhouses, etc., are on a hillside and what the ledge is like under. A better (but not complete) statement would advise putting the well or spring uphill from possible contaminents.

5. "You can use anything to wash with." As I said before, disease comes through open cuts as well as the mouth. Also, one coldwater rinse of a coffeecup with semi-sewage could start a bug.

Dead animals, crap, and the like aren't intrinsically bad; there are certain bacteria that do appear when manure or bodies rot; if we ingest them our bodies reject them (nausea, diarrhea). But the real heavies in bad water are diseases transmitted by humans and their body waste: typhoid, dysentary, hep. Farm animals don't often get the same kinds of these diseases humans get; but they can transmit them. Cows drinking bad water have passed typhoid in their milk. You shouldn't feed water to your animals you wouldn't drink yourself. So, half of the story is finding good water; the other half is keeping it good.

If you don't have a permanent water supply for man and beast, get a dowser, then build a spring or well with the following principles in mind. If you have a water supply that gives you cloudy, smelly, excessively taste-y water, if you have occasionally had diarrhea go through your house, if you tend to have crashers (or even visiting friends), if your water corrodes or discolors metallic utensils and fixtures, if you carry drinking (including cattle) or washing water, THEN (1) get a water test, (2) check the symptom/cause/cure table, (3) do something about it.

THE TEST. State health departments test private water supplies for coliform bacteria (fecal bacteria) without any hassle (see my Appendix 5 for information), as long as you get the sample to them in a couple of days. But the trick is to get a complete test of the water: for acidity, alkalinits, dissolved sodium, iron, manganese copper, lead, fluoride (yes, too much fluoride rots your teeth), sulphur, chlorine, ammonia, nitrate, nitrite, and calcium carbonate and magnesium (hardness).

If the test shows that your water has more per liter (N.B.: parts per million (ppm)=milligrams per liter (mg/1) than *a*) 10 coliform bacteria, *b*) .01 milligrams of ammonia, *c*) .05 milligrams of albuminoid nitrogen, *d*) 0 milligrams of nitrite salt, *e*) 2 milligrams of nitrate salt, start looking for sources of local seepage into your water supply. All of these things indicate sewage, manure, animal, or vegetable decay.

SANITATION FOR SMALL RURAL GROUPS

THE TABLE. Even without a chemical test you can spot some water problems.

Symptom	Cause	Cure
Water is cloudy, esp. after a rain	Groundwater seepage	Cover, ditch around the source and see my Appendices 3–5
Metallic taste (1) like rotten egg	Lots of iron, sulpher or manganese	Water often undrinkable before unsafe, but see my Appendix 2
Metallic taste (2) with blue-green stains on fixtures	Copper salts	Dangerous where staining is extreme; change water source, but avoid springs or wells near, or water from, streams with blue-green rocks.
Rapid corrosion of iron, steel, and copper	Acidity usually from rotting plants	Move well or spring away from swamp or stagnant water
Test indicates small excess of *a* or any two of *b–e*	Minor sewage contamination	Make a filter (see my Appendix 2)
Test indicates lots of *a* or more than two of *b–e*	Major contamination from surface drainage; dead animal; drainage from barn septic tank, out-house	Protect top of well, ditch, remove the carcass and disinfect the water supply, move well or source (see my Appendices 3–5)

"Nitrate-nitrite (combined) concentrations that approach 10 milligrams per liter will cause severe (often fatal) sickness in children under a year of age. Because the commercial and natural contaminents that contain these salts vary seasonally, you should test your water at three month intervals for a year if there is any nitrogen contamination other than coliform bacteria."

Hard water (presence of calcium and magnesium salts) is an indirect health problem . . . you can't get things very clean without using harsh and environmentally disastrous detergents. Washing soda (sodium bicarbonate) usually "softens" water by replacing the calcium in solution with sodium, which doesn't affect washing. Or go old timey, put up gutters, and collect rainwater, nature's softest.

THE DOING. Check with the Appendix for your kind of source. When a major change is necessary, it may be easier to move or rebuild the source of contamination, which is the business of the next section. A problem that is peculiar to collectives that take over an old house originally built 50 to 150 years ago for one family, is that the well, outhouse, barnyard, and cesspool were all put in by someone who didn't know too much about underground seepage, or that they have too little capacity for a collective. In this case it is usually better to move the well at least 100 feet away and uphill from the house, barn, outhouse, and pasture.

DISINFECTION. After you get done with cleaning, rebuilding, or moving your well, spring, filter tank, or any of that stuff, disinfect it. This is especially necessary if you take a dead animal out of your well. After cleaning the well and tank, add either 4 ounces of chloride of lime or one pint of clorox per 1000 gallons of water (there are about 8 gallons per cubic foot). Stir. Don't draw any water for several days. If the well and tank are open to the air, you can probably flush out the disinfectant in three days. If they are covered, wait till five, then draw a glass of water from the tank or well. If it smells like a swimming pool (chlorine), let it wait a couple more days. When the smell disappears, pump the well dry, and let it fill again. Give it the nose test again. If it doesn't smell, it can be used. This applies to a spring also.

IF YOU CARRY WATER . . . Dipping water in buckets and carrying it to the kitchen is bad news. But when the pipes freeze or the regular well dries up, you have to do it. So here's how to make it less lethal:

1. Use a special dipper left at the well that won't put any ground contamination into the well.
2. Pour the water into a covered container in the house, a new 20 gallon plastic garbage pail will do. (Avoid "odor-free" or green plastic garbage pails, since they are treated with chlorine salts that affect the taste of water stored in them.)
3. Dip with one dipper that stays inside the container when not being used; do not drink from this dipper.
4. Wash the pails frequently, and store them upsidedown, not inside of each other.

If you carry water normally, consider putting in a hand pump in the house. A pitcher-mouth pump, 100 feet of 1-inch plastic pipe, and a pipe strainer cost about $25, not much more than pails, dippers, and garbage cans. If you can't bury the pipe to protect it from frost, lay it so that it drains back into the well, then lift the pump handle all the way up when you are done drawing water. This allows the water to drain out so it won't freeze. Keep enough water to prime the pump for the next time. If the pipe won't drain, a three foot layer of hay, evergreen branches, or even snow over the pipe will usually keep it from freezing.

WASTE

The other half of the water story is keeping your waste out of it. But you have to think of more than your own safety when you dig your next shitpit. The environmental protection laws for Vermont fill a large box; for New Hampshire it is a smaller box, and for New York a much small box. But each state has very specific regulations for domestic waste. They have complicated the problem of sanitary waste disposal for collectives, since local towns can implement them for political as well as sanitary reasons. The best thing to do to avoid hassle is to visit your friendly local health inspector, building inspector, planning board chairman, or zoning board chairman (whichever is most powerful), make friends, and find out the regulations you could get nailed

SANITATION FOR SMALL RURAL GROUPS

with. Hold him responsible for the information you get.

Probably you are in one of two situations now: you are planning to make an adequate, sanitary, and environmentally homogenous disposal setup (congratulations), or you have inherited an old sewer system that occasionally clogs, and goes where you don't know (too bad). If, however, you know where everything drains and it's OK, skip this section.

Human and animal manure, garbage, and washwater cause two distinct problems: being wet, they can carry water-born diseases down to the water table; being highly organic, they make great fly hatcheries (more on flies in "The Kitchen," below). So it would seem reasonable to keep all waste dry and covered until the active bacteria in it has digested it and broken down the viruses. Flush toilets, garbage disposals, and septic tanks keep waste very wet so that it will flow through pipes. According to the Canadian Department of National Health and Welfare, "Household sewage disposal systems . . . are relatively expensive, seldom entirely satisfactory, and often a public health menace." On the other hand, ". . . properly constructed and maintained privies are one of the safest sewage disposal methods." If you want the specifics of wet and dry disposal methods, see my Appendix 6. Here are some principles for safe composting, drywell construction, sewer maintenance (if you must), and other waste considerations.

COMPOSTING. Whether or not you are into gardening, a compost toilet is probably one of the best things going. You might even be able to convince town officials in more congested areas that it is better than a septic tank and leaching field.

1. As far as possible, centralize your waste. One big toilet works better than several smaller ones.
2. Locate on high ground, where surface water flows away, off of, or well above ledge, and where subsoil drainage is good (see my Appendix 7).
3. Dig a hole at least four feet deep; the bottom should have an area of at least 2 square feet per person using it.
4. If you plan to retrieve the compost, dig two holes, or one big hole with a watertight divider, preferably on a slope to make removal easier. You'll be using one hole, or one division of the big hole, at a time (while the other cures). Also build a watertight lining at least half way up the side of the hole (this will retain most of the nitrogen).
5. Build a solid house which makes a relatively airtight cover for the hole inside the house. Put a ground level vent into the hole, and also a flue vent to let out odors. Build a solid house. Screen all openings. If you don't plan to empty the hole, make the house portable.
6. Don't build a bench. In addition to allowing total elimination, squat toilets do not transmit diseases through seat contact. The hole in the floor can be about the size of a toilet seat, but more oblong. It should have a tight cover. Make the hole part of a larger lid that can be lifted to pour in garbage and other organic waste.

There are graphic designs for two kinds of toilets in my Appendix 8 and sources of information on proper ingredients in Appendix 9. [see also section VII of "Commune Medics Guide" and diagrams following.] Everything organic—including garbage, garden wastes, spent animal litter, cuttings, manure—should go into the toilet. Although you might think that it would fill up very fast, the extra matter and fiber increases the decomposition rate. As much as 80% of what goes into the hole blows away as gas or vapor, or seeps away.

Avoid using chemical bucket toilets. They are smelly, messy, and environmentally undesirable since the chemicals kill a lot of useful bacteria that make the compost toilet work. The convenience of shitting in a nice warm house is not worth a burnt ass (from splashed chemicals) or the mess of carrying 5 gallons of putrid slop through your front parlor. In any case, don't mix it with your garden compost.

DRYWELLS. In almost every way a *dry* well—in which you dump water—is opposite from a *wet* well—from which you get water. If you use a compost toilet, you will need a separate place to safely get rid of washwater, even if you don't have a sink and drain.

1. Unlike a toilet, several drywells are better than one.
2. Locate on high ground, protected from surface drainage, off of ledge, and where there is good subsurface drainage (make a percolation test—see my Appendix 7).
3. Be particularly careful to locate away from wells and springs, or brooks and ponds (state sanitation laws set specific distances from bodies of water).
4. Dig a hole that is at least 6 inches deeper than the deepest known frost for your area; for northern New England 4 feet is deep enough. The area of the bottom depends on the number of people in your family (see my Appendix 10).
5. Line the bottom with field stone or coarse gravel.
6. Cover the hole tightly to keep surface drainage out. If your drain pipe is small (2 inches or less), include a vent pipe that rises above probable snow level and is screened. If you use wood for the cover, thoroughly creosote it.

Unlike the toilet, little decomposition takes place in a dry well. Therefore it is important to keep solids, like bits of food, out of the drain. If the well is big enough, at least six feet above the water table, and isolated from the water supply, it should never back up, and should safely dispose of dirty, potentially diseased water.

SEWER MAINTENANCE. If you inherited flush toilets, the disposal system probably isn't big enough for your family. On the other end of that sewer pipe there can be an outlet into a river or lake, a cesspool (just a big dry well), or a septic tank and leaching field. If you have one of the first two, you are due for a bust by the state health board; so start thinking about compost toilets before they come. In the meantime guard against backing up with a can of lye. A third of a can of this deadly, corrosive stuff poured down a cleanout hole will clear any grease or other organic matter. A cleanout is a Y in the soil pipe (usually in the cellar) with a removable plug in one of the branches. Don't let anything go down the drain while the lye works.

A leaky toilet is a distinct health hazard, but it is easy to fix. Flush the toilet, then loosen the two acorn nuts on the base of the stool. You may also have to disconnect the tank from the stool. Lift the stool free. Around the hole in the floor is a greasy seal; this is the problem, usually. Clean any grit from the neck of the hole and also the outlet of the stool, then replace with a new seal (sometimes called a bowl seal in hardware stores).

If you have a septic tank and field, at least explore it. Try to find out how big the tank is; 600 gallons is standard for a one family house, and is good for up to 12 people if they aren't very extravagant with water. Find out also the area of the leaching field. This is what drains the tank; its capacity isn't as stretchable as the tank's (see chart in Appendix 11); since it is buried, it is hardest to fix when it gets clogged or overused. If you are going to stick with the system, add some more branches to the leaching system.

The septic tank will occasionally have to be pumped out. Toilet paper, tampax, and other inorganic solids that don't decompose into a liquid effluent settle to the bottom of the tank; after a while this sludge piles up and blocks the flow.

Bear in mind that most septic tanks and connecting pipes are leaky, and therefore potentially dangerous to wells.

OTHER WASTES. As I have often mentioned, barns and pastures can drain into water. Indiscriminate pissing near even a deep well should be checked. Burning of rubbish or brush near a water supply can quickly alkalize it. Liming a field near a water supply can do it, too. If you use a separate compost pile or manure pit, keep them covered: (1) flies breed in open piles of rotting organic matter; (2) rain leaching through the pile may contaminate the water supply; (3) preventing leaching will preserve the nutritive value of the matter.

THE KITCHEN

There are lots of disease sources wherever there is food. The chances of any of them acting seems to increase geometrically with the number of people trucking around the kitchen. Although everybody likes to stir the soup and taste the pudding, someone better be cook for a day and yell "Get the hell outta the kitchen!"

In building a kitchen or just moving furniture, try to make a distant separation of food storage, cooking, and washing areas. This allows several people to work without walking on each other, as well as isolating disease-laden traffic from cooking, and especially, stored food.

COOKING PRACTICES. Although keeping vitamins in food usually goes with good sanitation, I'll leave that rap to someone else; also the stuff on safe canning and food poisons. I will lay on one cooking tip: cook all meat, including homegrown, and especially pork, well to kill trichinae and other parasites in the tissue (see "Commune Medics Guide"). Other things to be conscious of:
    1. Hands that touch everybody's food have to be clean. If you are into tacking up "Wash Yr Hands" signs, put them over the stove or the kitchen table, not the sink; they would insult the intelligence of anyone who makes it that far. Also, wash in clean, warm (if

possible) water. If you use old dishwater or someone else's washwater, you might as well not wash.

2. People with colds, hay fever, infections of any sort, running sores, lots of pimples, boils, and carbuncles can contribute staphylococcus organisms to the menu, especially starchy things. Cooking doesn't necessarily kill the toxins. The organisms move slyly along a mixing spoon, through the air. Keep them out of the kitchen.

3. Wash garden vegetables and fruit that have been recently (two weeks) fertilized (organic or not) especially carefully.

4. Avoid cooking anything acid (tomatoes and other fruits) in aluminum, since harmful salts can occur.

5. Keep leftovers cool and covered. Staph bacteria grow and bloom in four hours at room temperature.

DISHWASHING. The policy in some houses of everybody-wash-their-own doesn't make it sanitationally. It puts everybody's grimy hands in the dishpan, which dirties and sometimes contaminates the water quickly. The water gets filthy and cold, and the next one in line isn't about to lay himself out to dump it and fill the pan.

Everybody can get their hands in the pan, but one or two to a meal, please. Here are some principles:

1. Use as hot a washwater as you can stand.

2. Either use scalding hot rinse water (tongs or a wire basket will get the dishes out of the water), or use a disinfectant in the rinsewater. A teaspoon of Clorox or ½ teaspoon of Iodophor per 5 gallons is enough. A second rinsewater is necessary to rinse off the disinfectant, which in both cases is poisonous. The scalding rinsewater method is better.

3. *Never* wipe dishes. If the rinse water is hot enough, they will dry themselves.

4. It is better to wash silverware and drinking vessels first when the water is cleanest, plates, bowls, and serving dishes next, pots last.

STORAGE. Hanging is probably the cleanest way to store pots. Putting them inside of each other introduces stove soot and general grime to the insides of pots. Hanging is also good for kitchen tools, since drawers tend to accumulate junk and dirt, and rarely get soaped down.

Cover *everything* eatable. And garbage, too. Flies, mice, cats will walk around in your rice without bothering to wash beforehand. It is usually better nutritionally, since many grains lose food value if exposed to light and oxygen. Also, clean the refrigerator or larder as soon as it begins to smell. Molds and bacteria do grow at 35 degrees F.

FLIES. Although malaria isn't very common around here, other fly-borne diseases are. Any virus transmitted by body waste or the mouth is fair game for flies, since they tend to breed in shit, walk in garbage, and snack in your kitchen. Even if your disposal is fly-tight, your garbage sealed, and your dishes sterilized, flies will still buzz your kitchens, and tromp through your food after they've explored someone else's spent Kleenex.

   1. Screen them out. This actually works; but it works better if the kitchen isn't the only entrance into the house.
   2. Flypaper isn't exactly organic, but it beats DDT; it is also safer than those yellow Shell strips, which are now banned from food areas for being toxic. Put flypaper where flies congregate, but not in sunlight or drafts, since these dry out the paper too soon.
   3. Avoid burning lights in the kitchen during fly season; incandescent (including gas and kerosene) light attracts flies.
   4. Flies often lay their eggs in open, warm, moist places like the kitchen ceiling. Wash it with a disinfectant like lysol; that will kill larvae and maggots, and eliminate a whole fly generation.

The war against maggots and flies goes on all year; a fly is buzzing above my lamp now in January. (See "Hepatitis" for more reasons for and tips on fly control).

We have found that hens offer good fly control if you let them out to scratch for themselves. In a pasture near our house they eagerly peck the fly larvae out of the fresh cow shit. The hens are healthy and give bigger eggs. A few venture into the garden to steal bean bugs and other vegetarians.

ANIMALS

Meat and milk animals and poultry can get a variety of diseases that injure the food they produce. Household pets pass things like fleas and worms on to us, because we handle them so much. Sometimes animals get sick from the water they drink; it ought to be as pure as the water you drink. Spoiled or infested food often lays them down. Dirty, wet litter and bedding spreads parasites. Appendix 13 lists animal diseases that directly affect man. To keep disease out of the barn and off your table, you have to treat the animals as brothers and sisters.

The variety of animal diseases is greater than human diseases; so I will mention only general types and principles that will reduce their spread.

WATER-BORNE GERMS AND INFECTION. Each animal has its own variety of water-borne disease; other animals aren't generally susceptible to them. For example, dogs get hepatitis, but not the kind that humans get. However, TB comes to humans through the milk of afflicted cows; other diseases can cause bad effects in people who eat animal produce.

Mastitis is a common udder infection in cows and goats that often spreads viruses to humans. It is usually caused by vaginal discharge flowing onto the animal's tits (teats), her lying in shit, or some physical injury to the udder. Calves can cause it by roughly butting the bag before sucking—this is instinct. There are a variety of cures depending on the degree of infection; the important thing to remember is that as soon as you notice any change in the feel of the tit, the pliability to the bag, or the color and texture of the milk, something is usually wrong, and the milk should not

be used. Other milking and milk-handling considerations:
1. Wash the tits before milking. A drop of Iodophor in a pint of warm water is strong enough.
2. Take one squirt from each tit into a small cup to check for curds, stringyness, yellowish, or bloody milk—signs of infection. If these are present, milk the animal to remove the infected material and *discard the milk.*
3. Milk into an easily cleaned bucket (plastic will do), partially covered, if possible, to keep bedding and flies out.
4. When finished stripping, dip each tit into the Iodophor solution. This protects against infection as the tit contracts.
5. Quickly strain the milk and cool it. If you strain with cloth, use a clean one for each milking.
6. Wash the milk pail as you would a drinking glass.

There is controversy in the straight world about the value of pasteurization. This heating destroys some of the B vitamins, vitamin C (there *is* some in raw milk), and vitamin D (that's why they have to add it). The two major diseases—TB and brucellosis (undulant fever in man)—killed by pasteurization have been generally checked by state testing and inoculation programs; goats rarely get TB. Your animals aren't likely to get them, unless you swap and truck them around a lot. Pasteurization properly done does destroy disease bacteria in milk but it does not replace good milkroom sanitation. More on pasteurization in Appendix 12.

INTESTINAL PARASITES. These are worms trichinae, and others that cause dysentery. Grazing animals get them by eating grass that a mildly infested animal (including wild animals) has dumped on. Pigs fed raw slaughter waste often get them. Dogs get them by eating carcasses left by hunters. Every cowpie is a potential hatchery for both parasites and flies that could carry the larvae into your kitchen. Some larvae are so small that they blow around in the air, easily inhaled. The life cycle varies by species and season; but it ranges from several days to two weeks. That is the amount of time you have to act when you first spot parasites. When an animal eats without looking healthy, check its shit. Here are some ways to avoid the parasite cycle:
1. Milk in a clean place away from where animals are likely to dump; a closed or at least screened room is better. Use flypaper over the stanchion.
2. Feed animals in mangers and troughs, not where the feed can be mixed with bedding.
3. Rotate pastures frequently—every 4 to 5 days; some farmers have found that this alone almost eliminates worms.
4. Avoid using the area around the house, outhouse, or water supply for pasturage.

Rare cooked meat—pork especially—is a great source of worms.

FLEAS, LICE, CRABS AND TICS. Dogs, cats and most other hairy animals get fleas and tics. Cows, goats, and hens get lice. They can all give them to you if you handle them, or even walk near them. Crabs are pretty much a human-to-human thing, since they can hardly crawl on their own; but they are a louse's first cousin, and can be taken care of the same way. Fresh bedding in the barn, good housekeeping, and personal cleanliness are about the only preventatives. A thorough delousing procedure is described in "The Commune Medic's Guide."

If you come across tics (they are not very common in New England) dab them with kerosene before you try to pull them off; try to do it with tweezers so that the head does not stay in and infect the skin. Derris root powder will kill them, too.

POSTSCRIPT

Most of the information that I have used in this article is based on conditions we have seen in various collectives in the Vermont–New Hampshire area, as well as our own experience living in groups, on a farm. I have referred to technical sources for the exact number of something or a chart useful for situations beyond experience. I have suggested the use of disinfectants hesitantly because I know that they are equally poisonous to humans as to germs. If anyone knows alternatives to these dangerous chemicals, or has seen a bum steer in what I have written, or has a situation that needs discussion, please write me, so that I can improve future issues of this article.

Owen Lindsay
L'Chaim
Passumpsic, Vt. 05861

APPENDIX 1

DAILY REQUIREMENTS OF WATER for various animals (adapted from *Farm Water Supplies,* circular 133, Vt. Extension Service)

Human (washing, drinking, kitchen in a house with piped water, flush toilets, showers, etc.)	50–75 gallons
Cow, horse, steer (drinking only)	12 gallons
Servicing a milk animal (probably less if milking is not mechanized).	20 gallons
Goat or sheep	2 gallons
Hog	4 gallons
100 Chickens or hens	5–10 gallons
100 Ducks or turkeys	10–18 gallons
Human (washing, drinking, kitchen in a house with only hand-drawn water, no toilets).	15 gallons

APPENDIX 2

A SAND BARREL FILTER will reduce or eliminate the effect of minor sewage contamination, or some cloudiness from small particles suspended in the water. It works best with a continuous flow spring, but can be adapted to any situation, as long as you are willing to pour water into the top of the barrel. Use a watertight 55-gallon drum to which you can attach a filter screen and tap at the bottom. Line the bottom 6-10 inches with coarse gravel, fill up to about 6 inches from the top with fine river sand. Be sure to keep the top of the barrel covered to keep bugs, leaves, and other crud out of the water. This will filter about 3-5 gallons per minute, depending on the sand.

APPENDIX 3

DEEP WELLS are usually driven right next to the house (unless that is in a valley floor). They are costly to build ($10-15 per foot) but are usually reliable through droughts. They are only as safe as their casing and cap are tight. Seepage from a leaky septic tank can easily get into the casing. It is easier to move the septic tank, outhouse, etc. Before you replace the cap, disinfect the casing (see DISINFECTION, p. 68). In this case, dilute the chlorine with about five gallons of water, and pour it down the casing, making sure it drips down all the sides.

APPENDIX 4

SHALLOW WELLS AND SPRINGS are sensitive to local contamination, because they feed on streams near the surface. But for that reason they are easy to relocate, away from the barn, drainage field, etc. Get a dowser and head uphill from the sources of contamination. Shallow streams are usually easiest to find on the sides of hills. If you have an old well or spring sufficiently protected from seepage, it may have to be covered tightly to keep ground runoff, leaves, bug larvae, and small animals out. If you are rebuilding the casing, raise it two feet above the ground, ditch around it, and put a tight cover on it with all openings screened.

APPENDIX 5

WATER TEST and REFERENCES: Circular 133 of the Vermont Extension Service thoroughly describes the effects of various contaminants and pollutants, as well as many mechanical, chemical, and wholly orthodox ways of getting rid of them. Water testing sample bottles can be obtained by writing (Vermont) Dept. of Health, 115 Colchester Avenue, Burlington Vermont or (New Hampshire) New Hampshire Department of Health, Concord, New Hampshire. I don't know the address for New York or Massachusetts. Supposedly Vermont will test private water supplies thoroughly (not just coliform) once a year, but you have to press for this. Sometimes water softener salesmen can get your water tested for minerals if you talk sweetly.

Other sources of information:

Water Supply for Rural Areas and Small Communities, E. G. Wagner and J. N. Lanoix, pub. by the World Health Organization, 1959.

Sanitation Manual for Isolated Regions, Dept. of National Health and Welfare (Canada) 1967. This has a good section on hard water.

APPENDIX 6

WET VS. DRY DISPOSAL—the technical names are *anaerobic* (wet) and *aerobic* (dry) decomposition. Actually the difference is in the amount of air that can circulate through the decomposing matter. Under water and in a sealed septic tank the matter has little of the oxygen necessary to aid the chemical reaction that builds up tremendous quantities of heat that in turn kill many disease organisms. The dry aerobic method allows the pile to reach temperatures of 140 degrees, 160 degrees, which is the temperature Pasteur found killed bad things.

APPENDIX 7

A PERCOLATION TEST is just a way you can see if the ground can absorb moisture. Dig a post hole through to top soil, or go down about 18 inches. It is best to do this in a wet season; if it doesn't work then, your dry well will back up in the spring thaw. Line the bottom of the hole with gravel, then fill the hole with water. The percolation rate is the number of inches the level of the water drops per hour. (See Appendix 10 for table for a dry well and Appendix 11 for a leaching field).

APPENDIX 8

DESIGNS FOR A COMPOST TOILET AND REGULAR TOILET

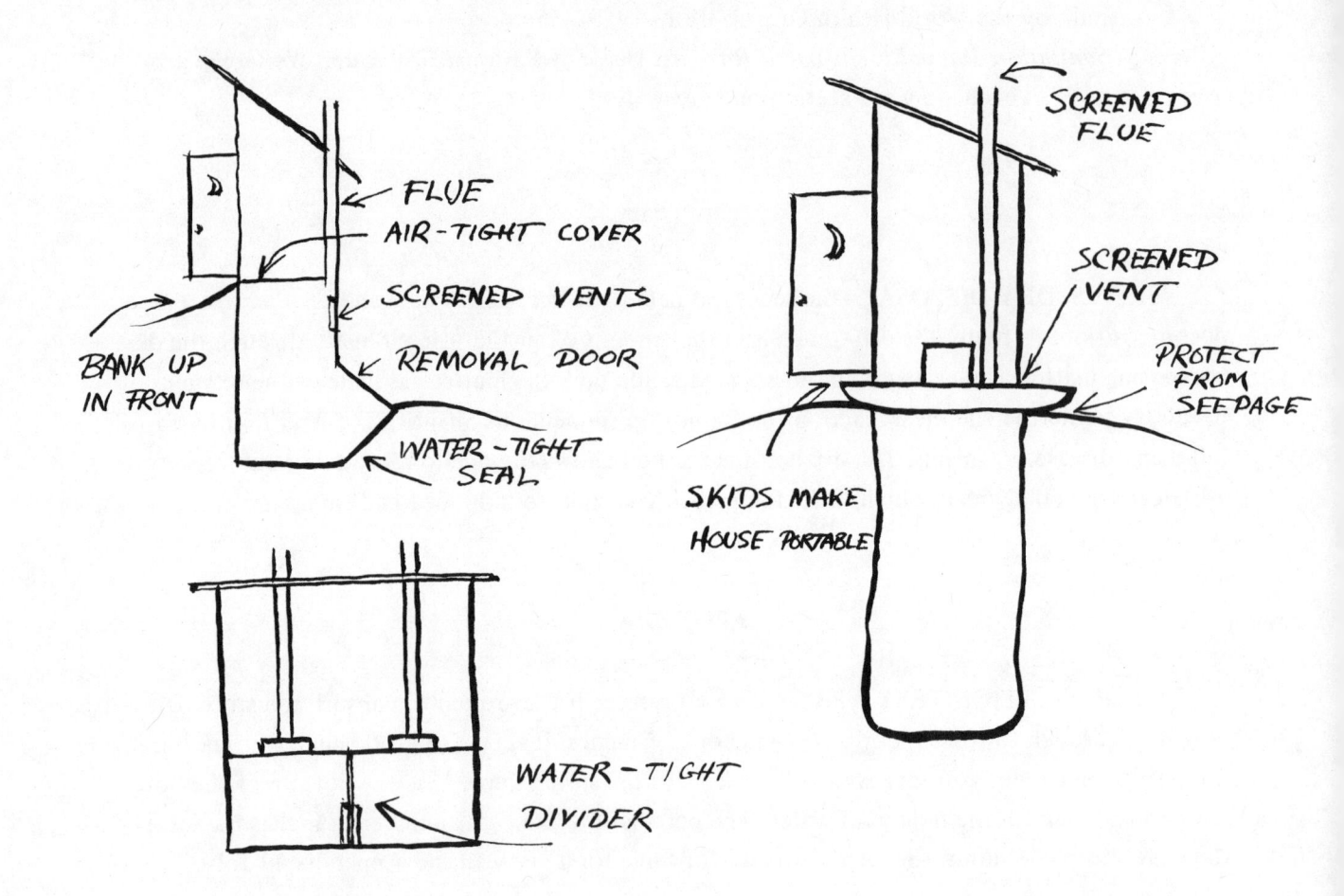

APPENDIX 9

INFORMATION ON SAFE COMPOSTING

Composting, H. B. Gotaas and *Excreta Disposal for Rural Areas and Small Communities*, Wagner & Lanois, World Health Organization, 1958.

"Compost toilet" by Ken Kern in the *Mother Earth News* No. 6. Good discussion of the principles involved.

The Encyclopedia of Organic Gardening, J. T. Rodale and staff, Rodale Press. Believe it or not, this lists the nutritive content of every imaginable organic substance, and would help you work out the carbon-nitrogen ratio that Kern stresses.

SANITATION FOR SMALL RURAL GROUPS

APPENDIX 10

DRY WELL AREA: Before you can use this chart you need to make a percolation test (See Appendix 7). A percolation rate of less than 2 inches per hour isn't good for much of anything. Hunt for a spot where the soil is sandy and well above any known subsurface streams. Often how fast the water seeps down is related to the hydrologic effect, that is, the distance above any underground water—it's like an upside down lamp wick.

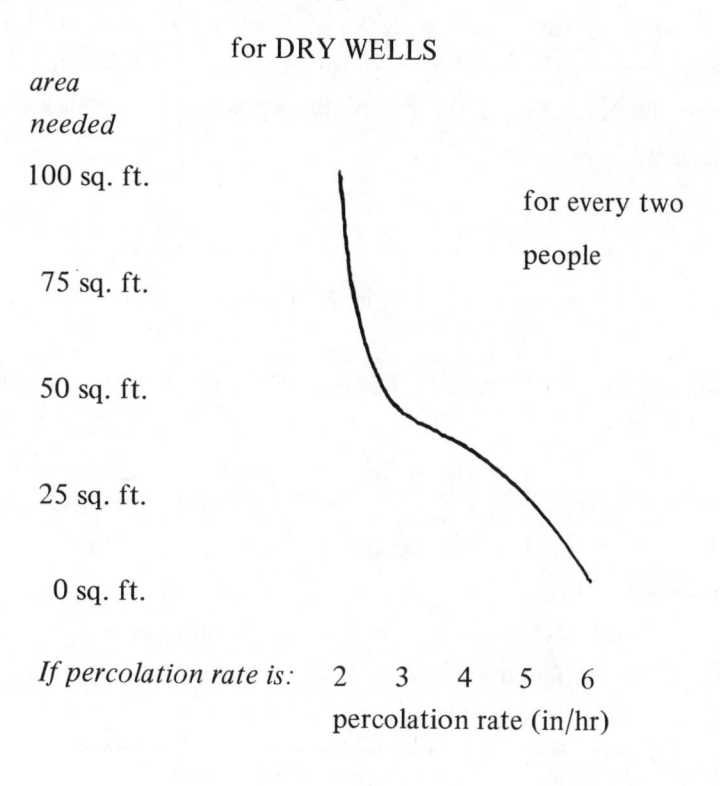

for DRY WELLS

area needed

100 sq. ft.

for every two people

75 sq. ft.

50 sq. ft.

25 sq. ft.

0 sq. ft.

If percolation rate is: 2 3 4 5 6

percolation rate (in/hr)

APPENDIX 11

LEACHING FIELD AREA: This too, requires a percolation test. This chart and the one above come from *Soils Suitable for Septic Tank Filter Fields,* USDA Soil Conservation Service bulletin No. 243, which has good tips on selecting a site for both dry wells and leaching fields.

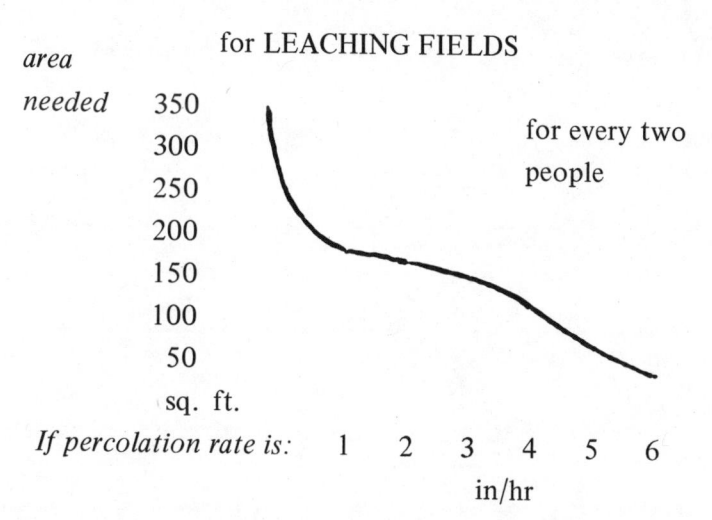

for LEACHING FIELDS

area needed

350
300
250
200
150
100
50
sq. ft.

for every two people

If percolation rate is: 1 2 3 4 5 6

in/hr

APPENDIX 12

PASTEURIZATION pros can be had at any milk dealer's or farm agent's office. The cons are harder to come by, but I found ten in the *Health Finder* by J. I. Rodale and the diverse writings of that original organic milk freak, Adelle Davis. But it is a good idea if your cow or goat has a cold or a minor case of mastitis. Here's how it works: *over water*—set a stainless-steel, glass, or unchipped enamel pan of milk in a dishpan of water, for example—quickly heat the milk (stir to prevent burning if you don't do it over water) to 170 degrees F. and hold it there for 30 seconds. (Or heat it to 145 degrees F. and hold it there for 30 minutes.) You can use a meat, jelly, or maple syrup thermometer. Then cool the milk as rapidly as possible in a cold water bath to 40 degrees F. That's all there is to it.

APPENDIX 13

ANIMAL DISEASES THAT AFFECT MAN: here are the most common and the animals that normally harbor them.

Dogs and cats	*Cows, goats and sheep*	*Hogs* (in addition to most bovine diseases)	*Poultry*
rabies	tuberculosis (cows)		salmonellosis
tic borne diseases	brucellosis		psittacosis
leptospirosis	cowpox	trichinosis	
ringworm	ringworm	cystercercosis	
tape worm	Q-fever		
cat scratch fever			

Owen Lindsay

NOTES

SAFE CANNING
(and Freezing)

When you are wondering how to keep fruits and vegetables over the winter, plan to store as many as possible whole. The processing of foods (canning, freezing, etc.) takes time, deprives foods of some of the valuable vitamins, and may result in food spoiling without easily being noticed. Cabbages, onions, late squashes, pears, apples, leeks, brussel sprouts, and all root crops will keep over the winter if stored properly. Enzymes, which cause decay after plants are picked, are increasingly active at warm temperatures. Therefore, gather the crops at a cool time of the day and store them immediately. Another good way of storing plants is by drying them. Peas, various beans, many fruits, leaves for teas and herbes, and some other vegetables can be dried and kept for long periods of time. These methods of storage are not in the scope of a canning rap, but read several of the following articles and you'll get a good idea of how it is done.

1. J. I. Rodale's *Encyclopedia of Organic Gardening.* (see Storage; Dried fruits and vegetables)
2. Bruce Lowther's *Wood Heat Quarterly No. 2.* (see Winter Food Storage)
3. *Storing of Vegetables and Fruits in basements, cellars, outbuildings and pits.* Home and Garden bulletin No. 119; U.S.D.A. Send 15 cents to Superintendant of Documents, U.S. Government printing office, Washington, D.C., 20402. Or get it free at a local Agricultural extension service.
4. (If you are carnivorous) E. Jaeger's *Wildwood Wisdom,* pp. 220–226; info on Smoking meat, Jerky and Corned meat.
5. Scott and Helen Nearing, *Living the Good Life.*

You will be amazed at how easily these foods are stored and how well they keep if you follow the suggestions of people who have done it before.

Tomatoes, berries, asparagus, swiss chard, and other foods can be stored over the winter cheaply and easily by canning. "Canning" is a term referring to the packing and processing of foods in airtight containers. Commercial canned foods come in tin cans (actually coated steel) or in glass jars with vacuum sealed lids. Home canning is generally done in mason jars (Ball, Kerr...) with a two-part metal lid. Some jars have glass lids. We prefer the two-part metal lids because they are easy to test for seal. If the lid is flexible, it hasn't sealed. If it is rigid and makes a "ping" when you tap it with a spoon, it has. The lid consists of a band or ring and a dome lid. Bands used during processing may be taken off once the jar has sealed and cooled. They may be reused as long as they are not rusty, warped, or worn. The dome lid seals the jar and must be in perfect condition. Use each dome lid only once. Notice that the rubber ring attached to the dome lid will have a raised ridge after you pry it off a sealed jar. This indicates that the jar did seal. You can buy a variety of mason jars with bands and dome lids, and boxes of just bands and/or dome lids in most markets.

SAFE CANNING (AND FREEZING)

TYPES OF SPOILAGE IN CANNING

Many of us who are somewhat unfamiliar with canning connect it with "ptomaine poisoning" and botulism. The idea of a food poisoning developing that is tasteless and odorless is enough to scare anyone from canning or eating home-canned foods. Here, I will describe various types of spoilage in canning, what causes them, and how to recognise them. The important thing is this: spoilage will not occur if canning procedures are followed carefully.

There are three types of organisms (all are plants) that cause spoilage in canning: molds, yeasts, and bacteria. Molds are a common fungus that are useful in making penicillin and other antibiotics; roquefort, camembert, and other cheeses. In canning they usually grow on the surface of acid foods such as fruits and tomatoes (tomatoes *are* technically fruits). Since it requires oxygen and moisture to grow, mold on a jar indicates that it didn't seal. Boiling will easily kill molds. I have never heard of molds themselves being poisonous. (Molds are the cause of ring worm and other skin diseases, but this has nothing to do with canning). However, since molds indicate that a jar didn't seal, bacteria can enter and food can start to spoil. So it's a good idea to disgard canned food with mold in it. Exception: jams, jellies, and syrups have large amounts of sugar which reduce the chance of spoilage. I have scraped the mold off these foods, boiled them, and used them—no problem.

Yeasts, like molds, are found most everywhere. They are the chief agents in fermentation: the process by which simple sugars are turned into alcohol and carbon dioxide. Like molds, yeasts are most apt to grow in acid foods, and like molds they are easily killed by boiling. Fermented foods have a sour odor, bubble, and the carbon dioxide released will cause the dome lid to release. Fermented canned foods mean that the food was not processed (cooked in the jar) long enough. Some bacteria also cause fermentation. Do not try and use fermented canned foods.

Bacteria, the third cause of spoilage, is more complicated to understand and control. Certain types of bacteria produce toxins that are highly resistant to heat and will not be killed by normal processing. Many bacteria are anaerobic, which means they grow best in the warm airless situation of a canning jar. It is therefore essential to get rid of bacteria by:

1. Carefully washing all foods to be canned *before* cutting them, paring them, or pulling out the hulls (strawberries). Otherwise the bacteria can get inside. Berries are best washed by LIFTING them out of the water, so that dirt will settle to the bottom.
2. Wash jars in hot soapy water, rinse in scalding water, and drain. Dome lids should remain in scalding water until used.
3. Wipe top of jar with a clean damp rag after filling so that no berry seed, etc., can interfere with the seal.
4. Process exactly as recommended. All non-acid foods such as vegetables, meats, fish, should be processed in a pressure cooker. Add 1 minute to processing time for each thousand feet elevation if the time called for is 20 minutes or less. Add 2 minutes per thousand feet elevation if the time called for is more than 20 minutes.

BOTULISM. Soil particles everywhere contain the bacteria Clostridium Botulinium. Everyone swallows these spores and bacteria on fresh fruits and vegetables. These are not harmful. But if canned foods contain these spores, and since these heat-resistant devils are unlikely to be killed during processing, they may develop and produce a deadly toxin, botulism.

It is not always easy to notice when a jar contains this poison. Most types of botulism produce a gas that would eventually cause the jar seal to release, but I have never heard that this *always* happens. Generally there is a "cheesy, gassy, sharp, bitter" off odor, and the food is foamy and faintly rancid. These characteristics are more noticeable when the food is heated. Botulism is more apt to develop in the less acid foods (vegetables, meat, fish), but in the acid foods any off odor is harder to detect. You cannot get rid of the toxin by washing the food. The only way to destroy the toxin is by boiling the food five to ten minutes. It is a good precaution to boil canned vegetables and meats seven minutes before serving them. Smell the hot food for any off odor. If you suspect Botulism, destroy the food without tasting it. G.M. Dack (*Food Poisoning*) suggests mixing the food with several spoonfuls of lye and letting it stand 24 hours, and washing the jar out with a lye solution. Never taste canned food with an off odor. Extremely small amounts are lethal.

(brief digression)

GENERAL FIRST AID FOR POISONING
(except: strong acids, alkalis, strychnine, kerosine)

1. Dilute the poison by giving water or milk.
2. Induce vomiting with several teaspoons baking soda in half a glass of water or milk or magnesia.
3. Give 2 parts crumbled burned toast in 1 part tea and 1 part milk of magnesia.
4. Call a doctor.

NOTE: Do NOT give liquids to or induce vomiting in a person who is unconscious or having convulsions.

Antitoxins for botulism have been developed, but since symptoms of botulism are so slow in developing, they and first aid can rarely be given in time. Nausea and vomiting usually occur in 12-36 hours, but may not occur for 2-4 days. There is pain in the abdomen, difficulty in muscular coordination, diarrhea followed by constipation, double vision, and dry mouth. These poisonings are often fatal.

Flat Sour Spoilage is also caused by soil bacteria. The jar seal does not release because no gas is produced. When opened the food has a bad acid odor. There may be a white sediment at the bottom of the jar. Flat sour spoilage takes place at 130-150 degrees F. This means that when you take jars out of the canner, set them on racks where air can circulate around them and they can cool past this temperature as quickly as possible. For the same reason, food packed hot should not stand before processing. If you suspect spoilage in any canned food, discard it.

SAFE CANNING (AND FREEZING)

There are other types of food poisoning, not found in canning, which have symptoms similar to botulism, but they appear and disappear more rapidly. Staphylococus food poisoning is the most common. It appears in cured and salt meats, bakery goods, and unrefrigerated milk or cream. Symptoms appear in 1-3 hours. Recovery is in 1-3 days. The bacteria grow best at room temperature, so this type of food poisoning is easy to control by heat or refrigeration.

Salmonella food poisoning comes from the meat or milk of diseased animals.

"Ptomaine poisoning" is a misnomer. Ptomaines are the products of decayed foods and do not themselves cause disease. It is rather the toxins produced by the bacteria that cause illness. Except for botulism, food poisoning by bacteria is rarely fatal.

REFERENCES ON FOOD POISONING.
1. G. M. Dack, *Food Poisoning,* U. of Chicago Press, 1943, 1956.
2. E. B. Dewberry, *Food Poisoning,* 1959.
3. Most canning booklets have a section on spoilage.

(back to canning)

FOOD FOR CANNING

Fruits should be fresh, ripe, firm. Pick over berries carefully. Discarded fruit is great for jams and jellies.

Vegetables should be young and tender. Older ones take longer processing to prevent spoilage. Wash food carefully.

As with any food to be stored, the quicker you gather the food and store it away, the better. Some booklets say "Two hours from garden to jar;" others say one hour. Whichever it is, don't gather more crops than you can handle in a short time. Have your processing equipment and fire ready to go. Don't let the enzymes destroy valuable nutrients.

Meats should be from healthy animals and thoroughly cool before canning (no body heat).

METHODS OF PACKING JARS

Raw or Cold Pack is used for most fruits and tomatoes. Pour boiling liquid (water, syrup, or fruit juices) on top of tightly packed raw fruit. Process the jars in a boiling water bath for the recommended time. Be sure to leave the suggested head space at the top of the jar. It is generally ½ inch for acid foods.

Hot Pack is used for the non-acid foods (vegetables, meats, fish). Boil the foods for a short time before packing them in jars. Then process the jars in a pressure canner. Check one of the booklets for the precooking and processing times. It varies depending on the type of food and jar size. Non-acid foods generally require 1 inch head space.

The Open Kettle method is used only for jams, jellies, butters, pickles and other foods which have enough sugar or vinegar to prevent spoilage. Boil the jars for 15 minutes. Fill each jar with the boiling food to be canned. Seal the jars immediately. You do not have to process these foods further.

METHODS OF PROCESSING

BOILING WATER BATH (for acid foods). Place the jars on a rack in a kettle of *boiling* water; the jars should not touch each other. The water should be 1 inch over the jar tops. Process the foods for the recommended time, starting after the food has come to a boil again.

PRESSURE COOKER METHOD (for non-acid foods). Place the jars on a rack in the cooker, not touching. A pressure cooker is a large pot holding 7 quart jars. A pressure sauce pan is a 4-6 quart pan that will hold a few pint jars. If you are using a pressure sauce pan for canning, add 20 minutes to the processing time, because these small pots heat up and cool off more rapidly than the larger ones. Let the steam vent 10 minutes before putting on the petcock, so the pressure in the canner will be even to start. Let the pressure in the canner reach zero *naturally*. (Do NOT run cold water over the canner to reduce the pressure.)

SOME FINAL TIPS ON CANNING

Knife out air bubbles before sealing the jar.
Clean the top of the jar and threads with a clean, damp cloth.
Screw the band on until it is just tight.
Fill only as many jars as will fit in the canner.
Always use recommended time and method of processing. Get one of the booklets listed under "Canning and Freezing References."
Let the jars cool on a rack in a well-ventilated, but not cold or drafty, area. See *Flat Sour Spoilage* discussion above.
Test the seal with a spoon or by pressing it.
Store the jars in a cool, dark, dry place.
Plan to use the cans within a year. After that they start to lose their vitamins.

SAFE CANNING (AND FREEZING)

FREEZING

If you have access to a freezer, this is also an excellent way of storing food. Having had no experience with this myself, I will simply list some of the tips I have read. As in canning, certain precautions have to be taken in order to avoid spoilage and growth of bacteria.

1. Choose foods that freeze well. Berries, asparagus, corn and meats freeze well. Tomatoes and pears do not.

2. Choose foods that are at their peak of ripeness. Again two hours garden to freezer is advisable.

3. Fruits should be washed in cool water, but never allowed to stand in it. Drain them thoroughly before packing.

4. ALL vegetables except green peppers should be blanched; that is, scald them by boiling water or steam. Time according to charts. If steam is used (better from a nutritional standpoint) add two minutes to blanching time.

5. Freeze foods rapidly to zero degrees F. or colder. Don't put any more foods in a freezer than will freeze in 24 hours.

6. Frozen foods begin to deteriorate after 6 months or a year depending on the type of food and freezing temperature.

REFERENCES ON CANNING AND FREEZING (*indicates booklets we got free at the Agricultural Extension Service. In Vermont there is one in every county)

Blue Book (info on canning and freezing)
Box 2005, Muncie, Indiana (35 cents)

Kerr Home Canning Book (includes freezing)
Kerr Glass MFG Corporation
Department 998
Sand Springs, Oklahoma (35 cents)

*10 Short Lessons in Canning and Freezing
Kerr Field Services Department
Sand Springs, Oklahoma

*Making Pickles and Relishes at Home
Home and Garden Bulletin No. 92
U.S.D.A. (United States Dept. of Agriculture)

*Home Canning of Fruits and Vegetables
Home and Garden Bulletin No. 8
U.S.D.A.
Or send 20 cents to: Superintendent of Documents
U.S. Government Printing Office
Washington, D.C. 20402

*How to Make Jellies, Jams, and Preserves at Home
Home and Garden bulletin No. 56
Or send 15 cents to the Superintendent of Documents (above)

Storing food for the winter is not difficult once you have done it and understand it. Last summer we canned blackberries, raspberries, applesauce, apple juice, cherry juice, cherry soup, tomato sauce, and cucumber pickle. You don't have to can berries in a sugar syrup. We prefer them canned with boiling water. We also boxed hundreds of apples in sand, but many spoiled and we wished we had stored them in leaves or between layers of newspapers. This fall we are again canning only the acid foods. The other vegetables and grains we store by drying or packing carefully in our root cellar.

Arie Lindsay

NOTES

HEALTH AND NUTRITION

EDITORS' NOTE. There is an old German fairy tale about a baker who made his bread with the ingredients used in disappearing ink. The bread was delicious, and the townspeople ate and ate and ate; and were wasting away to nothing until the baker's secret was discovered.

Americans are facing the same problem as the inhabitants of the German Town in the fairy tale. We have instant hamburgers and hotdogs that contain less protein than a teaspoonful of peanut butter; we have sugar-coated sawdust for breakfast, grease-coated instant chicken for lunch, and, then, to be sure we're getting enough proteins and vitamins, gorge ourselves with huge dinners of cholesterol-laden steaks and potatoes.

Eating should be:
1. Simple
2. Nutritious
3. Sacred
4. Pleasurable

It can be!

This article contains two sections, one (for your body) concerned primarily with problems of eating a healthy and nutritive meal, the other (for your head and your body) emphasing the simplicity and sacredness of eating.

"What kind of a Revolution would it be," someone said, "if all the people in the world could sit in a big circle and eat together."

His Revolution is inadequate. We need a revolution where all the people in the world could sit in a big circle and eat *good* food together.

FOR YOUR BODY

INTRODUCTION: Eating an adequate diet is one of the most important preventive medicine measures a person can take to keep healthy.

A well-nourished person has a far better chance of warding off infections and illness than a poorly nourished person. Poor nutrition affects every system of the physical body and can affect a person's emotional well-being as well. A person who is tired and rundown or irritable may be poorly nourished.

There is growing evidence that nutrition affects intellectual and behavioral as well as physical growth. The brain may be damaged by various influences during the period of its fastest growth, which in human beings occurs from about five months before to about ten months after birth. Severe malnutrition in a pregnant woman may affect the unborn child by reducing the nutrients available to it for normal cell growth. Severe malnutrition during the first six months of the infant's life further reduces the number of brain cells the baby will develop.

It's relatively easy for a person who eats eggs, milk, cereals and breads, fruits and vegetables to be well-nourished. But a person who is on a vegetarian diet must be careful to make up all the necessary amino acids (found in proteins) and Vitamin B_{12}.

A person who eats heartily and feels thoroughly satisfied stands as much a chance of being deficient in an essential nutrient as a person who eats close to nothing. It is by no means how much a person consumes, but *what* he eats that counts. Simply eating to fill a cavity or for the love of eating will not keep a person from being malnourished, unless the person maintains a balanced intake of all the nutrients essential to the body's well-being.

Maintenance of a well-balanced diet can be accomplished by following the allowances of the "Basic Four Daily Food Guide," which contains the necessary daily nutritional allotments for the average person. The following is a brief sketch of the chart:

1. *Milk Group:* Made up of milk and related dairy products—cheese, ice cream, cream, yogurt, etc. On the average, children should have the equivalent of 3 to 4 cups of milk per day; teenagers, 4 or more and adults, 2 or more. Lactating and pregnant women need more.
2. *Meat Group:* All age groups should consume 2 or more daily servings—beef, veal, lamb, etc. These can be replaced with equivalent protein foods, such as eggs, combination dry beans, combination dry peas, nuts (peanut butter), etc.
3. *Bread Cereal Group:* For all ages, 4 or more servings should be eaten. The most nutritious are whole-grain products from wheat, oats, barley, rice (brown is best), etc.
4. *Vegetable, fruit Group:* Again, 4 or more servings. These include fruits such as oranges, grapefruits, bananas, melons, and vegetables of both the dark green and deep yellow varieties such as spinach, parsley, beans, carrots, squash.

MAJOR NUTRIENTS. To enable a person to analyse his dietary intake, on a more specific basis, the following is an explanation of the major nutrients, their major sources, and functions. Understanding will allow a person to be sure of eating the daily requirements by way of food substitution. A person on a vegetarian diet, for instance, must make up many of the amino acids and B vitamins which he would get primarily in meat proteins. Measuring against the allowances shown in the chart on pp. 98–99, the only "complete protein" (all necessary amino acids) vegetable is the soy bean. In such a diet, all but Vitamin B_{12} can be substituted and, for the latter, either dairy products, eggs, or some type of capsule from dietary supplement can make up the deficiency. Anyone attempting to raise a child without giving him milk, eggs, or meat should work with a medic or a physician in planning the diet and carefully watch the child's development.

The "Key Nutrients" are the fundamental three which make up the substance of the ingested food. These are proteins, fats and carbohydrates.

1. *Proteins* form the building blocks of all tissues and play a major role in repair in case of breakdown. They're important in blood building and for normal function of the white blood cells,

HEALTH AND NUTRITION

which are essential in fighting infection.

The major protein sources are meats, fish, poultry, eggs, and milk with all its related dairy products. Also good sources are certain dried beans and peas such as soy beans, lentils, red beans, etc. Nuts, peanut butter and most grains—rye, wheat, barley, oats—are good sources.

Proteins are made up of 18 chemical blocks called *amino acids.* For the body to utilize these amino acids, it must consume all 18 of them at once. Most animal protein contains all 18 amino acids, while most vegetable protein is incomplete and must be consumed in variety to make up the full number of essential amino acids. The only "complete protein" vegetable has been found to be the soy bean, which can, of itself, totally replace meat foods.

2. *Fat's* major purpose is as energy supplier: a very small amount gives off a large quantity of heat. Fats also supply fatty acids which help to maintain healthy skin. All butters, oils, creams, meat fats, etc., are almost completely fat.

3. *Carbohydrates* make up most of the consumed bulk. They supply energy and are, at the same time, a main source for many other nutrients. Cereals are made up of high protein grains, dried fruits contain vitamins, etc. Other foods high in carbohydrates are potatoes, cookies, chick peas, etc.

Minerals are the next largest classification of nutrients. They come in minute quantities, but play an essential part in body metabolism.

1. Calcium is essential in building bones and teeth and also in helping blood to clot. The major source is milk and related dairy products—cheese, ice cream, etc. Some vegetables also contain calcium: mustard greens, turnips, collards, broccoli and kale, among others.

2. Iron combines with protein to make hemoglobin—the red part of the blood which carries oxygen to the cells. It is found primarily in organ meats, liver, kidneys, etc. Egg yolks are a very good source, as are dried beans and peas. Green leafy vegetables like spinach, cabbage and certain fruits: prunes, raisins and dried apricots contain much iron. Some grains are also good.

3. Iodine helps control the rate at which the body uses energy. The best suppliers are sea foods and plants grown near the sea. People out of reach of the sea or sea food can rely on iodized salt.

Vitamins are the third large nutrient classification. They are important for disease prevention, and aid in regulation of body processes. Although they themselves do not enter into reactions, they must be present for the reactions to take place. Very minute quantities are needed of most vitamins; yet their absence could cause many types of dangerous diseases such as beriberi, scurvy, pellagra, and others.

There are at least 14 different vitamins that are essential to man. The following explanation will consider 7 of the major ones.

1. *Vitamin A:* Important in controlling bone growth, preventing night blindness and maintaining clear and smooth skin. It also helps keep mucous membranes firm and resistant to infection.

The major sources are liver and egg yolks. Particularly high in Vitamin A are dark green leafy and yellow vegetables such as spinach and carrots. Also good are yellow fruits such as cantaloupe and dairy products.

2. *Thiamine or Vitamin B₁* is important for the nervous system: it helps to keep it healthy. It also promotes normal appetite and digestion and helps the body to release energy from food.

Pork is by far the best supplier, but it can also be obtained from other meats, fish and poultry. Eggs, grains such as wheat germ and rice polish, and dried beans and peas are good, too.

3. *Riboflavin* helps cells use oxygen. Some of the first signs of deficiency are scaly greasy skin around the mouth and nose. Dairy products, fish, poultry, eggs and many meats are good sources.

4. *Ascorbic Acid or Vitamin C* makes a cement-like material which holds body cells together. It helps keep walls of blood vessels strong and helps in healing wounds and broken bones. It may help in preventing colds.

Dangers of Vitamin C overdose include: painful kidney stones in humans, false readings in diabetic urine testing, changes of bone structure in test animals, and altered reproductive ability in some animals, including dead fetuses, and decreased chance of conception.

The major sources are citrus fruits—oranges, grapefruit, lemons, etc. Strawberries, cantaloupes, tomatoes, green pepper, broccoli, raw greens and cabbage.

5. *Niacin* is important for keeping nervous system, skin, mouth, tongue, and digestive tract healthy. It also helps cells use other nutrients.

It's found in nuts (peanut butter), meat, fish, poultry, milk and various grains.

6. *Vitamin D* helps absorb calcium from the digestive tract and builds calcium and phosphorus into bones. The best sources are milk, fish, liver, oils and sunshine.

7. *Vitamin B₁₂* has been newly discovered to be an antipernicious anemia factor—it is an important factor in blood production.

It is *only* found in animal products: no plants carry it. Best sources are organ meats and fish such as oysters and clams. Eggs and dairy products also contain B_{12}. A vegetarian diet can easily result in a deficiency in B_{12}, one which can be remediated with weekly dosages in capsule form.

A lack of any vitamin causes the reversal of what its presence does.

Linda Fried

SAMPLE WEEK'S MENU FOR AN ADULT VEGETARIAN DIET
INCLUDING DAIRY AND EGG PRODUCTS

	Breakfast	Lunch	Supper
Mon.	orange juice wheatena whole wheat toast butter milk, coffee, tea	egg salad sandwich milk tomato soup ice cream	lentil casserole tossed salad broccoli brown rice baked apple milk
Tues.	grapefruit half fried eggs ww toast milk	peanut butter sandwich vegetable soup apple pie milk	spinach soy beans brown rice fruit salad milk
Wed.	orange juice hard boiled eggs ww toast milk	pizza green salad sherbet milk	egg souffle cole slaw strawberries milk
Thurs.	grapefruit juice oatmeal brown sugar ww toast milk	tomato omelet toast oatmeal cookies milk	macaroni and cheese green beans tossed salad spice cake milk

Fri.	orange
	scrambled eggs
	ww toast
	milk
		grilled cheese
		carrot & celery
		    sticks
		gelatin w/ fruit
			stuffed peppers w/ rice
			    and tomatoes
			brussels sprouts
			tossed salad
			ice cream
			milk

Sat.	orange pancakes w/ syrup milk	tomato juice western sandwich succotash fruit salad milk	baked beans cole slaw Indian pudding milk
Sun.	grapefruit half french toast milk	split pea soup ww toast oatmeal date bars milk	vegetable chop suey brown rice cherry pie milk

AN ADEQUATE ADULT ALL VEGETARIAN WEEK'S MENU
(almost no dairy or egg products)

	Breakfast	Lunch	Supper
Mon.	orange juice familia ww bread honey coffee or tea	pea soup ww bread tomato slices fruit salad	soy bean loaf spinach baked potato lemon cornstarch pudding
Tues.	grapefruit wheatena ww bread w/jelly coffee or tea	peanut butter & jelly sandwich vegetable soup *Oatmeal-Date Bars	baked beans tossed salad broccoli apple pie
Wed.	orange slices oatmeal w/brown sugar ww toast coffee or tea	lettuce & tomato sandwich fried corn, green pepper & onion baked apple	*Curried Lentils brown rice cole slaw *Oatmeal Peach Betty
Thurs.	grapefruit juice *Crispy Oatmeal Slices coffee or tea	tomato soup *Peanut-Butter Soy Patties pineapple	*Chick Peas w/Tomatoes mashed potatoes green beans cherry pie
Fri.	orange juice ww bread w/honey grits coffee or tea	*Curried Lentil Patties lettuce & tomato fruit salad	*Baked Soy Beans mustard greens macaroni w/parsley apple sauce
Sat.	Maypo ww bread orange coffee or tea	*Vegetable Stew french fries rhubarb sauce	*Pasta Fagioli tossed salad fried eggplant baked bananas
Sun.	grapefruit Cream of Wheat ww toast coffee or tea	*Cold Bean Salad onion soup apple pie	spaghetti w/mushrooms kale pecan pie

*Recipes for starred dishes on following pages.

HEALTH AND NUTRITION

OATMEAL DATE BARS

Mix I	Mix II
1 c. brown sugar	1¼ c. chopped dates
1 c. whole wheat flour	½ c. hot water
1 c. oats	
½ c. oil	
1 tsp. soda	
¼ tsp. salt	

Put Mix II into a small pan, cover tight and simmer until dates are soft. (5 minutes) Mash.

Stir together all ingredients in Mix I, put half crumbs at bottom of 9 inch pan. Spread date mix over it and sprinkle with remaining crumbs. Bake at 350 degrees for 30 minutes. *Makes 3 dozen date bars.*

+ + + + + +

CURRIED LENTILS

Add small amount of water and 1 teaspoon curry to one pint of lentils. Cook with onions—serve on rice. *Serves 8 to 10.*

+ + + + + +

OATMEAL PEACH BETTY

2/3 c. all purpose flour	2 tbls. lemon juice
¼ tsp. salt	¼ tsp. cinnamon
¼ tsp. baking soda	1/3 c. brown sugar
2/3 c. quick-cooking oats	½ tsp. vanilla
¼ c. melted shortening (or oil)	
2 c. canned sliced peaches (or other fruit of same consistency)	

Sift together first 3 ingredients. Mix oats into flour. Put fruit in buttered casserole. Sprinkle with lemon juice and cinnamon. Add brown sugar to melted shortening and then add flour mixture. Stir until crumbly. Add vanilla and spread mixture over fruit. Bake at 375 degrees for 45 minutes. *Serves 4 to 6.*

+ + + + + +

CRISPY OATMEAL SLICES

2 c. quick-cooking oats	3 c. boiling water
1¼ tsp. salt	oil

Stir oats & salt into boiling water. Cook 1 minute, stirring occasionally. Cover pan; remove from heat & let stand 5 minutes. Turn into a loaf pan; chill several hours. Turn out, cut in ½ inch thick slices. Brown in butter (oil) over medium heat, turning once. Serve with syrup. *Serves 4 to 6.*

+ + + + + +

PEANUT-BUTTER SOY PATTIES

    1 c. mashed soy beans
    2 tbls. peanut butter
    4 tbls. dry bread crumbs

Mix all together. Shape into small patties. Roll in bread crumbs and place in oiled pan. Brown in 350 degree oven. *Serves 4.*

+ + + + + +

CHICK PEAS WITH TOMATOES

Fry garlic in oil. Add can of tomatoes and simmer for 15 minutes. Add a can of chick peas. Serve on brown rice in 5 minutes. *Serves 4.*

+ + + + + +

CURRIED LENTIL PATTIES

Mix Curried Lentils (see above) with leftover rice. Shape into patties; dip in milk or water and then in dry bread crumbs and fry.

+ + + + + +

BAKED SOY BEANS

    2 c. dry soy beans
    6 c. water
    2 tbls. salt

    2 tbls. molasses
    1 tbl. powdered vegetable broth
    or ¼ c. finely minced celery

Soak beans overnight in salted water. Cook until almost done—drain water. Place beans in casserole. Add molasses and broth plus enough water to almost cover. Cover and bake 2 to 3 hours in moderate oven. *Serves 4 to 6.*

+ + + + + +

HEALTH AND NUTRITION

VEGETABLE STEW

Cut up all sorts of vegetables in cubes and allow to steam in little water with garlic, salt, and pepper.

+ + + + + +

PASTA FAGIOLI

      8 oz. macaroni   1 No. 2 can red kidney beans
      olive oil   wine vinegar

Cook macaroni and drain. Heat beans till hot. Mix together with 3 tablespoons olive oil and wine vinegar to taste. *Serves 4 to 6.*

+ + + + + +

COLD BEAN SALAD

Mix different cooked beans together and season with olive oil, vinegar, salt and pepper.

+ + + + + +

NOTES

Part No. 1

RECOMMENDED DAILY DIETARY ALLOWANCES[1]

(Revised 1968)*

	AGE[2] YEARS From–To	WEIGHT Kg. Lbs.	HEIGHT cm in.	K Calories	PROTEIN gm	CALCIUM gm	IRON mg	VIT. A I.U.	THIA. mg.	RIBO. mg	NIA.[5] (equiv) mg	VIT. C mg	VIT. D I.U.
INFANTS	0 – 1/6	4 9	55 22	kg x 1200	kg x 2.2[3]	0.4	6	1500	0.2	0.4	5	35	400
	1/6 – 1/2	7 15	63 25	kg x 110	kg x 2.0[3]	0.5	10	1500	0.4	0.5	7	35	400
	1/2 – 1	9 20	72 28	kg x 100	kg. x 1.8[3]	0.6	15	1500	0.5	0.6	8	35	400
CHILDREN	1 – 2	12 26	81 32	1100	25	0.7	15	2000	0.6	0.6	8	40	400
	2 – 3	14 31	91 36	1250	25	0.8	15	2000	0.6	0.7	8	40	400
	3 – 4	16 35	100 39	1400	30	0.8	10	2500	0.7	0.8	9	40	400
	4 – 6	19 42	110 43	1600	30	0.8	10	2500	0.8	0.9	11	40	400
	6 – 8	23 51	121 48	2000	35	0.9	10	3500	1.0	1.1	13	40	400
	8 –10	28 62	131 52	2200	40	1.0	10	3500	1.1	1.2	15	40	400
MALES	10 – 12	35 77	140 55	2500	45	1.2	10	4500	1.3	1.3	17	40	400
	12 – 14	45 95	151 59	2700	50	1.4	18	5000	1.4	1.4	18	45	400
	14 – 18	59 130	170 67	3000	60	1.4	18	5000	1.5	1.5	20	55	400
	18 – 22	67 147	175 69	2800	60	0.8	10	5000	1.4	1.6	18	60	400
	22 – 35	70 154	175 69	2800	65	0.8	10	5000	1.4	1.7	18	60	---
	35 – 55	70 154	173 68	2600	65	0.8	10	5000	1.3	1.7	17	60	---
	55 – 75+	70 154	171 67	2400	65	0.8	10	5000	1.2	1.7	14	60	---
FEMALES	10 – 12	35 77	142 56	2250	50	1.2	18	4500	1.1	1.3	15	40	400
	12 – 14	44 97	154 61	2300	50	1.3	18	5000	1.2	1.4	15	45	400
	14 – 16	52 114	157 62	2400	55	1.3	18	5000	1.2	1.4	16	50	400
	16 – 18	54 119	160 63	2300	55	1.3	18	5000	1.2	1.5	15	50	400
	18 – 22	58 128	163 64	2000	55	0.8	18	5000	1.0	1.5	13	55	400
	22 – 35	58 128	163 64	2000	55	0.8	18	5000	1.0	1.5	13	55	---
	35 – 55	58 128	160 63	1850	55	0.8	18	5000	0.9	1.5	12	55	---
	55 – 75+	58 128	157 62	1700	55	0.8	10	5000	0.9	1.5	10	55	---
PREGNANCY				+200	65	+0.4	18	6000	+0.1	1.8	15	60	400
LACTATION				+1000	75	+0.5	18	8000	+0.5	2.0	20	60	400

Part No. 2

	AGE [2] YEARS From–To	WEIGHT Kg.	WEIGHT Lbs.	HEIGHT cm	HEIGHT in.	VITAMIN E Activity I.U.	VITAMIN B6 mg	VITAMIN B12 mg	FOLACIN [4] mg	PHOSPHORUS gm	IODINE mg	MAGNESIUM mg
INFANTS	0 – 1/6	4	9	55	22	5	0.2	1.0	0.05	0.2	25	40
	1/6 – 1/2	7	15	63	25	5	0.3	1.5	0.05	0.4	40	60
	1/2 – 1	9	20	72	28	5	0.4	2.0	0.1	0.5	45	70
CHILDREN	1 – 2	12	26	81	32	10	0.5	2.0	0.1	0.7	55	100
	2 – 3	14	31	91	36	10	0.6	2.5	0.2	0.8	60	150
	3 – 4	16	35	100	39	10	0.7	3	0.2	0.8	70	200
	4 – 6	19	42	110	43	10	0.9	4	0.2	0.8	80	200
	6 – 8	23	51	121	48	15	1.0	4	0.2	0.9	100	250
	8 – 10	28	62	131	52	15	1.2	5	0.3	1.0	110	250
MALES	10 – 12	35	77	140	55	20	1.4	5	0.4	1.2	125	300
	12 – 14	43	95	151	59	20	1.6	5	0.4	1.4	135	350
	14 – 18	59	130	170	67	25	1.8	5	0.4	1.4	150	400
	18 – 22	67	147	175	69	30	2.0	5	0.4	0.8	140	400
	22 – 35	70	154	175	69	30	2.0	5	0.4	0.8	140	350
	35 – 55	70	154	173	68	30	2.0	5	0.4	0.8	125	350
	55 – 75+	70	154	171	67	30	2.0	6	0.4	0.8	110	350
FEMALES	10 – 12	35	77	142	56	20	1.4	5	0.4	1.2	110	300
	12 – 14	44	97	154	61	20	1.6	5	0.4	1.3	115	350
	14 – 16	52	114	157	62	25	1.8	5	0.4	1.3	120	350
	16 – 18	54	119	160	63	25	2.0	5	0.4	1.3	115	350
	18 – 22	58	128	163	64	25	2.0	5	0.4	0.8	100	350
	22 – 35	58	128	163	64	25	2.0	5	0.4	0.8	100	300
	35 – 55	58	128	160	63	25	2.0	5	0.4	0.8	90	300
	55 – 75+	58	128	157	62	25	2.0	6	0.4	0.8	80	300
PREGNANCY						30	2.5	8	0.8	+0.4	125	450
LACTATION						30	2.5	6	0.5	+0.5	150	450

1. Allowance levels are intended to cover individual variations among most normal persons as they live in the U.S. under usual environmental stresses. Recommended allowances can be attained with a variety of common foods, providing other nutrients for which human requirements have been less well defined.
2. Entries on lines for age range 22–35 represent reference man and woman age 22. All other entries represent allowances for the mid-point of the specified age range.
3. Assumes protein equivalent to human milk. For proteins not 100% utilized factors should be increased proportionately.
4. The folacin allowances refer to dietary sources as determined by Lactobacillus casei assay. Pure forms of folacin may be effective in doses less than ¼ of the RDA.
5. Niacin equivalents include dietary sources of the vitamin itself plus 1 mg equivalent for each 60 mg of dietary tryptophan.

*Tables on these two pages compiled by the National Academy of Sciences.

NOTES

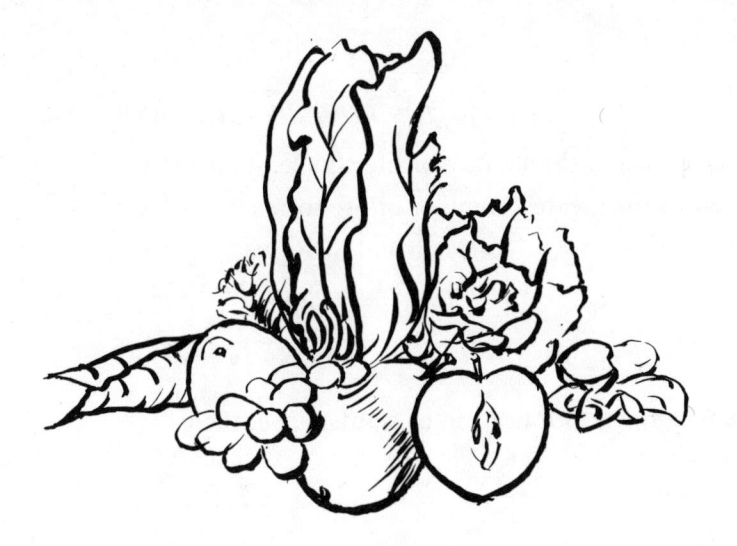

HEALTH and NUTRITION

FOR YOUR HEAD AND YOUR BODY

And God said, "Behold I have given you every plant yielding seed which is on the face of all the earth and every tree yielding seed in its fruit; you shall have them for food and . . . to everything that has the breath of life, I have given every green plant for food."

Genesis

The human practice of eating the dead bodies of fellow creatures has gone on for so long a time that it is regarded generally as normal.

Helen and Scott Nearing
Living the Good Life, 1954

One of the reasons for choosing to be an herbivore that eats low on the food chain— it is simply less wasteful. And, . . . herbivores are less likely to accumulate potentially harmful environmental contaminants than are carnivores.

Frances Moore Lappe
Diet for a Small Planet, 1971

I learned from my two years experiment that it would cost incredibly little trouble to obtain one's necessary food, even in this latitude; that many a man may use as simple a diet as the animals, and yet retain health and strength.

Henry Thoreau
Walden, 1854

The journey of a thousand miles begins with one step.

Lao Tzu

We were looking for a kindly, decent, clean and simple way of life: the least harm to the least number and the greatest good to the greatest number of life forms.

> Helen and Scott Nearing
> *Living the Good Life,* 1954

The essence of civilization consists not in the multiplication of wants but in their deliberate and voluntary renunciation.

> Gandhi

He who tells the truth says almost nothing.

> Porchia

How sensitive are you to your INNER ENVIRONMENT?

To eat little and of few things is a good guide for health and for simplicity.

> Helen and Scott Nearing
> *Living the Good Life,* 1954

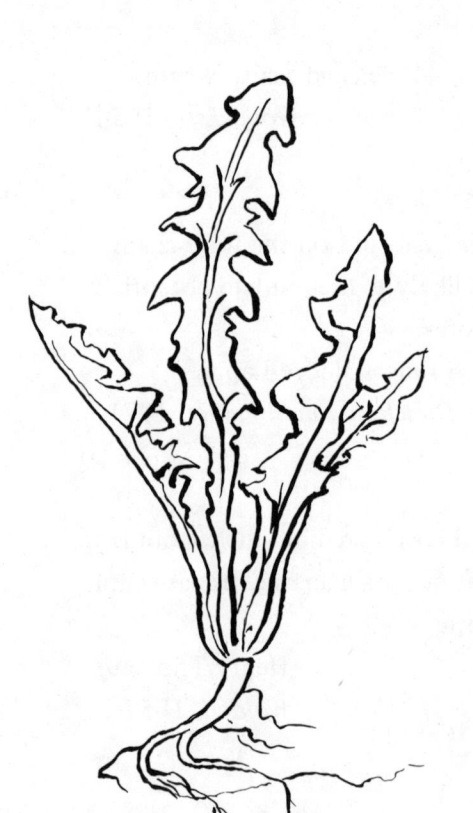

SIMPLICITY

THE BODY:
"A CLEAN, WELL-LIGHTED PLACE"

Your food shall be your remedies and your remedies your food.

> Hippocrates

HEALTH AND NUTRITION

THE SEVEN CONDITIONS OF HEALTH

No fatigue
    Good appetite
        Deep and good sleep
            Good memory
                Good humor
                    Clarity in thinking and doing
                        The mood of justice

                                George Ohsawa
                                Zen Macrobiotics, 1954

It is a just observation that he who lives by rule and wholesome diet, is a physician to himself.
    Helen and Scott Nearing
    Living the Good Life, 1954

Be concerned with the vibrations associated with the source, preparation and eating of foods.
    Baba Ram Dass
    Be Here Now, 1971

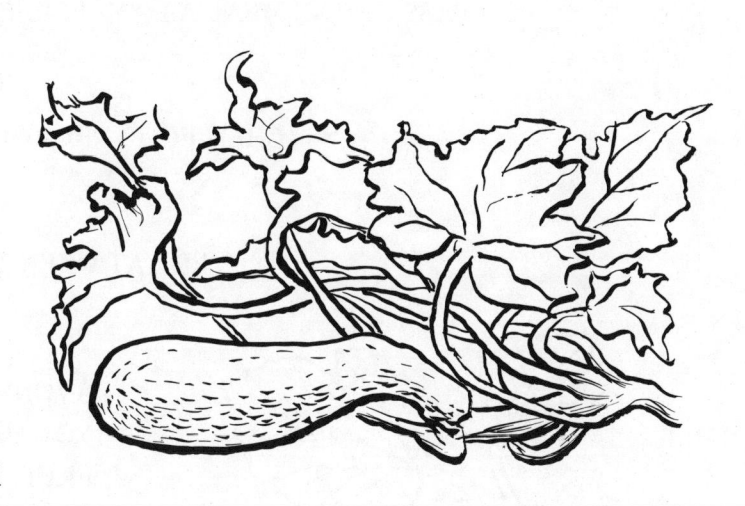

        When the sun rises, I go to work,
        When the sun goes down, I take my rest,
        I dig the well from which I drink,
        I farm the soil that yields my food,
        I shape creation, kings can do no more.
            Ancient Chinese, 2500 B.C.

SIMPLICITY

"NATURE IS THE GREATEST HEALER"

> Pursue a path whose goal is the unity between the individual and the way of nature herself, the creation of an equilibrium between man and his biological destiny.
>
> George Ohsawa
> *Zen Macrobiotics*, 1965

PROTECT YOUR HEALTH AND PROLONG YOUTHFUL VIGOR

EAT ONLY IF HUNGRY—TRUE HUNGER IS PHYSIOLOGICAL

PASS UP ONE MEAL A DAY—PREFERABLY BREAKFAST

CHEW FOOD THOROUGHLY

NEVER EAT WHEN TIRED

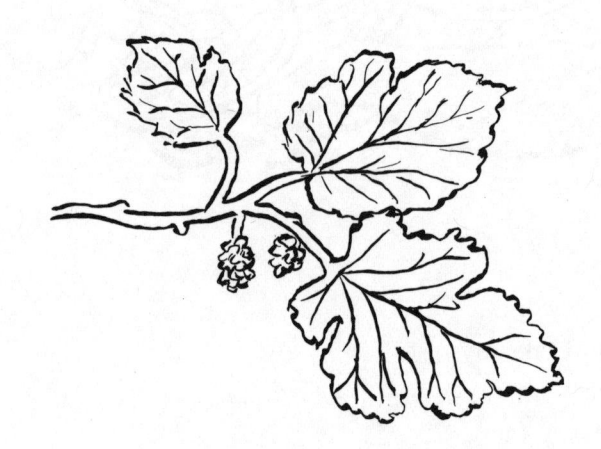

AVOID EATING BETWEEN MEALS UNLESS YOU HAVE FRUIT, JUICE, OR FRESH FRUIT

DO NOT EAT WHEN YOU ARE EMOTIONALLY UPSET

GET A GOOD NIGHTS SLEEP

GET SUNSHINE ON YOUR BODY AS MUCH AS POSSIBLE

BREATHE DEEPLY AND RHYTHMICALLY

GET EXERCISE EVERY DAY

ALWAYS EAT FRESH FRUITS AND VEGETABLES IN SEASON, PREFERABLY RAW

The foods we chose to live on were those that had the simplest, closest and most natural relationship to the soil.

>Helen and Scott Nearing
>*Living the Good Life,* 1954

Nutrition is one of the primary factors in determining the health, happiness and usefulness of every human being.
>Helen and Scott Nearing
>*Living the Good Life,* 1954

Diseases only attack those whose outer circumstances, particularly food, are faulty .... The prevention and banishment of disease are primarily matters of food.
>G. T. Wrench
>*Wheel of Health,* 1941

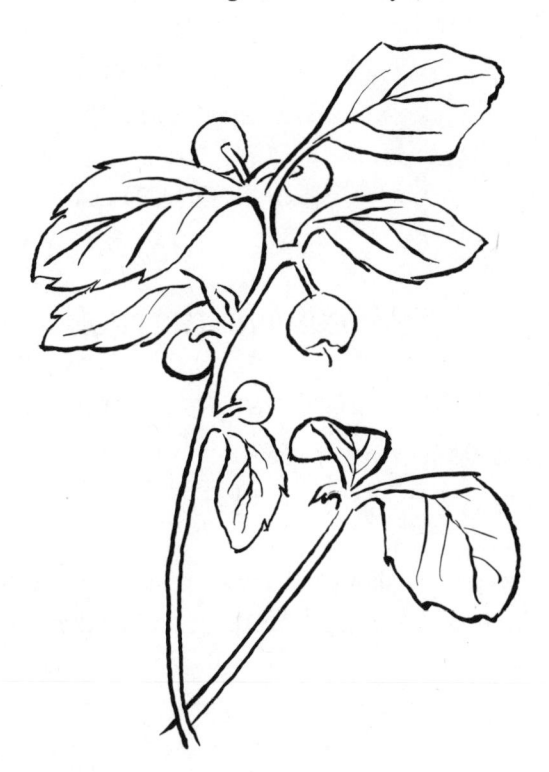

Our body has an inherent, automatic and practically unlimited power of renewal. If we regard life as something eternal and indestructible, it should be possible to remain both mentally young and physically fit indefinitely.

>Renee Taylor
>*Hunza Health Secrets,* 1969

SIMPLICITY

HEALTH
FOOD   DRINK
AIR
SUNSHINE
COSMIC ENERGY
THE NATURE OF THESE MATERIALS
DETERMINES
YOUR
INNER ENVIRONMENT

QUANTITY
VARIETY
QUALITY
COMBINE THE PROPER FOODS IN A PROPER DIET
AND
THE HEALTH-BALANCE IS MAINTAINED

Good food should be grown on whole soil, be eaten whole, unprocessed, and garden fresh. . . . Any modification at all is likely to reduce the nutritive value of a whole food.

> Helen and Scott Nearing
> *Living the Good Life,* 1954

SIMPLICITY

THOUGHTFULLY – AVOID – THOUGHTFULLY

REFINED SUGAR AND REFINED SUGAR PRODUCTS
REFINED WHITE FLOUR AND REFINED FLOUR PRODUCTS
HYDROGENATED OILS AND SATURATED FATS
ALL SALTED FOODS AND THE USE OF SALT—There is some salt in just about every food we eat, more than enough to meet the needs of the normal body.

FRIED FOODS – EXCESSIVE FATS
STIMULANTS SUCH AS COFFEE, TEAS, AND ALCOHOLIC BEVERAGES
TOBACCO DESENSITIZES YOUR TASTE BUDS

MEAT

The craving for concentrated protein foods is an acquired and a dangerous habit, in that it over-energizes the human organism and overloads the system with acid-forming elements.

> Helen and Scott Nearing
> *Living the Good Life,* 1954

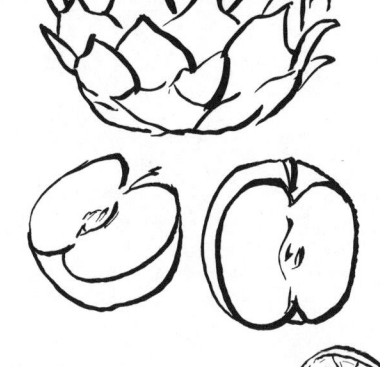

STRONG FOODS, SPICES, BAKING SODAS, BAKING POWDERS
FOODS USING CHEMICAL ADDITIVES IN THEIR PRODUCTION, PROCESSING, PRESERVATION, OR PACKAGING

Poisoned, processed and chemicalized foods result in malnutrition, since deficient foods, even when consumed in large quantities, upset the nutritional balance. Faulty nourishment has immediate effects, on body health, emotional stability and mental efficiency.

> Helen and Scott Nearing
> *Living the Good Life,* 1954

Modern practices tend to continually weaken the ability of the individual to assert the natural resistive qualities of his body.

> J. I. Rodale
> *The Complete Book of Food and Nutrition,* 1971

The statistics show that the people in the United States are suffering from breakdown of the vital tissues and organs. There is every reason to suppose that this breakdown is related to inadequacies in the food intake.

> Helen and Scott Nearing
> *Living the Good Life,* 1954

SIMPLICITY

No self-drugging
No aspirin
No antihistamines
No laxatives
No sleeping pills
No tranquilisers
No pain killers
etc., etc., etc.,

RIGHT DIET

Apply to vegetables and fruits the principles of wholeness, rawness, garden freshness, and one or few things at a meal, and you have the theory of our simple diet.

Helen and Scott Nearing
Living the Good Life, 1954

EAT ALL VEGETABLES—especially green leafy ones; eat less starchy ones.

ORDER FINEST QUALITY SEEDS
NICHOLS HERB AND RARE SEEDS
NICHOLS GARDEN NURSERY
1190 North Pacific Hwy.
Albany, Oregon 97321

YOUR OWN VEGETABLES YEAR-ROUND

Early in the Spring

Parsnips
Salsify
Celery Root
Parsley Root
Leeks
Chicory

Late in the Spring

Asparagus

HEALTH AND NUTRITION

> Dandelion
> Chives
> Multiplier Onions

Early Summer

> Spinach
> Radishes
> Mustard Greens
> Garden Cress
> Early Lettuce

Middle Summer

> Green Peas
> Beets
> Standard Lettuce
> String Beans
> Squash

Late Summer

> Corn
> Tomatoes
> Shellbeans
> Broccoli
> Cauliflower
> Celery

Autumn

> Cabbages
> Winter Squash
> Turnips
> Rutabagas
> Carrots
> Escarolle
> Chinese Cabbage
> Collards
> Cos Lettuce
> Fall Radishes
> Spinach
> Beets
> Potatoes
> Dried Beans

Root Cellar

> Cabbages
> Winter Squash
> Potatoes
> Beets
> Carrots
> Turnips

Onions
Rutabagas
Celery Root
Parsley Root

Complete information on freezing and canning
How to grow vegetables and fruits by the organic method

J. I. Rodale & Staff

Compost-grown fruits and vegetables taste better than the same products grown with commercial fertilizers or fresh animal manures.

Helen and Scott Nearing
Living the Good Life, 1954

EAT PLENTY OF FRUIT

The attractiveness, flavor and food value of fresh fruits should place them high on the preferred list of anybody's daily menu.

J. I. Rodale
Food and Nutrition, 1971

HAVE AN

| Apple | or | Apricot |
| Apricot | or | Avocado |

Why not a

Banana

Blackberries

Blueberries

A deep red cherry

maybe

Currants (dried)

Dates (dried)

Figs (dried)

Apricots (dried)

Raisins (dried)

or

FRESH

Grapefruit or Grapes
Lemons and Limes

Perhaps

Loganberries In the Tropics
A mango or papaya
Orange
Peaches and Pears
Persimmons or Pineapple
Plums
Prunes (dried)
Black Raspberries
Red Raspberries

Don't Forget

Strawberries & Tangerines

Sprout Seeds especially
    Alfalfa Seeds
    Mung Beans
    Wheat Berries
    Soy Beans

Use aromatic herbs, grow them in your garden, and dry them:
Basil
    Sage
        Thyme
            Summer Savory
                Marjoram
                    Parsley
                        Celery Leaves
                            Dill

Dry chamomile, peppermint, spearmint, raspberry and strawberry leaves for tea.

Protein sources include nuts

    Cashews
    Walnuts
    Almonds
    Peanuts
    Pecans
    And Nut Butters

Seeds

    Sunflower
    Pumpkin
    Sesame
    Flax
    Beans

Soy

    Moniezuma
    Kidney
    Garbanzo
    Shell

Cereal Grains

    Wheat
    Rye
    Oats
    Corn
    Barley

Remember, as activity and environment permit—
Use only pure vegetable oils cold pressed

Virgin	Olive
Safflower	Peanut
Soy	Sunflower
Corn	Sesame

HONEY OR MAPLE SYRUP
UNHEATED
YOUR ONLY SWEETNERS

Eat nuts with dried fruits; juicy fruits make nuts indigestible.
Nature's open book is simplicity. The fewer food mixtures the better.
Do not over-eat. Mother nature requires moderation in all things.

                          Arnold Ehret
                         Mucusuess Diet Healing System, 1922

HEALTH AND NUTRITION

MENU

BREAKFAST. Fit your meals to your needs and schedule. If you work outside your home you may have to follow the standards pattern of large breakfast, small lunch, large dinner.

If you work at home, experiment. Have a cup of herb tea on arising, work for a few hours, and then have breakfast. Have a large lunch followed by a nap, and a small dinner followed by a long walk.

The optimal arrangement of meals for you depends on your pattern of activity and rest. Try several arrangements and pick the simplest and most satisfying.

You may have:
- A healthful herb tea (Rose-Hips)
- Some fruit juice or small bowl of fruit with alfalfa sprouts
- Or bananas, apples, etc. dipped in honey or wheat germ or both or spread with nut butter
- Some dried fruit with some nuts and seeds—granola might serve this purpose—especially if you are active

Crunchy Granola

Mix

- 4 cups rolled oats
- 2 cups shredded unsweetened coconut
- 2 cups wheat germ
- 3 cups chopped nuts
- 2 cups hulled sunflower seeds
- ½ cup flax seed
- ½ cup sesame seed
- 1 cup pumpkin seeds
- ½ cup bran
- 1 cup ground roasted soybeans

Heat

- ½ cup oil
- ½ cup honey
- ½ tsp vanilla

Add

Honey-oil mixture to dry ingredients and mix (mixture will be very dry)

Spread

Mixture on oiled cookie sheet, preferably with sides and bake at 325 degrees about 15 minutes or until mixture is *light* brown.

All measurements are approximate and it's nice to improvise with ingredients, too. Important! Turning granola on the cookie sheets is most important near the end of the 15 minute cooking period.

As weight and activity permit, try some toasted whole grain bread with honey or nut butters.

In cold climates perhaps a little whole grain cereal.

About Yogurt: "Yogurt is basically milk. But we are convinced that the changes wrought in its composition by the culture mitigate many of the bad features of milk, . . ., and offer many excellent ones. Such as increased benign intestinal flora and decreased bowel putrefaction."

J. I. Rodale & Staff
*The Complete Book of Food
and Nutrition*, 1971

"Yogurt offers . . . A "factory" of hardworking bacteria willing to produce B vitamins for future needs."

Adelle Davis
Let's Eat Right to Keep Fit

LUNCH. Some fruit definitely, and give it a little time for digestion. Green salad with oil dressing, a little lemon juice, and some herbs or yogurt dressing

    ½ pint (1 cup) yogurt
    Juice of ½ lemon
    1/3 cup oil
    ¼ cup apple cider vinegar
    basil, dill, celery seeds, oregano, thyme, pepper
    2 tbls. wheat germ

Avoid the use of too much vinegar, but use only an organic apple cider vinegar.
Rose hip extract (vitamin C) can also be added to dressings
Or cole slaw seasoned with home-made mayonnaise and herbs
IMPORTANT: Use fertile eggs exclusively (if possible); their vital nutrients far surpass commercial eggs.
A baked or stewed vegetable or steamed preferably.

The fire is kept small, giving the food a chance to simmer in its own juices instead of boiling them away. Very little water is added, and if so the water in which the vegetables are cooked is served with it, or drunk later, but it is never thrown away.

Renee Taylor
Hunza Health Secrets

HEALTH AND NUTRITION

On sprouting: "Seeds contain the elements necessary to grow new plants when given heat and moisture. They become rich in vitamins, particularly B complex."

"Select clean, whole seeds, grains or beans."

¼ cup dried — ½ cup soaked — 2 cups sprouted

soak overnight

Simplest method:

Soak seeds in quart jar covered with double thickness of cheesecloth (rubber band).

Next morning, drain off water and reserve as stock if desired.

Rinse seeds a few times and then store jars on their sides in a ventilated, moist, warm and dark cupboard.

Rinse sprouts several times a day and they will be ready to eat in 3 to 6 days.

Beatrice Trum Hunter
The Natural Foods Cookbook, 1961

As activity permits, use toasted whole grain breads, brown rice and bean recipes. Also dried fruits and nuts and nut butters.

SUPPER. Some stewed fruit such as apple sauce, apricots, prunes, peaches or very ripe bananas, or some fresh fruit—and remember to pause for digestion.

A large combination salad or cole slaw including some dried fruit and nuts.

One or more cooked vegetables, starchless and steamed preferably.

In season bake winter squash and potatoes.

As activity and climate permits use toasted whole grain breads, brown rice and bean recipes.

Yogurt (Better than any commercial variety)

Beat

2 cups tepid water

2 cups non-instant powdered skim milk (organic source)

Yogurt culture or 3 tbsp. commercial yogurt

Add

1 quart tepid water

1 large can evaporated milk

Pour into jars and incubate in water bath; bring water level to rim of glasses or jars. Cover pan, and set over pilot light or in warming oven where a temperature of 100 to 120 degrees can be maintained for 3–5 hours. Chill immediately after milk thickens.

Adelle Davis
Let's Eat Right to Keep Fit, 1954

RECIPES

PLEASE SEE:
The Natural Foods Cookbook   Beatrice Trum Hunter
Diet for a Small Planet   Frances Moore Lappe
Zen Cookery—Practical Macrobiotics: The Philosophy of Oriental Culture I   Lima Ohsawa

SIMPLICITY

SENSITIVITY

THOUGHTFULNESS

The Tassajara Bread Book   Edward Espe Brown
SECONDARY SOURCES
Mucusless Diet Healing System   Prof. Arnold Ehret
Hunza Health Secrests   Renee Taylor
The Soybean Cookbook   Dorothea Van Gundy Jones
The Complete Bean Cookbook   Victor Bennett
Mrs. Rorer's Vegetable Cookery and Meat Substitutes   Sarah Tyson Rorer

BIBLIOGRAPHY

Living the Good Life   Helen and Scott Nearing
   An authentic handbook for living simply including valuable information on gardening, composting, mulching, diet, root-cellar storage, canning and much, much more.
Diet for a Small Planet   Frances Moore Lappe
   This book is about protein—how we as a nation are caught in a pattern that squanders it. And how you can choose the opposite—a way of eating that makes the most of the earth's capacitiy to supply this vital nutrient.
Mucusless Diet Healing System
Rational Fasting for Physical, Mental and Spiritual Rejuvenation   Prof. Arnold Ehret
   These two books describe a logical, simple, and natural nutritional philosophy based on a diet of fresh and dried fruits and starchless green leafy vegetables and cooked vegetables.
   Emphasis is placed on the mono-diet and on the disciplined use of fasting to eliminate toxic substances in the system, which are the root cause of disease.
Zen Macrobiotics—The Philosophy of Oriental Medicine Vol. 1   George Ohsawa
The Book of Judgment—The Philosophy of Oriental Medicine Vol. 11   Georges Ohsawa

HEALTH AND NUTRITION

A valuable discussion of oriental medicine whose goal has been the unity between the individual and the way of nature herself, the creation of an equilibrium between man and his biological destiny.

The aim is happiness through health through nutrition.

Hunza Health Secrets   Rennee Taylor

The Hunzas are the healthiest people on earth who have never used western processed poisoned foods; they are free from the degenerative diseases that afflict western man. Their simple life-philosophy creates lasting youth and long life.

The book emphasizes their acquired knowledge of relaxation, peace of mind and long life and includes their simple diet and valuable recipes.

The Complete Book of Food and Nutrition   J. I. Rodale and Staff

A heavily researched work filled with invaluable information on almost everything and anything consumable.

Learn the nutritional facts about cereals, dairy products, fruits, nuts, seeds, sweets, vegetables, food supplements, cooking, processing, chemicals in food and much, much more.

Prevention (Periodical) Rodale Press, Inc., Emmaus, Pa. 18049 (Subscription: 33 East Minor Street, Emmaus, Pa. 18049; 1 yr. $5.85)

The latest information on nutritional research and health.

Let's Eat Right to Keep Fit   Adelle Davis

Let's Cook It Right   Adelle Davis

Let's Have Healthy Children   Adelle Davis

Although Adelle overemphasizes the role of protein in the diet, the use of milk and dairy products, and the necessity of a big breakfast, she gives valuable information on vitamins, minerals, fats, carbohydrates, right diet and recipes.

How to Grow Vegetables and Fruits by the Organic Method   J. I. Rodale and Staff

To quote the author, "How to grow vegetables and fruits by the organic method is the biggest gold mine of information in existence for organic gardeners—Now and for years to come."

THE BOOK TELLS ALL

- Planning the vegetable garden
- Improving your soil
- Starting plants from seed
- Watering and irrigation
- Harvesting
- Storing surplus
- Green houses
- Fruits

etc., etc., etc.

Organic Gardening and Farming (Periodical)   Robert Rodale and Staff. Rodale Press, Inc., Emmaus, Pa. 18049 (Subscription: 33 East Minor Street, Emmaus, Pa. 18049; 1 yr. $5.85)

You guessed it: the latest research and information on organic gardening.

Stalking the Wild Asparagus   Euell Gibbons
Stalking the Blue-Eyed Scallop   Euell Gibbons
Stalking the Healthful Herbs   Euell Gibbons

There is enough food growing wild to meet all our needs, and it is to be had for the taking. Let Euell Gibbons guide you.

"Each time I am in the presence of the work of nature, I enjoy and admire the simplicity of her means."   Will Rogers

Spiritual Diet   Baba Ram Dass
Be Here Now   Baba Ram Dass
Meditation in Action   Chogyam Trungpa Rinpoche
Integral Yoga Hatha   Yogiraj Sri Swame Satchidananoa

Michael Beale

NOTES

DENTAL HEALTH

One problem common to all rural folks is bad teeth. Most of us in Vermont know people in their 20's or 30's whose mouths look like our grandparents'; and some of us are beginning to look that way, too.

Most people see the dentist as a repairman to the inevitable breaking down of their teeth. Much of this fatalistic viewpoint is based on a misconception that natural teeth are not strong enough to last a lifetime. This is not true!! Dental disease can be prevented, and it is up to *you*, not the dentist.

Dental decay, periodontitis (pyorrhea), and gingivitis (bleeding gums) are all infectious, contagious diseases caused by certain strains of streptococcal bacteria. These strep are normally found in the mouths of 98% of the entire American population. They are transmitted via droplet and spray much as are cold and flu viruses. Normally, these strep are freely floating about in the saliva. In this condition they can do no damage.

Everyday, throughout our entire lives, dental plaque forms anew on all tooth surfaces and gums. This plaque is a combination of saliva and food debris (the fuzz or fur you can feel on your teeth). It is a perfect culture medium for the disease-causing strep. The freely floating strep attach themselves to the plaque and colonize, multiplying at a tremendous rate. These strep colonies can best metabolize one food substance—sucrose (table sugar). The metabolic end products of these strep colonies are acids, enzymes and toxins. The acid is produced within 20 seconds after sucrose is in your mouth and continues to be produced until the bacteria have no more food (about 20 minutes). The acids decalcify tooth structure, producing cavities; the enzymes and toxins break down the proteins and irritate the tissues of the gums, producing gingivitis (bleeding gums) and periodontitis (phorrhea). Part of this is because of bad nutrition (candy bars, sugar coated breakfast cereals, etc.) but at least part of it is because we don't brush our teeth properly.

The strep cannot colonize on a clean tooth surface; if they cannot colonize, they cannot multiply to the point where metabolic end products can be produced in amounts necessary to produce dental diseases. If the amount of sucrose is limited, the strep have less to feed on. Therefore, a good method of controlling dental disease is to prevent the formation of plaque and to control the intake of sucrose. (The following foods have large amounts of sucrose: chocolate, maple syrup, jello, molasses, soda, white bread, candy, cookies, cake, jams and jellies, pastries, honey, gum, pastries, canned and frozen sweetened fruits.)

Diet controls sucrose; thorough brushing with a soft-bristled toothbrush removes the plaque and polishes tooth surfaces. Thorough brushing in the morning and in the evening is good, but after each meal is best. Angle the brush up into the teeth and gums of the upper teeth and down into the teeth and gums of the lower teeth. Use a circular (rotary) stroke with the brush. Do this on the outside of the teeth, the inside, and back and forth on the chewing surfaces.

You can use baking soda and salt sometimes when you brush. Or you can use hydrogen peroxide or a commercial toothpaste. Just using water is okay too.

Daily toothbrushing is important, but it does not do the thorough job necessary to prevent plaque build-up. A toothbrush helps to remove plaque from exposed surfaces, but it does not reach the hidden corners or areas between the teeth. Only dental floss can do this. Dental floss can dislodge and break up the bacterial colonies in between teeth and under gum lines, the exact areas where many cavities occur and gum disease starts.

When you brush your teeth, use your brush to massage your gums to toughen them and help keep them healthy. If a toothbrush is not available after you eat, swishing your mouth with water helps to dilute the sucrose.

If you want to keep your teeth for life, you must *yourself* give them the daily home care that your dentist cannot provide. You stand a good chance of preventing cavities and gum disease if you clean your teeth thoroughly every day, so that the plaque does not accumulate and organize.

Your teeth need to be thoroughly cleaned once every 24 hours, and only *you* can do it. This program of home care coupled with regular dental examinations can find your repair trips to the dental chair greatly reduced—along with the size of your dental bill. It may be a way to keep every one of your natural teeth for as long as you live.

However, if your teeth do get decayed, pain will result. Here is some first aid for your dental distress:

In the case of recurrent or persistent bleeding after a tooth has been extracted, place a hot tea bag over the bleeding socket and apply pressure. A piece of clean cloth can be used when a tea bag is not available. Also avoid rinsing the mouth at this time.

Most gum or mouth sores can be relieved by rinsing with a salt water solution of ½ teaspoon of salt in a glass of warm water.

Toothache can be relieved to some extent by applying either hot or cold compresses over the area of pain; sometimes it helps to apply something cold directly on the aching tooth.

In the case of an aching tooth with a visible cavity, some relief can be obtained when air and food is excluded by filling the cavity with a small plug of cotton or whatever other material is available, such as yarn, paraffin, candle wax, string, etc. Cotton moistened with eugenol, vanilla extract, or oil of cloves will also give some degree of relief when inserted in the cavity.

Dental pain that does not respond to aspirin requires professional attention. An aspirin tablet should not be placed in or around the aching tooth because it irritates and burns the gums, causing increased discomfort and pain.

John G. Long

NOTES

A PEOPLE'S HERBAL

The age of natural healing cannot be forgotten! Our ancestors relied on herbal remedies to keep them hearty and well. The gathering of herbs, roots, barks and berries was an integral part of the Indian's way of life. Preparations were passed on from one generation to the next. Their effectiveness was proven over hundreds of years of careful trial and use: It only made sense in that day that organic substances had the power to cure the human body.

The modern herbalist's approach to health is like that of the Indians. The herbalist believes that within each individual exists a life impulse, being the body's natural urge to heal itself. Consistent with this premise is the rejection of inorganic materials as a means of subsistance and curing one's ills. Many drugs commonly taken, such as aspirin, tranquilizers, and antihistamines treat only symptoms, while increasing the body's intake of artificial substances. The build-up of these substances can often be a cause rather than a cure. Botanical agents when taken help to expel poisons present in the body, and strengthen the body's existing vital forces. Herbalism becomes a way of life with the awareness that organic foods, herbal preparations, exercise, and fasting all contribute toward good health. Hence, perhaps the most important aspect of herbal medicine is prevention of disease. Many of the preparations that follow can be taken each day and will help build the body's resistance.

Led on by pervasive drug advertising, the narrow-mindedness of modern medicine, drug manufacturers' monopolies, and the rat race created by our technological society, today's consumer is often hoodwinked into over-the-counter instant cures and the prescription syndrome. We live in an age when each day humankind becomes further and further removed from a natural

Editors' note: We believe very much in the reexploration and revival of herbalism. There is no question that drugs are greatly overused in contemporary culture and counter-culture, and that herbalism can help reduce the overuse of drugs. As we begin to explore the uses of herbs, however, it is important to keep the following points in mind.

1) Herbalism was at the height of its development at a time when the diagnosis and understanding of disease was much cruder than at present. As we begin to experiment with herbs it is important to incorporate our more exact and differentiated diagnoses into our ideas on therapeutics. We now recognize, for example, several forms of arthritis. Many are still treated with medicines based on herbal remedies; some, however, may be more effectively treated with special diets (which are often part of herbal treatments) or new remedies.

2) It is important to remember that herbal strength varies tremendously. Studies of marijuana have shown that leaves from some plants have almost no effects while leaves from other plants have very powerful effects. Soil conditions, rainfall and amount of sunlight all affect the strength of an herb.

Commercially prepared medications such as digitalis leaf are standardized using biological assays, and hence desired dosages may be safely described.

When using local herbs, proper dosage must be a matter of careful trial and error.

3) We are beginning to learn that different people react differently to the same dose of a medicine.

The fact that a given dose of an herb worked for one person does not imply that that dose is appropriate for everyone.

4) In cases of serious or potentially serious illness, the use of prescription medicines, herbs, and other treatments must be weighed. Medical advice should be sought.

Use herbs instead of over-the-counter medicines when you have flu, gastrointestinal upset, or headaches. However, if symptoms continue, do not hesitate in consulting your local medic or physician.

We know of no herbs that will prevent rheumatic fever when people have sore throats caused by streptoccocus. Antibiotics are required. Nor are there herbs to treat many other infectious or metabolic diseases which once were incurable.

5) It is important to realize that our culture uses herbs: People drink enormous quantities of coffee and tea, and ignore the effects these infusions have on their emotional and physical balance.

You can begin to study herbs quite simply by eliminating your evening cup of coffee and replacing it with mint tea, vervain tea, or other infusions mentioned in the following article.

environment. Many of us have a groping awareness that now is the time to rediscover what was once a human union with nature.

We want this article to be useful to the reader. Therefore, this presentation is based on common health problems. Herbs are presented under the specific areas where they are most helpful. We have limited the array of herbs to encompass those which are safe, easily recognized, have many uses, and are common to our area (New England). We have also included instructions for gathering and preparing herbs and a brief guide to identifying plants.

Many of the treatments prescribed in this article may seem foreign to the reader. However, we strongly encourage you to try them and give them a fair test. What is here is only a beginning. We hope that it interests you enough to learn more on your own.

GATHERING AND STORING

You'll want to collect the desired part of the herb at the time when its essence is most concentrated. It is best to collect on a sunny day in the early afternoon. Avoid roadside picking or any area with residues of exhaust fumes, smoke stacks, etc. When you are collecting the whole plant, it should be picked just before and during flowering. It is at this time that the energy of the plant is culminating in the blossom. The herbs should be tied together at the base of the stems and hung upside down to dry in a dark, warm, and dry place. Once dried, they should be stored in opaque, air-tight containers.

Roots are best collected after the plant has flowered, but before it dies back. It is at this time that the plant's energy retreats back into the root. The next best time to collect roots is in the early spring before the plant blossoms. Roots should be thoroughly washed and dried in the oven at a low temperature. They are ready if they easily snap when broken. Use the same procedure as for storing herbs mentioned above.

The inner barks of trees and shrubs are collected in the early spring before the life-giving sap goes into the buds and leaves, or in the autumn as the tree once again draws its energy inward. The inner bark is just under the rough outer bark and is the desired part. It is easiest to peel off this bark in the early spring when the sap is flowing. The bark can be grated, or cut into pieces. It can be dried either in the oven or in a hot, dry place. Store as above.

Renew the herbs in your medicine chest each year to insure their healing powers.

PREPARATIONS

The most common herbal preparation is a *standard infusion* (st. inf.). Take a generous pinch of the desired herb and pour one (1) pint of boiling water over the herb (s). Take off heat, cover, and let steep for 10–20 minutes. In most instances, leaves, stems, and blossoms are infused, in accordance with their delicate nature, whereas roots, barks, and seeds are decocted.

The *standard decoction* is prepared with the same proportions of herb to water as for a standard infusion. The difference between an infusion and a decoction is that on the latter the herb is *boiled* for 10–20 minutes. Never boil the herb when an infusion is instructed.

Honey can be added to most preparations to make them more palatable. To make a longer-lasting preparation, wine or brandy can be added to the infusion or decoction. However, each additional process will weaken the potency of the preparation.

HERBAL TREATMENTS

COLDS, FEVER AND THE FLU. The herbal treatment for the common cold is based on the theory that fever, runny nose and phlegm are the body's way of curing itself. Whereas over-the-counter cold remedies suppress the symptoms, the appropriate herbal treatment will help the body cure itself.

At the onset of a cold or flu, we suggest a short, fast and immediate use of the following preparation: natural sources of Vitamin C: an infusion of rose hips, white pine needles, spruce twigs.

To bring down fever:

(1) Infuse a combination of 2 parts yarrow, 1 part boneset and ½ part of peppermint. Drink hot and add honey if desired.

(2) Equal parts elder blossoms and peppermint infused. Also, drink hot.

These preparations will produce sweating, bring down the fever and relieve aches and pains.

Sore throats:

(1) Raspberry leaf infusion taken as a gargle (more effective with hot vinegar added).

(2) Spoonful of honey.

These will act to soothe and coat the throat.

UPPER RESPIRATORY SYSTEM. Bronchitis and Prolonged Chest Colds:

(1) Garlic:

  a. Can be taken as a tea—infuse one chopped clove to 1 part water and add honey. Take as frequently as possible.

  b. Grate one bulb garlic into one cup of honey. Take over a period of 24 hours. Take courage and swallow quickly. It *really* helps.

Garlic is a natural antibiotic. It also acts as an expectorant. Raw garlic taken every day will help prevent bronchial complaints.

(2) Mullein: a st. inf. of leaves and flowers. Mullein acts as an expectorant and will also soothe the afflicted area.

CHRONIC ASTHMA AND ASTHMATIC BRONCHITIS. Preparation:

(1) Equal parts pleurisy root, elecampagne root, and comfrey root decocted. Take 3 or

4 times a day in wineglassful doses.

(2) Mullein, pearly-everlasting corn silk and/or coltsfoot can be smoked to relieve constriction.

For asthmatic allergic reactions, either of the above may be used for relief. For severe or persistent asthmatic reactions, a medic or physician should be consulted.

STOMACH AILMENTS. Acid Indigestion: St. inf. of meadowsweet

Nervous stomach: St. inf. of either peppermint, catnip or chamomile.

Gas: Many common house-hold cooking herbs can be used to alleviate this problem. St. inf. of ginger, spearmint, peppermint, cloves, rosemary, sage or anise.

ELIMINATIVE COMPLAINTS. Diarrhea: Adult treatment: 1 tbsp. ground mullein leaves boiled in 1 pint of milk for 1–15 minutes. Take ½ cup every 15 min. for first ½ hour, then once every ½ hour until the mixture is gone. Do not repeat for 12 hours. Mullein acts as an astringent which binds as well as a demulcent to soothe the mucous membranes.

Children: A standard decoction of blackberry root or blackberry leaves.

Infants: St. inf. of strawberry leaves.

NOTE: For severe or persistant diarrhea, see a medic or physician. To help evaluate the seriousness of the diarrhea in children, see George Little's "A Word About Routine Pediatric Care."

Constipation: Instead of coffee, a standard infusion of dandelion root. Pumpkin seeds are also helpful. For children, a st. inf. of violet flowers.

Hemorrhoids or Piles: Fresh leaves of plantain or burdock boiled in oil and applied locally as an ointment. Maybe helpful.

GENERATIVE SYSTEM. Women: Problems with the menstrual cycle: The agent used to bring on a period is called an *emmenagogue*. Emmenagogues often act as nervines which will alleviate cramping at the onset of menstruation.

(1) Painful menses: A st. inf. of catnip or peppermint combined with raspberry leaves. Add ginger to speed the effect.

(2) Profuse menses: (a) a st. inf. of raspberry leaves.

(b) decoction of cramp bark.

CAUTION: Under no circumstances should peppermint or catnip or any emmenagogue be taken during pregnancy. This could lead to miscarriage.

Pregnancy and Lactation: Raspberry leaf tea—St. inf. taken every day and through lactation will help prevent nausea and miscarriage. They are an excellent source of calcium, and this is especially important during lactation. Castor oil rubbed into the breast and wiped off before nursing will help to increase lactation.

Men: Prostate Gland: St. inf. of squaw-vine will strengthen this gland and also acts as a tonic for the male reproductive system.

Children: A st. inf. of calendula, raspberry, yarrow, or chamomile are common and safe herbs to use for minor illnesses. They are also aids during eruptive diseases (i.e., measles, scarlet fever, chicken pox). Peppermint and/or honey will improve the taste.

NERVES. Nervous ailments are treated with the class of agents called *nervines*. They act not only to soothe, but to strengthen the nerves.

Headaches: Often symptoms of a more serious illness. If they persist, for a long period of time, see a medic or physician for help in determining their cause.

(1) Valerian root—decocted, combined with peppermint as it steeps—is an effective nervine for headaches and facial neuralgia.

CAUTION: Valerian root must be used in small, but frequent doses. In larger doses, it will cause vomiting.

(2) Blue vervain—an anti-spasmodic nervine good for insomina and hypertension.

Other common nervines are catnip, chamomile, sage, peppermint, and spearmint.

SKIN AILMENTS. Herbal theory believes many skin diseases are caused by impurities and/or imbalances in the blood stream. Therefore, the herbalist treats these problems with *alterants*, agents which are thought to gradually cleanse and change the character of the blood. Alterants are commonly used for acne, eczema, psoriasis and other chronic skin conditions. Some of the best herbs to be used in these instances are yellow dock root and burdock seeds. A lotion can be made by boiling the root or seeds in water. Apply locally. Make fresh every twenty-four hours. Also, red clover heads can be infused and taken as a tea. A few blossoms can be added to other regular teas. It must be remembered that alterants act slowly and must be taken over a long period of time.

WOUNDS, CUTS, SPRAINS. Two of the best common wound herbs are daisy and comfrey. Upon injury, either herb should be infused and taken cold for the duration of the healing process. Also, simultaneously apply either herb to the wound using a cloth bandage soaked in the infusion.

For cuts, apply cider vinegar or calendula. These act as excellent antiseptics when applied locally.

TONICS. These herbal agents strengthen the system internally. They supply the necessary vitamins and trace minerals for a healthy body.

Meadowsweet, alfalfa, or nettles can be infused into a tea.

Meadowsweet beer is a great drink and body-builder. Take 2 oz. of each of the following, dried: meadowsweet, raspberry leaves, agrimony and nettles. Boil these in 2 gallons of water for 15 minutes. Strain. Add 1 lb. of honey. Let stand until nearly cool. Bottle and cap securely. This recipe does not need yeast. Keep in cool place several weeks before using.

POTHERBS. Many delicious plants can be gleaned for good eating. Collect young shoots or leaves

A PEOPLE'S HERBAL

of any of the following: fresh nettles, cowslips, horseradish, plantain, pigweed, milkweed, fiddleheads (ostrich fern), watercress, wild asparagus, yellow dock, burdock, dandelion, cattails and tiger lily. Cook like greens. Some herbs are bitter, especially cowslips, fiddleheads, and dandelions and must be boiled in several waters. Test before eating.

POISONOUS PLANTS. Some of the following plants are very dangerous and should be avoided. A dose as small as one berry could be fatal. For this reason, we stress the importance of proper identification. *Never* taste a plant without first knowing what it is.

PARTIAL LISTING OF COMMON PLANTS WITH INDICATION OF THE PARTS WHICH ARE CONSIDERED DANGEROUS

Plants	Dangerous Parts of the Plant
Avens	all parts
Azaleas	all parts
Baneberry (Doll's Eyes)	(see addenda)
Bittersweet**	berries, juice
†Black Locust	bark, foliage, seeds (not fatal)
Blue Flag	(see addenda)
Buckthorn Berries	(see addenda)
Burning Bush*	leaves
†Buttercups	all parts, acid, unpaletable
Castor Bean*	seeds
Christmas Rose*	whole plant, all parts
†Crocus, Autumn*	bulbs
Cyclamen*	tubers
†Daphne	berries
Dieffenbachia* (dumb cane)	all parts
Delphinium*	leaves
†Deadly Nightshade	berries
Dogbane	(see addenda)
Doll's Eyes (Baneberry)	(see addenda)
Elephant Ear*	all parts
†Elderberry (see Red Elderberry)	leaves, bark, twigs, all green parts
(Note: berries are edible, and are source of Vitamin C)	
Fox Glove**	leaves (source of digitalis)
Golden Chain*	capsules
†Hemlock (water)	all parts (see addenda); also poison hemlock
†Horse Chestnut	nuts, leaves
Hydrangea*	leaves

Listing partially adapted from "Preventing Accidental Poisoning in the Home" (Cooperative Extension Service—W.V.U. Circular 437)
 * = cultivated as house/garden ornamentals; not usually ingested except by children
 ** = these have important medicinal uses, but not for ingestion randomly!
  X = not found in Vermont, or at least not common here
  † = yes, common and dangerous

Plants	Dangerous Parts of the Plant
Indian Poke (White Hellebore)	(see addenda)
Iris*	underground stems
Ivy, most kinds	leaves
(only English Ivy leaves are poison)	(see addenda) (Va. Creeper berries are dangerous)
†Jack-in-the-Pulpit	all parts
Jessamine*	berries
†Jimsonweed	all parts
Larkspur	young plants, seeds
†Laurels	all parts
Lily of the Valley**	all parts (contains cardiac agent)
Lupins	leaves, seeds
Mayapple^X	root
(fruit is edible but not seeds)	
Mistletoe*	berries
†Monkshood	all parts
†Moonseed	berries
†Mountain Laurel	all parts
†Narcissus (also daffodils and snowdrops)	bulbs
†Nightshade	all parts, esp. unripe berries
Oaks	foliage, acorns (contain much tannin, but this is not a real poison; some edible when tannin leached)
Oleander*	all parts
Poinsettia	(see addenda)
Poison Hemlock	(see addenda)
†Potato	green tubers, sprouts (all green parts contain selenium)
Privet*	leaves, berries
Philodendron*	stems, leaves
†Red Elderberry	sheets, leaves, bark, berry
Rhododendron* (not common in Vermont)	all parts
Rosary Pea*	seeds
Rhubarb	leaves (all green parts contain Oxalic acid)
Snow-on-the-Mountains	(see addenda)
†Tobacco	all parts
White Hellebore (Indian Poke)	(see addenda)
†Wild Black Cherry (all cherries)	wilted leaves contain prussic acid seeds also contain prussic acid
†Yew*	*all* parts

ADDENDA

1. *"Doll's eyes" or Baneberry* (Actaea sp.) A common plant of the deep woods. Has a plume of white flowers in spring, followed in fall by fleshy-stemmed berries—either white or red—with large black spot in center; hence the name "doll's eyes." These berries are poisonous to children (who are often attracted to them). The plant is also poisonous and a relative

A PEOPLE'S HERBAL

of monkshood, etc.

2. *White Hellbore, Indian Poke* (Veratrum viride). A very strong medical plant, is still purchased by pharmaceutical companies as a heart agent. Very common in our area in stream borders. Has a very strong-ribbed leaf which comes up folded in the spring. Almost every year a family or group ends up in the hospital for picking and eating these, thinking they are Skunk Cabbage. Also common in mountainous regions such as Mt. Mansfield toll road.

3. *Dogbane* (apocynum. sp.) A very violent heart agent. Cousin of Milkweed family.

4. *Blue Flag* (the wild iris) grows beside streams. Has a violent action. Sometimes dug by mistake when seeking other streamside plants such as Sweet Flag.

5. *Poison Hemlock* A different plant from the Water Hemlock, but also virulently poison. This was the potion Socrates drank for his execution. This whole family of Umbelliferae have some of the most dangerous plants known to man (outside of some of the fungi) and people should exert great care in not mistaking them for Wild Caraway (or Wild carrot), which they resemble closely.

6. *Buckthorn Berries* (Rhamnus cathatica) Source of our cascara laxative is the bark of a kindred tree—are violently cathartic. Not deadly, but very uncomfortable. Very common everywhere in Vermont. Black berries on small tree.

(A note on the Virginia Creeper, mentioned under IVY). The berries of this resemble wild grapes, especially when the leaves are off the vines; and unfortunately the two grow often together, even intertwined. Can be distinguished if care is used. *English Ivy* is poisonous in all its parts, but doesn't grow far north in Vermont.)

Elder (mentioned in listing): Berries are edible, but should be cooked; and contain much vitamin C. But not the RED ELDERBERRY, which has a reputation for being poisonous. Elder leaves, shoots, etc. are apparently dangerous, and children who use the pithy elder stems for blowguns have sometimes had reactions. A brew of the leaves is used to kill blowfly maggots in hides of cattle!)

7. *"Snow on the Mountains"* another ornamental plant with white-edged leaves, much used on the borders of flower beds. Dangerous in all its parts.

Other: caution against any fungi (except Giant Puffballs) unless shown by an expert.

Poison Ivy, etc. and nettles can cause skin rashes, sometimes serious, but are not otherwise "poisonous," internally.

8. *Poinsettia:* house plant given at Christmas time. Dangerous: a 2-year-old child died after eating one leaf. Relative of "Snow on the Mountain."

IDENTIFYING PLANTS

Proper identification is a must!

When in the field, there are many different features to be noted on each plant. For instance, for flowering plants, note the design of the blossom; flower arrangements; number of petals, pistils, stamens; the shape and surface of stem (is it hairy, thorny, smooth?); shape of leaf (simple or compound); whether stem is present on leaf; if the arrangement of leaves is alternate, opposite, whorled or leaf rosettes, edges of leaf (serrated or smooth). Also, note color of each part of the plant. Recognize seedpods and shape of the root, bud formation. These are only some of the distinguishing characteristics of plants. Trees are just as tricky. For this reason, we feel that we cannot give accurate descriptions of all the plants we have mentioned in this article. However, we would like to point out a few of the herbs you may want to try.

1. Peppermint: Labiatae or Mint family.

Gives off an aromatic fragrance. Pinch leaf and smell. Flowers are pale violet or pink-purple. The lower petal is lip-like in form. Rings of flowers are around stems and in interrupted clusters forming a terminal spike. Usually a pair of leaves below each ring of flowers. The stem is square and usually purplish. Leaves stalked, opposite one another, 2–3 inches long, serrated slightly but not visibly hairy. The plant stands ½–3 feet high. Peppermint is commonly found in damp places.

2. Yarrow: Composite or Daisy Family.

Flowers are usually white and sometimes pink. Flowerheads are minutely daisy-like in flattened clusters. Usually many flower clusters to a plant. Leaves are lacy, alternate, aromatic, 3–4 inches long. Leaves clasp stalk lacking leaf stem. Stalk is ridged and rough. Plant grows 1–3 feet high. Common to pastures and roadsides.

3. Great Mullein:

A very tall plant. 5-petaled flowers are yellow, all blossoming at different times along the terminal spike of the plant which grows 2–6 feet high. Frequently the plant has present more than one terminal spike. Leaves feel like flannel, 6–8 inches long, stemless, smooth-edged, and the vasal leaves grow in a rosette.

4. Meadowsweet: Rose Family.

Also called Queen-of-the-Meadow. Common to overgrown pastures and young forests. Blossom is pale pink or white, 5-petaled flowers in clusters branching off a terminal spike. Stems red-brown in color. Leaves coarsely toothed, some large with smaller leaves interspersed. Top surface of leaf is darker green than the underside. Small shrub appearance growing 2–5 feet high.

5. Ginger:

Roots crawl along ground surface with leaf stalks growing off them paired. Large, full, heart-shaped leaves, with long stems. In the crotch of the leaf stems there is a beautiful deep red flower, hollow and bulb-like with three lobes. Stems are hairy. Plant 6–12 inches high. Very aromatic. Common to limestone ledges and found in beech-birch-maple forests.

6. Plantain:

Totally green plant found in waste areas and on roadsides. Rosette of vasal leaves; leaves broad, smooth-edged and blunt; leaves 4–8 inches long, 3–6 inches wide; vein parallel throughout length of leaf. Many four-parted flowers head the terminal spike. Whole plant stands 6–10 inches high.

A PEOPLE'S HERBAL   131

Stinging Nettle
(*Urtica dioica*)

Wild Ginger
(*Asarum canadense*)

Peppermint
(*Mentha piperita*)

132 THE HOME HEALTH HANDBOOK

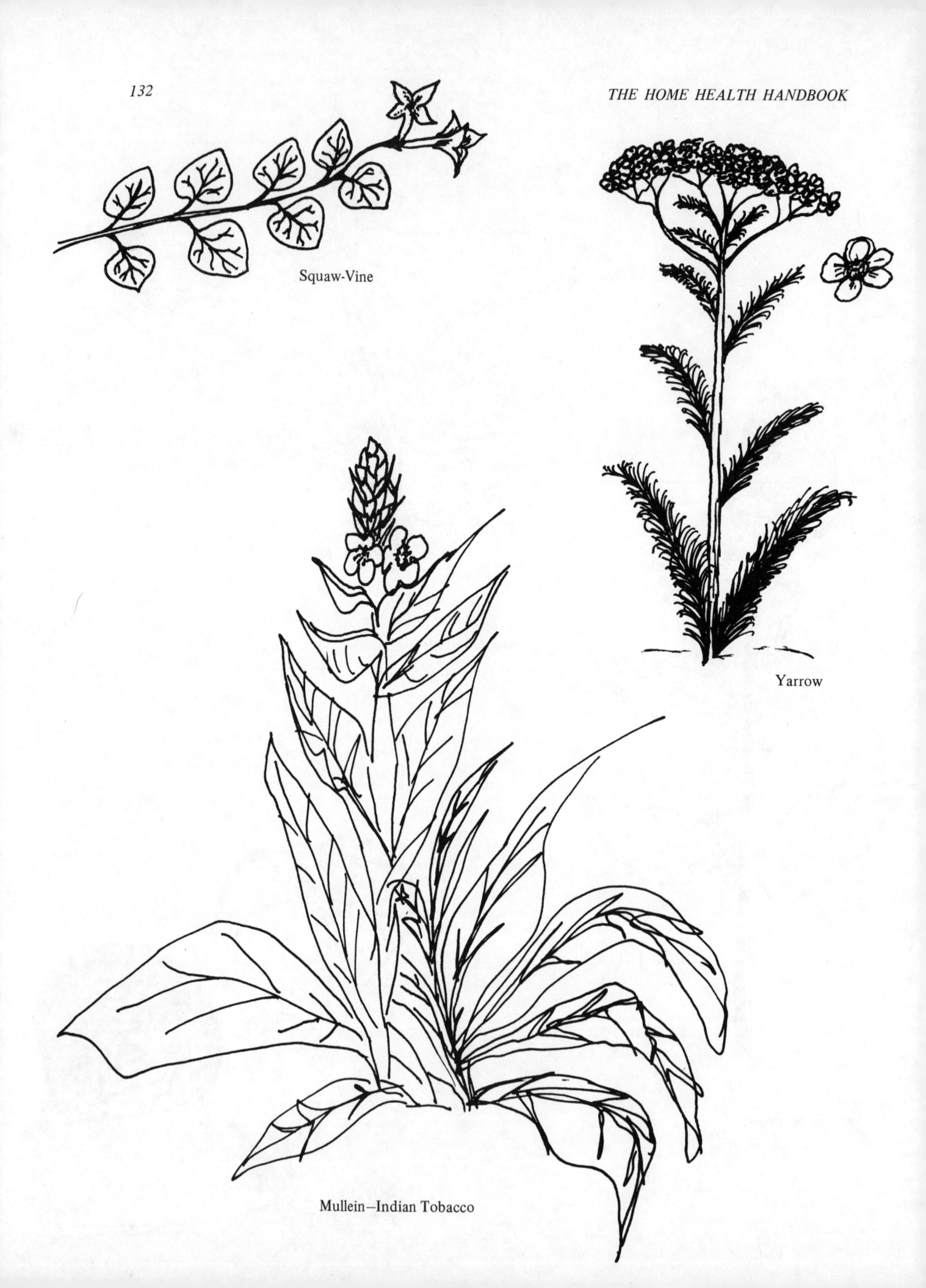

Squaw-Vine

Yarrow

Mullein—Indian Tobacco

A PEOPLE'S HERBAL

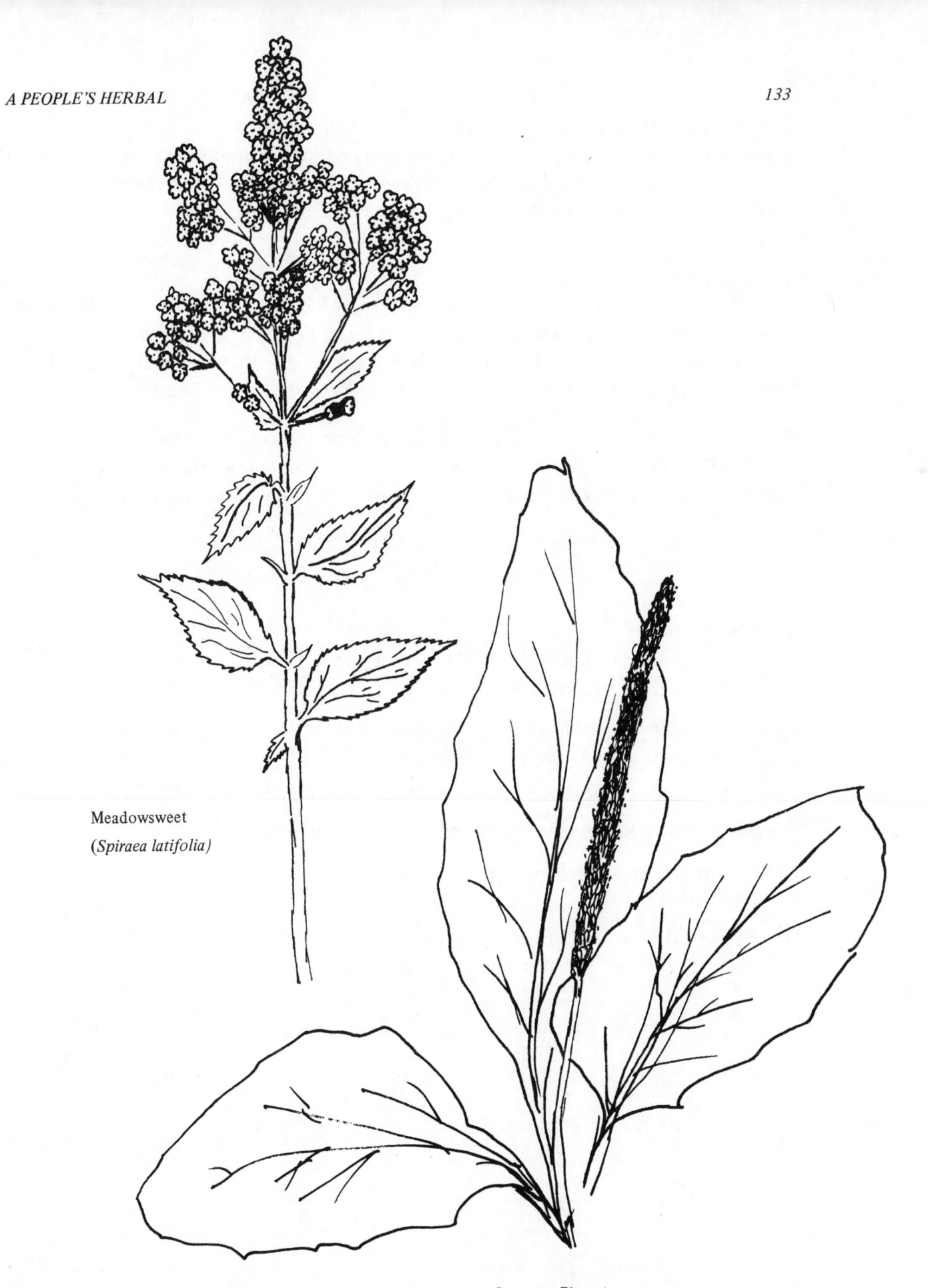

Meadowsweet
(*Spiraea latifolia*)

Common Plantain

7. Squaw Vine: Also called Partridge Berry.

Vine which crawls along the ground, common to evergreen forests. Leaves are shiny, evergreen-colored, with white vein down the center, paired, rounded and broad with short stems. Flowers are white or pink, 4 petals, bearded inside, paired at vine's end. Bears red berries each having 4 seeds.

8. Stinging Nettle:

Found on roadsides and in waste plains. Leaves are stalked, opposite, sharply toothed, elongated heart-shape. Flowers are greenish growing out of leaf axils. Female flowers dangle, male flowers are erect. Plant grows 2–3 feet high. Stem is four-sided, covered with stinging hairs. CAUTION: If stung, rub plantain leaf, if available, or any other safe green plant onto afflicted area.

NOTE: Readers are referred to R.T. Peterson and Margaret McKenny's *A FIELD GUIDE TO WILD FLOWERS*, 1968, published by Houghton Mifflin Co. of Boston. This guide covers over 1300 species with illustrations. This is an excellent source for beginners.

SUGGESTED SOURCES:

Fernald, Merritt Lyndon, & Kinsey, Alfred Charles, *Edible Wild Plants of Eastern North America,* 1958, Harper & Row, New York.

Gibbons, Euell, *Stalking the Healthful Herbs* and *Stalking the Wild Asparagus,* 1966, David McKay Company, Inc., New York.

Grieve, M., *A Modern Herbal,* in 2 volumes, 1971, Dover Publications, Inc., New York.

Harris, Ben Charles, *Eat the Weeds,* 1969, Barre Publishers, Barre, Mass.

Lucas, Richard, *Common and Uncommon Uses of Herbs for Healthful Living,* 1969, ACR Books, New York.

Potter's New Cyclopaedia of Medicinal Herbs and Preparations, re-edited and enlarged by R. W. Wren, 1972, Harper Colophon Books, Harper and Row, New York.

In Good Health,
Janet Young
Elizabeth Baer

NOTES

DRUGS

Drugs are like anything else: if you're going to be involved directly or indirectly, you should know something about them.

The following chapter is a series of short discussions on:
- I. General information
- II. Stimulants
- III. Depressants
- IV. Hallucinogens
- V. Common signs and symptoms
- VI. Treatment for various drug problems
- VII. Crisis centers in Vermont
- VIII. Comments on some drug laws in Vermont

I. GENERAL INFORMATION

A drug is any chemical substance that affects the mind or body—it's that simple. The end result of taking the substance is determined basically by three parameters: pharmacological, psychological, and environmental.

PHARMACOLOGICAL. Your reaction to a drug is effected by just what chemical it is, by what route you take it, how much you take, at what rate it is taken, and then by the many involved ways the body handles the drug. Not all bodies are the same in this regard; age, sex, nutritional status, preexisting diseases, genetic abnormalities, tolerance and reserve tolerance, other drugs—all play a part in determining the effect the drug will have on a person.

PSYCHOLOGICAL. Psychological factors are of course a big determinant. If you have specific expectations (what you are looking for in this particular drug experience), and reliable factual education (do you have any idea what is going to happen or is the whole experience going to be a surprise?), then as the effects come on you are more likely to avoid panic, fear, and anxiety. General expectations are also important: compare being uptight about getting raided with feeling safe and secure. Finally, you have to consider preexisting disorders and diseases. The latent schizophrenic is going to take off a lot differently from most of us.

ENVIRONMENTAL. Then you must consider the peripheral business of what kind of day it has been, who you're with, where you are, music, etc., all told—the personal and physical environment in which you are acting.

Now a word or two about how a drug relationship develops. This relationship is basically a reinforcement and reward phenomenon which can lead to varying degrees of dependence. If the effect the drug has is positive, and multiple trials result in continued reinforcement, then the continued use constitutes *primary psychological dependence*—wanting to continue use of the drug for the end obtained. This category of primary psychological dependence applies to most of the drugs society has accepted socially: caffeine in coffee, nicotine in cigarettes, alcohol, betel (a kind of bean) chewed in Southeast Asia, khat (an African plant), etc. All of the drugs used in this fashion have the potential for physical and psychological harm, but the relationship is controlled and their use has an accepted place in our society as a whole. Ups, downs, and hallucinogens cause a primary psychological dependence, but are separate, since they possess in the most cases the potential for other problems. Not that our parents drugs don't have some liabilities (for example, alcohol and liver disease, tobacco and lung cancer, caffeine and heart disease); it's just that the problems of hallucinogens are different and we as a society lack long-term experience in dealing with their attendant difficulties. They are also separated for legal reasons.

II. STIMULANTS
(Ups, Pep Pills, Dexies, Bennies, Co-pilots, Meth, Coke, Snow, Happy Dust, etc.)

The stimulants or ups (usually the amphetamine class of chemicals) increase alertness, reduce hunger and may produce a feeling of well-being. Their medical benefits are minimal except for two rare conditions—hyperkinetic children and narcolepsy. They have been prescribed for suppression of hunger and reduction of depression, but it is generally agreed that there are now better and less dangerous drugs for these purposes. Cocaine, benzedrine (bennies) Dexedrine (dexies), methamphetamine (Meth) are the most common stimulants—collectively called "speed."

Speed works by increasing the concentration of the chemicals in the body that make the connections between nerve cells. This stimulates many body processes. Speed can be taken orally, sniffed, or injected intravenously. In varying degrees it dilates pupils, increases heart rate and blood pressure, drys up the mouth, increases muscle tone, and increases sweating.

In ordinary small amounts the amphetamines provide a sense of alertness and well-being. Hunger is diminished and short-term performance may be enhanced in the fatigued person. When amphetamines are taken intravenously in large amount, an ecstatic high occurs which decreases over a few hours. Reinjection of them is then necessary to reproduce the stimulation. Shakiness, itching, chills, muscle pains and tension are common side effects of this high. Upon withdrawal many speed users feel terribly depressed and lethargic. A rebound depression occurs such that if the individual was depressed before the high, the subsequent crash can be to an even lower level of depression.

Reinjection of speed relieves the symptoms. Increased doses are usually required, tolerance develops, and large amounts of amphetamines are considered physically addicting. Small amounts are psychologically habituating or cause primary psychological dependence. Many people use speed in small amounts or on an intermittent basis and enjoy their highs without encountering many serious side effects—but many have problems. In addition to the disease associated with the use of unsterile needles (hepatitis, endocarditis, etc.) other medical complications can occur. Liver damage, heart rhythm abnormalities, drastic increases in blood pressure, drastic weight reduction, malnutrition, and psychiatric problems are all possible with prolonged use of speed.

Medical complications can arise when even small amounts of speed are used, since speed can help precipitate active diabetes, convulsions, active heart disease, and ruptured blood vessels in the brain. Granted, many speed users never encounter these problems—but some do. While under the influence of speed the individual usually becomes overactive and talkative. He can also become irritable, paranoid, and sometimes violent.

Most people who use speed do not suffer side effects after the effects of the drug have worn off, but panicked paranoid states can develop which linger on for variable periods of time.

The speed freak with a problem poses special consideration in terms of being helped. His high often prevents him from recognizing certain things about himself. Speed can prevent him from realizing he is talking too much, becoming irritable, not keeping even reasonably clean, and seriously neglecting his health. As a result, the speed freak is often very hard to live with or help, and he can wind up turning a lot of people off, as well as slowly (and speedily) destroying his body and his mind.

III. DEPRESSANTS (Downers)

The depressants include many drugs of several categories, which act upon the central nervous system to relieve pain, reduce anxiety, or cause sleep. All the depressant drugs, with rare exceptions, are capable of producing physical and possible psychological dependence. The physiological dependency develops along with tolerance to the drug so that the individual develops a continuous need for a drug, and withdrawal symptoms occur when that drug is discontinued. The withdrawal reaction may be severe, particularly in the case of dependence on barbiturates and other sedatives.

NARCOTICS (Smack, Junk, Horse, Skag, Etc.) A narcotic is a depressant drug that relieves pain and causes drowsiness or sleep. Drugs in this category include morphine and codeine, which come from opium. Heroin, which is six times stronger than morphine, is produced by a chemical alteration of the morphine base.

The depressant effect of the narcotics produces drowsiness, sleep and a lessening of physical activity. Some common side effects include nausea and vomiting, constipation, itching, flushing, constriction of the pupils and respiratory depression. Narcotics produce more than an indifference to pain. They reduce sensitivity to both psychological and physical stimuli and also repress the inner drives that motivate an individual to satisfy hunger, find identity, seek sexual gratification, and respond to provocation with anger. Therefore, they seem to develop a state of "total drive satiation"; that is, nothing needs to be done because all things are as they should be. For some people, such a state of euphoria (well-being) is very pleasant. With daily use of narcotics, tolerance develops and the amount of drug needed to get high increases. As tolerance increases both the pleasure and side effects may diminish, and anxiety often develops over obtaining sufficient drug supply to avoid withdrawal sickness.

The severity of withdrawal symptoms varies with the degree of physiological dependence and the drug. This in turn is related to the amount of drug normally taken. (In Vermont the percentage of heroin per bag ranges between 0% to 5%, while in the boroughs of New York City it may be from 0% to 10% or more). This variation in strength makes it difficult to take a constant daily dose, and occasionally leads to death, due to overdosage. The normal withdrawal symptoms consist of yawning, shakes, anxiety, sweating, running eyes, pupil enlargement, gooseflesh, vomiting and diarrhea, muscle aches and jerks, abdominal pain, chills, and backache; hallucinations and delusions can also develop. Typically the onset of symptoms occurs about 8–12 hours after the last dose. Thereafter, the symptoms increase in intensity, reach a peak between 36–72 hours, and gradually diminish over the next few days. Some symptoms such as weakness, insomnia, nervousness, and muscular aches and pains may continue for several weeks. The symptoms eventually subside spontaneously, but may be relieved with an injection of a narcotic or by withdrawal under medical supervision. In rare cases death may result from the absence of medical treatment.

The following serious problems arise for the non-medical users of narcotics who inject the drug using non-sterile syringes, needles and solutions: Tetanus, viral hepatitis, bacterial infection, inflammation of the heart valves, and skin abscesses; inflammation and scarring of veins (track marks) may occur. Since heroin is cut with many different types of diluents (lactose, quinine etc.) and the small particles are not properly put into solution, they can accumulate in the lungs, causing hypertension.

BARBITURATES (Nembutal–"Yellow Jackets"; Seconal–"Red Birds"; Amytal–"Blue Heavens"; Luminal–"Purple Hearts") The barbiturates are among the most widely used depressant drugs available and are increasing in popularity as street drugs. Medically they are used for epilepsy, insomnia, and in the treatment of emotional disorders. A person on barbiturates (downers) may have a staggering walk and slurred speech. His reactions may be sluggish. He is emotionally labile and can be easily moved to tears or laughter. Quite often, he is irritable and antagonistic. He has feelings of being in a cloud and euphoric.

Accidental overdosing may occur for many reasons:
People often take too much of the drug, especially when no physiological tolerance has been built up.
Overdose often occurs because of the many different types of barbiturates and their variability in onset of action and potency. Some barbiturates will last in activity for 3–4 hours, others from 6–8, and still others upward of 12 hours. The barbiturates also have a range of activity from several minutes to upwards of an hour before any drug activity is noticed.
Mixing alcohol and barbiturates can be fatal. Their action is additive, and depending upon

many variables (dose of both drugs, time for metabolisms, etc.), mixing them may result in fatal depression of respiratory and cardiovascular systems.

Continuous misuse of barbiturates leads to the development of tolerance and physiological and psychological dependency. Physiological dependence seems to develop only after continued use with doses somewhat higher than the normal medical doses. With physiological dependence on sedatives, abrupt withdrawal is extremely dangerous and should be supervised by an experienced physician. In withdrawal the person appears to improve 8–12 hours after his last dose. Later, signs of increasing nervousness, headache, anxiety, muscle twitching, weakness, tremor, insomnia, nauseas develop. A person may experience a sudden drop in blood pressure when he stands up. For 24 hours these symptoms are quite severe. There are changes in the EEG reading, and within 36–72 hours a convulsion resembling epileptic seizures can develop. Such convulsions may occur as early as the sixteenth hour of withdrawal or as late as the eighth day. Convulsions can be fatal and are an ever-present danger with barbiturate withdrawal. This makes barbiturate withdrawal more dangerous than narcotic withdrawal. There may also be a period of mental confusion, delirium, and hallucination. Delirium may be accompanied by an extreme agitation causing exhaustion. It may develop early in withdrawal or last for several days followed by long periods of sleep.

Withdrawal thereapy usually involves substitution of another drug and gradual decreased dosage over a period of many days or weeks.

IV. HALLUCINOGENS
(Pot, Grass, Mary Jane, Tea, Acid, Hawk, "The Chief," etc.)

This group of drugs, including LSD, DMT, STP, mescaline, psilocybin, and THC (THC is the most active chemical in marijuana, and in large enough dosage acts as a hallucinogen) is capable of causing changes in sensation, thinking, self-awareness and emotion.

How this group of drugs affects the central nervous system is still a mystery, but a possible hypothesis shall be explained. The brain receives and sorts through hundreds of millions of sensory inputs per second, and these inputs pass through filters which group together the necessary inputs needed for survival. These drugs somehow disrupt or temporarily disable the filters and allow many more sensory inputs through. This floods the brain with an excess of information (hence the term *mind-expanding*) and therefore sometimes drastically changes an individual's normal perception of the world, as well as his mood, thoughts, and activities.

The hallucinogenic experience varies greatly, from no response to an overwhelming one, because of dosage, personality of the user, environment, and many other variables discussed earlier in the chapter.

Perceptual changes which may occur during the experience greatly affect the senses: Colors seem to intensify or change, spatial relationships become disoriented, objects can pulsate or appear to have auras surrounding them (visible vibrations). The senses can cross over and color may be tasted. Illusions and hallucinations can occur. Time seems to speed away, stop, slow down or even go backwards. Thoughts are many and free-flowing. There can be laughter, tears, or no emotion at all, all within a single experience.

INFORMATION ABOUT HALLUCINOGENS

1. Flashbacks are a recurrence of hallucinogenic-type experience after the drug effect has worn off (shortest activity is DMT, one half hour to several hours, and the longest is STP, which may last upwards of several days). It can be set off by physical or psychological stress and by other chemicals, but they only seem to occur in a very small percentage (5% or less) of regular users.
2. Conflicting reports of possible genetic (chromosomal) damage or organ damage due to hallucinogens is an unresolved question.
3. Creativity may seem enhanced, but probably is not.
4. Physiological effects may include dilated pupils, tremors, rise in temperature and heart rate, and a slight increase in blood pressure.
5. The use of hallucinogens is usually self-limiting because:
    a. No physiological dependency develops.
    b. Tolerance develops with daily use.
    c. Unreliability of street drugs. Studies have shown that drugs purchased on the street as LSD contained everything from pure LSD to none, plus speed (amphetamines), STP, strychine, MDA, and many combinations of drugs within this list. The amount of bad dope is usually dependent upon the economic law of supply and demand.
    d. Law of diminishing return comes into play. With continuing use, you don't always get off like you used to.

V. COMMON SIGNS AND SYMPTOMS OF PATIENTS WITH MIND/MOOD-ALTERING DRUG TOXICITY

SIGNS AND SYMPTOMS	Sedative–Hypnotics	Narcotics	Hallucinogens	Stimulants	Solvents	Tranquilizers
Coma in overdose	A	A			A	A
Convulsions	W					A
Depression	A			W		
Hallucinations	A		A	A		
Restlessness	W	W	A	A	A	W
Aggressive Behavior			A	A		
Paranoia Panic	W		A	A	A	
Psychosis	W		A	A	A	
Disorientation	A		A	A	A	
Lack of Muscle Coordination	A	A	A	A	A	A
Pain masking	A	A	A	A	A	A
Parkinsonism						A
Slurred speech	A	A			A	
Tear flow		W			A	
Rapid Side to Side Eye Movement	A					
Pupils: Pinpoint		A				
Dilated		W	A	A		
Normal	A				A	A
Runny nose		W			A	
Jaundice—Liver Damage	A	A		A	A	
Skin rash	Bromides			A		
Needle tracks	A	A		A		
Gooseflesh	W	W				
Resp. depression	A	A			A	A
Rapid Heart Action		W	A	A		
Cramps	W	W		W		
Fever				A		

A = Seen in acute intoxication
W = Seen in withdrawal phase
NOTE: This table is intended to list common signs. It does not preclude rare exceptions.

VI. TREATMENT

Whether or not you believe that the use of mind-altering drugs is dangerous or that their use should be prohibited is no longer the question. People use them. And now a few hints on how to handle some of the problems encountered in their use.

DEPRESSANTS. Overdoses occur when the body is simply overloaded and cannot handle the increased concentration of the drug in the blood stream and tissues. This can occur due to simply taking in too much: for example, the quality of the heroin hit is better than usual or the number of pills and their dose is more than the body can tolerate. Overdose can also occur when the rate of ingestion exceeds a manageable level. Drugs like phenobarbital act over a long period of time and may take 1 hour to take effect. Therefore, impatience may lead to taking too many. The signs and symptoms of overdose are decreased rate and depth of breathing, decreased pulse rate and intensity, and unresponsiveness. This last one is the key. Downs make people relaxed and sleepy, but at all times the individual should be able to be aroused; if he cannot be, he is in trouble.

(1) Shallow slow breathing, (2) weak slow pulse, and (3) unresponsiveness all point to a medical emergency. Death can occur in minutes. Support breathing by mouth-to-mouth respiration and get your buddy to a doctor immediately. Don't screw around with ups or stimulants.

WITHDRAWAL. Withdrawal is a group of body reactions signaling the body's need for more depressants. They can occur after prolonged regular use of any of the depressants. The symptoms include:

muscle twitching	anxiety	sweating
yawning	dizziness	stomach pain
runny nose	diarrhea	headache
chills	vomiting	backache

They can also go on to:

| convulsions | coma | death |

Again, don't screw around. This is a medical emergency. Get your buddy to a doctor immediately. If he becomes unresponsive, support his breathing with mouth-to-mouth respiration. The correct medical treatment of withdrawal often requires that a drug of the same class as the one he has been taking be substituted.

ANXIETY REACTIONS. Next some words on anxiety reactions including bad trips from acid. The following discussion can apply to anxiety reactions to stimulants, hallucinogens, and grass (yes, even grass). These pointers are useful for any situation involving acute anxiety—drug or non-drug.

Psychedelics create changes in the way our minds receive and interpret sensory input. These changes can be enjoyable, exhilarating, and beautiful, or they can be ugly and frightening, and result in panic. Only a small percentage of people have bad trips or anxiety reactions, but when they do they need help. People using a particular drug for the first time, or people using combinations unknowingly, are particularly suceptable. (See also earlier comments on what goes into a drug response.)

Drug-induced increased awareness can work both ways: increased enjoyment or increased suffering; additionally, the mind tends to fix on what otherwise might be disregarded. The clouds, a flower, a pleasant thought or a fear of insanity, police, or death. This is what I like to think of as hypersuggestability. From here anxiety and fear dig in and only increase the fixing mechanism and hypersuggestability. From the fear and anxiety comes loss of control and panic.

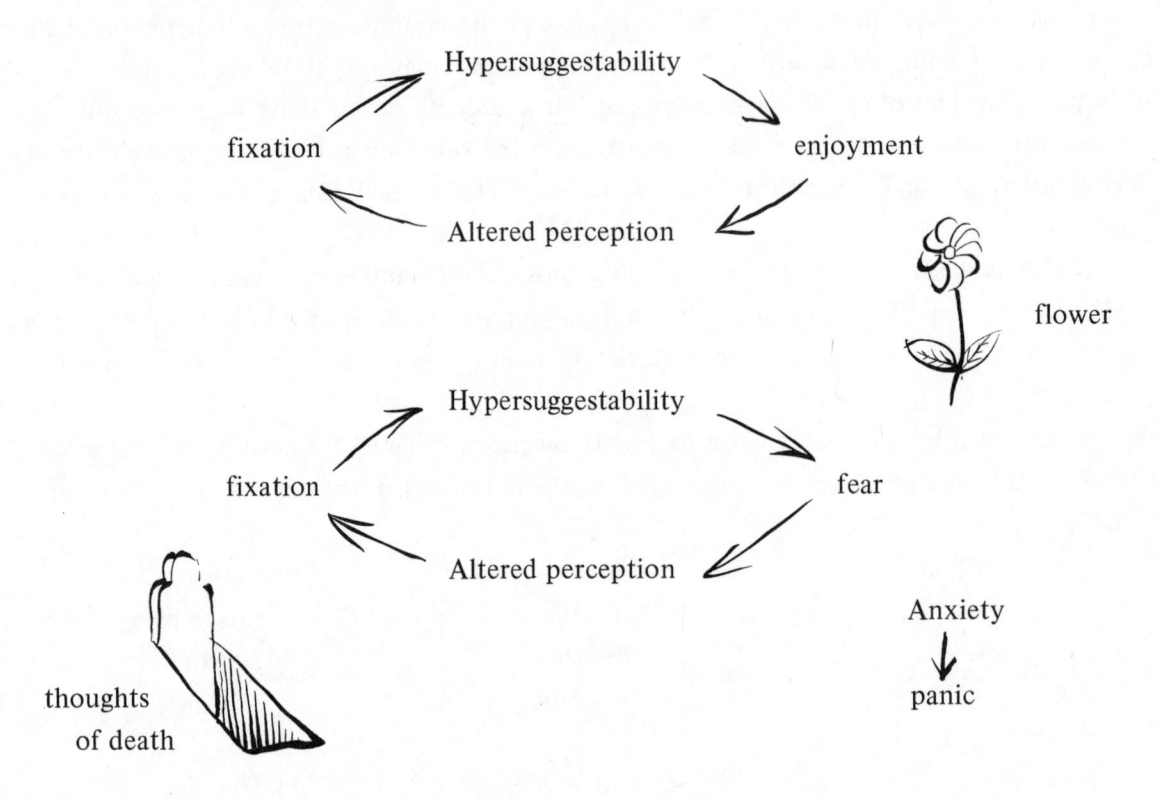

fixation → Hypersuggestability → enjoyment
Altered perception ←
flower

fixation → Hypersuggestability → fear
Altered perception ←
Anxiety ↓ panic

thoughts of death

This can also be accompanied by a feeling of infinite wisdom or strength which may lead to irrational acts such as trying to fly or stop cars.

EVALUATION
1) Protect the drugged person from physical or psychological harm to himself or others.
2) Friends can sometimes help as to what was taken and when, but don't rely on this too much—the information is rarely very helpful.
3) Wide variations are possible, from mild apprehensions to violent panic and suicide.
4) The most common fears that will touch off a bad trip are insanity and death. The loss of control of the mind and sensory input in a good trip can be terrifying to some and result in a fear of losing control forever. Loss of identity and body orientation can often wind up as death.

DRUGS

5) An important part of recognizing the severity of the anxiety reaction and evaluating it is finding out whether or not the individual knows he is on a bad trip. This is called ego disruption—his ability to see himself physically, with his eyes. Since he is real, his ability to see himself is an important touch with reality.

TREATMENT

1) Do not let the individual take any more drugs of any kind. This includes depressants.
2) Since the anxiety reaction was probably precipitated by some external sensory input, try to reduce the sensory input: quiet surroundings, few people, little commotion, dim lights, and so forth. But if he is alone and in the dark to start with, add some sensory input to distract him—but not too much.
3) Establish a bridge with him; between his unreality and your reality. Any one or combinations of the following:
    a) Verbal—repeat simple phrases or names over again. "You are John and I am Jim and we are in a house in Burlington."
    b) Tactile—feel my hand. Feel my hand. This is your hand. Do you feel it? Do you feel me touching it? (hands, books, balls, sticks, etc.)
    c) Visual—a little tougher to do but sometimes good. "See the ball. Watch the ball." (throw it up and down).
    d) Hearing—tap a stick repeatedly, or jingle some keys. Music can work sometimes but only if it is not too heavy.

Whatever you try, stick with it if it works and be patient—keep it up as long as it works. If it makes things worse, stop and try something else.

4) Get the guy to verbalize his fears—find out what is hassling him and react directly and simply to it. "John, you are not going to die. You are not going to die. I will stay with you and help you."

Get him to start building the bridge back to you with his own words. Stress safety and protection from injury—if he verbalizes these fears. "You are safe here. I will protect you."

5) You are essentially dealing with a child lost in a dark woods. Treat him as such.

A few general comments:

1) The reaction can last up to 15 hours. Any longer and you have to think of getting help.
2) Avoid hospitals if possible in situations of drug-induced acute anxiety—it is a real bummer. A fear of death and going crazy will only be confirmed by white coats, needles, and sirens. I also feel that talking someone down decreases his chances of having another bad trip. He will understand how he came down and next time he can prevent it or take himself down.
3) But if you're not making any headway, get help from a local crisis center or an experienced friend. If all else fails and your friend shows no signs of coming down after a long trial of help—the hospital may be needed. Call ahead first (no pun intended!).
4) Coming down is an on-again, off-again thing. Drifting in and out of the trip can be a problem in trying to determine when he is down. Don't leave him alone or let him drive a car for about 24 hours.

5) In summary: a confident, direct, simple approach directed towards re-establishing touch with reality will work. No special skills required except sensitivity and patience.

NOTE: Strychnine is terribly misunderstood. It is sometimes present but usually in only small amounts—but 15–30 micrograms can cause convulsions and even death by respiratory depression. Fast and expert medical attention (via emergency room) is the only thing that will help because death can occur within 20–30 minutes.

VII. CRISIS CENTERS IN VERMONT

BRATTLEBORO:
Hotline for Help, Inc. —————————— 257–7989
17 Elliot St., Brattleboro, 05301

BURLINGTON:
Place (24 hr. telephone service) ———————— 658–3812
260 College St., Burlington 05401

SHAC (Emergency Shelter) ————————— 864–7423
81 Maple St., Burlington 05401

CASTLETON:
Fifth Step ———————————————— 468–5555
Episcopal Church, Castleton 05735

MONTPELIER:
Another Way ——————————————— 223–3481
Drawer H, Montpelier 05602

NEWPORT:
Rooms ————————————————— –334–7952
90 Main St., Newport 05855

ST. JOHNSBURY:
Help, Inc. ————————————————– –748–8711
79 Railroad St., St. Johnsbury 05819   748–8712

VIII. COMMENTS ON SOME DRUG LAWS IN VERMONT

I. INTRODUCTION. This is an attempt to give a broad outline of the consequences of enforcement of Vermont drug laws on persons sixteen years or older who are in possession of or who sell "regulated drugs." Persons under sixteen are treated as juveniles.

DRUGS

A *regulated drug* is defined very broadly to be a narcotic drug, a depressant or stimulant drug, an hallucinogenic drug, or marijuana. Each of these five classes of drugs is defined much more specifically. However, the further definition is very technical. It tends to bore and confuse the non-scientist.

Some of the types of the above classes of drugs that laymen would be familiar with are morphine, heroine, and codeine (narcotic); sodium seconal or red devils (depressant); the amphetamines—dexedrine, benzedrine, and speed (stimulants); LSD or acid and STP (hallucinogenic); and weed or tea or pot or simply marijuana. This list by no means includes all of the types of regulated drugs. There are many, many more.

II. POLICY OF LAW. Vermont law is geared to punish a person who illegally pushes or sells drugs. It can also be said that it tends to encourage a person who uses drugs to receive the help necessary for him or her to stop using them.

This policy is indicated in three separate parts of the Vermont drug law. First, a first-offense possession of a regulated drug is a misdemeanor. Thus, a person convicted of such cannot be sentenced to the state prison. A person who has not voluntarily sought help can be required to do so by the courts. Subsequent possession offenses are felonies. Second, it is no longer the duty of a physician or hospital to report the names of those who seek treatment of a drug problem. Third, in 1971 the legislature made it possible for a minor twelve years or older to receive medical treatment for a drug problem, alcohol problem, or venereal disease without the consent of his or her parent or legal guardian. The statute only requires that the parent or legal guardian be informed about such treatment when immediate hospitalization is required.

III. LAW. In Vermont it is unlawful for a person to possess, prescribe, dispense, or sell a regulated drug unless he or she fits one of the following:

Exceptions

A. A manufacturer or wholesaler may sell a regulated drug on official orders to one of the following:
    1. a manufacturer, wholesaler or pharmacy
    2. a physician, dentist, or veterinarian
    3. a person in charge of a hospital or laboratory if
       (a) the hospital or laboratory has a certificate of approval
       (b) the drug is to be used for medical or scientific purposes
    4. a person in the employment of a government—federal, state, territory, district, county, or municipality—who should purchase, receive, possess, or dispense regulated drugs by reason of his official duties
    5. a person in charge of a ship or aircraft, which has no licensed physician on board, with an order form approved by a commissioned medical officer or an acting assistant surgeon of the U.S. Public Health Service.

B. A physician, dentist (for human beings) or veterinarian (only for animals) may prescribe, administer, or dispense regulated drugs if this is done:
1. in good faith, and
2. during the course of his professional practice.

C. A duly licensed pharmacist may sell a regulated drug if such sale is done:
1. in good faith, and
2. during the course of his profession, and
3. with a written or oral (reduced promptly to writing) prescription of a licensed physician, dentist or veterinarian.

D. Individuals may possess regulated drugs if:
1. they have obtained the drug for their own use or for the use of their animals
2. such drug was prescribed, sold, or dispensed by a licensed physician, dentist, pharmacist, or veterinarian.

IV. PENALTIES. On July 1, 1972, all drug offenses in Vermont became misdemeanors except for second and subsequent offenses of knowingly and unlawfully manufacturing, compounding, dispensing, administering, prescribing, selling for a consideration, or selling to a minor under the age of eighteen years, a regulated drug.

There are five different maximum penalties for unlawful possession and sale of regulated drugs. These maximum penalties and the offenses for which they can be imposed are as follows:

A. *Six Months Confinement, and/or $500 fine*

This penalty can be imposed for conviction of unlawful possession of the following types of regulated drugs—marijuana, depressants, or stimulants.

B. *One Year Confinement, and/or $1,000 fine*

This penalty can be imposed for conviction of unlawful possession of the following types of regulated drugs - a narcotic or an hallucinogenic.

C. *Two Years Confinement, and/or $2,000 fine*

This penalty can be imposed for the following drug offenses:
1. Second and subsequent convictions of possession of any regulated drug—whether it be marijuana, a depressant, a stimulant, a narcotic or an hallucinogenic
2. Conviction for unlawfully possessing a regulated drug with intent to sell the same
3. Unlawful possession of the following types of drugs in the following amounts:
   (a) 25 or more cigarettes of marijuana
   (b) one or more preparations, compounds, mixtures, or substances of an aggregate weight of: 1/8 oz. or more containing alkaloids or salts of heroin, morphine, or cocaine; 1/2 oz. or more containing marijuana; 1/2 oz. or more containing reae or prepared opium
   (c) 100 times the manufacturer's recommended maximum individual dose of a depressant or stimulant drug
   (d) 500 micrograms or more of lysergic acid diethylamide

DRUGS

        (e) 50 milligrams or more of psilocybin

        (f) 6 milligrams of methyl phenylethylamine

        (g) 200 milligrams of dimethylatriptamine

   D. *Five Years Confinement, and/or $5,000 fine*

      This penalty can be imposed for the following drug offenses:

     1. Conviction for unlawful possession of the following types of drugs in the following amounts:

        (a) 100 or more cigarettes of marijuana

        (b) one or more preparations, compounds, mixtures, or substances or an aggregate weight of: 1 oz. or more containing alkaloids or salts of heroin, morphine, or cocaine; 2 oz. or more containing marijuana; 2 oz. or more containing reae or prepared opium

        (c) 300 times the manufacturer's recommended maximum individual dose of a depressant or stimulant drug

        (d) 1000 micrograms or more of lysergic acid diethylamide

        (e) 100 milligrams or more of psylocybin

        (f) 12 milligrams or methyl phenylethylamine

        (g) 400 milligrams of dimethyltriptamine

     2. Conviction for unlawfully manufacturing, compounding, dispensing, administering, prescribing, selling for a consideration, or selling to a minor under the age of eighteen years, a regulated drug

   E. *Minimum of ten years, maximum of twenty-five years and/or $10,000 fine*

This penalty can be imposed for second and subsequent convictions for the offense set out above in D. 2. (above).

V. LAWS PERTAINING TO THE PURCHASE OF DRUGS FROM A PHARMACY

   1. Hypodermic syringes and needles:

      The State of Vermont has no laws or regulations pertaining to the purchase of syringes and needles. Any person with a legitimate use for these items may purchase them from a pharmacy. Be sure and answer all questions the pharmacist may ask you, as he will not sell these items to you if he thinks you might use them for illegal purposes.

   2. Cough syrups:

      There is a legitimate use for certain cough syrups which may contain a small amount of narcotic. These are called exempt narcotic cough syrups. You will be required to produce some identification and will be required to sign an exempt narcotic register. You are not permitted to purchase excessive quantities of these cough medicines; you have a right, however, to purchase such items within these limits. Don't let a druggist hassle you.

   3. Diarrhea preparations:

      There are available medicines for your use which contain very small quantities of narcotics for the control of diarrhea. The most popular is paregoric. This medicine may be obtained from a pharmacy by showing identification and signing an exempt narcotic register. You may not buy more than 2 ounces at a time.

4. Forged prescriptions:

There is a state law against forging prescriptions. Do not attempt to do this, as it is a sure way to get busted. The writing of a prescription is a very complicated procedure and many safeguards have been inserted into the filling of a prescription that will lead to your being caught and prosecuted.

Lynne Curtis	Jim Salander
Ed Croumey	David Giannuzzi
James Marmar	Francis Murray

NOTES

STRESS

Getting sick is almost never due to just one cause, and getting better should always involve the total picture of why a person is sick. Anyone who claims that all sickness is due to nutrition, or to the mind, is as blind as the person who blames it all on germs.

When people get sick, it's important to treat what's causing their sickness on all levels with medicines to help the body fight the disease, but also with lots of attention and care, good food, sanitation and rest. One theory that tries to tie these all together is Hans Selye's stress theory.

The stress theory is as important as Western medicine's attempt to quantify and define an organism's reactions to changes in the environment that require some adaptation within that organism. The theory recognizes the whole organism and deals with men and women and their diseases as complex interactions of the person, past and present, their society and family, their physical condition, their physical environment, and their contact with other's diseases.

The drawing below shows how I think of myself in the world.

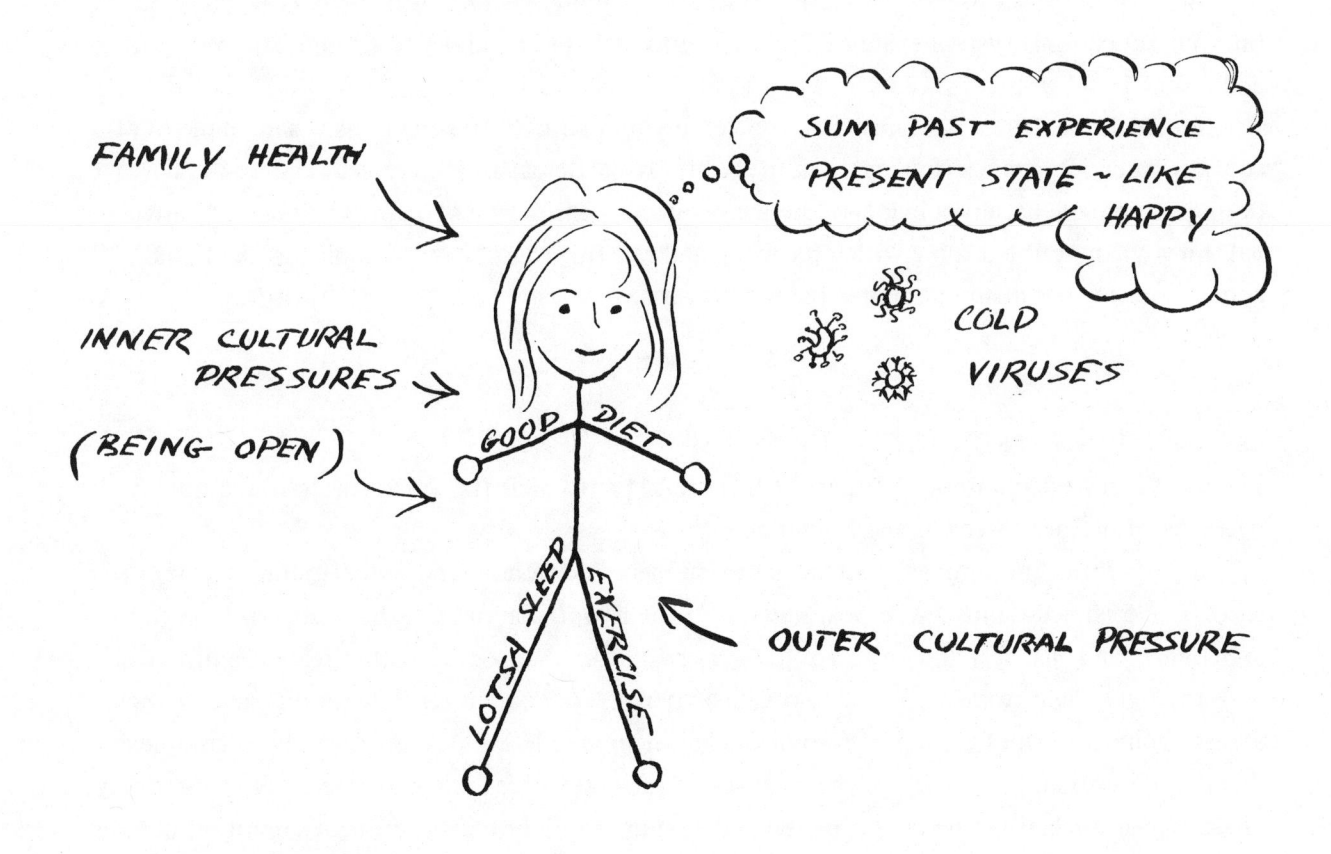

Any of those things acting on me or within me might be a stressor, and in combination with the other things might produce a disease state. *Disease* can be defined as "the sum total of the reactions, physical and mental, made by an organism to a noxious agent entering the body from without or arising from within." So disease is a whole and complex reaction of the body to various stressors and is dependent on many variables for its outcome. To further our understanding of disease, it is important to understand stress and how it affects the human organism.

STRESSORS

Stress as used herein means the reaction of an organism. *Stressor* is the acting agent which may produce the condition of stress in a person. There are many stressors. There are some, such as cold, heat, uncomfortable binding of the body, flashing bright lights, which might be thought of as universal stressors because most organisms react to them with stress patterns of high predictability. But an important component of other kinds of stressors is the person's interpretation of an input. In people, "threats and symbols of danger call forth reactions little different from those to assault." (Wolff, *Stress and Disease,* 1953). A living situation which is full of strife may be a kind of ongoing stressor, or a job, like in an insurance office or collecting agency.

Society can also produce stressors in its patterns and expectations of people. We have built into our educational system exam periods, and into male lives military draft and perhaps fighting and killing in the army.

Medical researchers have made some attempts to quantify stressors . . . so many degrees of cold, so much job strain as estimated numerically by participating employees. The results have been questionable because obviously the meaning and significance of a stressor is a very individual thing when you're dealing with a receiving and reacting organism as complex as the human being. Even to cold different people react with variance.

$$\text{Organism} \longleftrightarrow \text{Stress}$$

A. ENDOCRINE STRESS PATTERNS

The most complex and important part of the stress syndrome is the organism itself and how it perceives or defines a stressor and how it chooses to react.

The historical beginnings of stress theory in medicine were in endocrine studies, in the theories of a man named Cannon who postulated that the hypothalamus was the source of affective experience, and that fear and anger are the major emotions associated with disease. Cannon worked with the fight-flight reaction. When an organism perceives danger it reacts with fear and/or anger and a certain pattern of endocrine response from the body. The endocrine response is complex, much more so than I can pass on here. It involves the entire metabolism of the body in some way, especially through affecting the hormonal and enzyme regulations of the various bodily functions. The following diagram is oversimplified, but perhaps helpful:

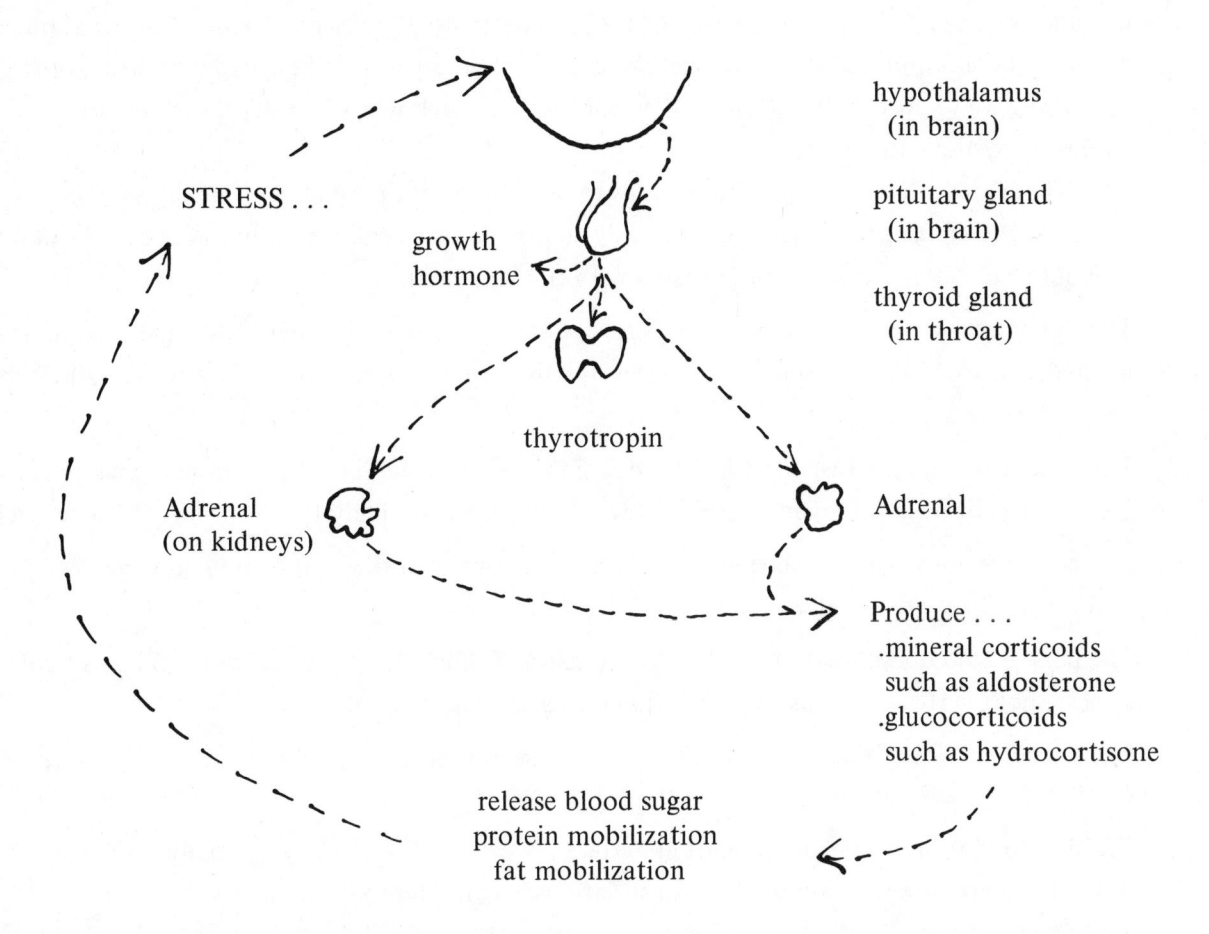

```
                    STRESS ...
                         growth
                         hormone
                                              hypothalamus
                                                (in brain)
                                              pituitary gland
                                                (in brain)
                                              thyroid gland
                                                (in throat)

                         thyrotropin

        Adrenal                              Adrenal
        (on kidneys)

                                             Produce ...
                                               .mineral corticoids
                                                 such as aldosterone
                                               .glucocorticoids
                                                 such as hydrocortisone

              release blood sugar
              protein mobilization
              fat mobilization
```

In addition to the mechanisms shown in the drawing, the fight-or-flight reaction also stimulates heart rate, breathing rate, closes down blood vessels in the periphery, in the stomach and intestines, and shunts blood to the muscles, the heart and the brain. As shown, it stimulates the production of minerals corticoids and glucocorticoids in the adrenal glands so that there is plenty of blood sugar available for metabolism into energy. The body is then ready to take on some challenge actively . . . like running from a bear.

Selye took these beginnings further to say that this whole mechanism, or *parts* of it, can be stimulated by other things than overt physical danger, anger, or fear. There is a specific reaction to a topical stressor, such as a burn on the hand, which brings forth a *local adaptation syndrome* of inflammation. (Inflammation is caused partly by mineral corticoids, and growth hormones are also involved.)

Selye also describes a *general adaptation syndrome* to a non-specific stressor, such as anxiety. In this pattern, the body has nothing concrete to work against and so responds with some combination of any of the above described reactions. Sometimes these reactions may be inappropriate and if longterm will cause functional disorder and disease.

B. PERSONALITY AND STRESS PATTERNS

The human mind—we're all somewhat familiar with how that works or doesn't work. The importance of a person's past, his attitudes, his perception of his present situation, his loved ones, his mental condition in determining his response to stressors cannot be overemphasized, but is something we've all seen in action. The person who gets sick when he's depressed, or tired and lethargic when confused.

There seem to be some generalizations to be made about personality, and stress. Some types of personalities react to stressors with grossly similar patterns and certainly the same person tends to react to different non-specific stressors with the same pattern.

The hypertensive person (one who reacts to stressful situations with high diastolic blood pressure) is usually meek, over-conscientious, frequently unable to act because caught between self-doubt and self-assertion.

The executive who has responsibility for decisions over the lives of other people, under constant pressure to control in frequently competitive environment, is likely to get ulcers of the stomach.

The person who is highly ambitious, self-disciplined, over-working and restrained in aggressive outbursts is likely to develop a bad heart.

The person who doesn't suffer from chronic malfunctioning due to stress seems to be easygoing, affable, not overly ambitious, satisfied, quick to anger and to cool.

When a person doesn't want to face things in a situation, he may become lethargic and sleep a whole lot.

Families tend to have similar adaptation patterns. Work has been done, especially on twins, to show that a specific reaction to stressful situations is common to both parties.

The person who has developed bowel problems is characteristically outwardly calm, superficially peaceful person of more than usual dependence. But underneath may lie unexpressed resentment, hostility and guilt.

Tense, dissatisfied, resentful people may complain of headaches, backaches because of muscle tension caused by their heads.

Severe and recurring headaches seem coupled with anger and striving.

Any of these patterns and more not mentioned may not be chronic and therefore may not produce organic disorder; they are also used situationally by healthy people who do not repeat them again and again.

One pattern may predominate for a long time only to be wiped out by another reactive stress pattern to a new and more powerful stressor. Jewish businessmen, in a German concentration camp, lost their ulcers in a situation of deprivation in which they had no control. When they returned to take up their pre-war lives, after the war was over, peptic ulcers resumed in many.

Stressors can have a cumulative affect. Like I could badly burn my hand, over-tire myself, and when meeting with hostility from a close friend, might react with a severe headache, succumb to a cold, and get an infection in the burned hand.

There are times when whole populations seem more susceptible to disease when the stress-producing factors are a common cultural experience. The American Indians on reservations died in large numbers from smallpox, malnutrition, alcoholism, and TB. Still are, for that matter. Because of persecution, isolation, poverty and uprootedness. The Irish migration showed a much higher incidence of TB in Irish migrant populations in the U.S. as compared to those who stayed in Ireland. Economically, the populations were comparable, and the American-Irish retained much of their cultural integrity in their new environment.

APPLICATION

The stress studies can be important on many levels.

Simple nursing techniques require a treatment of the stress component of disease in healing the disease. This means dispensing affection, consideration, and support to the sick person.

In communal living situations, I have frequently observed the cutting off of a sick person, refusal to recognize illness when it exists, as we are a people who have been brought up with relatively little illness in our antiseptic, isolated family homes where the doctor was frequently called to dispense wonder drugs. Thus, we've tended to develop distrust of illness, impatience with sick people, especially the chronically ill person or the "psychosomatic." It is then extremely important in our directions to include awareness and acceptance of illness and disease, and the ability to give the needed emotional and intellectual support to the patient—doing these things both to bolster the ill person's strength and to *not* add another stressor, that of your anger and impatience, to the disease pattern.

In so many ways group living situations add to the weight of stressors acting on us:
- a) contagion is increased when we have close physical and psychological contact with numbers of people in and out of our lives
- b) sanitation is more difficult when large numbers of people have poor health consciousness and a blithe unconcern with and even resistance to cleanliness as it relates to sanitation
- c) poverty makes it difficult to keep sewage systems working properly, and makes it hard to get needed medical attention
- d) group living may produce an emotional environment that is frequently chaotic and questioning
- e) the whole group-living environment may be so stimulating that getting enough rest is difficult
- f) overcrowded living conditions, which sometimes means not enough space for quiet and isolation, may have an important effect on our health. Certainly studies on animals have shown that crowding produces unhealthy effects in individual animals.

Since we are unlikely to give up our group living conditions, we must do the best we can to reduce the stressors, as collectives and as families. Mostly this requires heightened consciousness of illness and living situations and learning to channel energy in good ways to meet the discovered needs.

The medical profession has worked on approaches to stressor alleviation. Nursing schools now include large units on stress and how to work with it at the nursing level. There is beginning to be emphasis on the whole human in medical schooling, and an ending to the separation of mind and body.

Psychiatry and psychology have long recognized the whole person as their emphasis. But they can usually deal with that person only in *isolation* and cannot reach that person's environment much at all.

And today that environment is increasingly difficult and hard for any one or isolated few of us to reach in U.S.A. 1972

    a) with no FAMILY unit of any strength so leading to isolation and loneliness.

    b) as citizens of the U.S. which is currently killing thousands of people each day in Vietnam, supporting oppressive governments all over the world, and using the giant's share of the world's materials. This must produce isolation, alienation, frustration, and maybe guilt.

    c) coupled with growing awareness of the ECOLOGICAL disaster looming not so far ahead.

    d) all aggravated by extended MEDIA coverage so that all the world is condensed into our awareness and we share the disasters of the whole planet.

Maintaining our health when we're conscious and conscientious human beings is going to get harder and harder in light of the above. Recognition of stress and the responsibility we each carry for our own health and the health of those around us is a matter of life and death.

Barbara McIntosh

NOTES

MENTAL HEALTH CLINICS IN VERMONT

If you are black and your car happens to break down around 11 P.M. near one of the more racially prejudiced fraternal organizations in Vermont, you may be in for a little stress.

If you happen to have a visit from the Neighborhood Improvement Association, who go on a bill-mounting inspection of your home and present you with a list of violations that need to be erased through your expenditures of X dollars, you may wonder what actual legal steps they would take if you ignored them.

If you have ever watched legislators react to a gallery-full of long hairs draping a flag over the rail, you realize that paranoia goes beyond the walls of Waterbury, that the legislator shooting out the rear door of the state house to avoid the protestor is avoiding reality as neatly as the alleged mentally ill person at the state hospital.

There are eleven community mental health centers in Vermont, plus the state hospital in Waterbury, and the Brandon Training School for the retarded. Together they form the mental health system in Vermont, a system that is good for the standard stuff—therapy, counseling, aftercare for ex-patients from Waterbury, and some drug rehabilitation. They are heavy on crisis intervention, which means if you're anything less than suicidal, you may have to wait a week or three to be seen. They consult with schools and parole officers, provide activity programs for retarded people and offer the sorts of service that they can be reimbursed for through federal programs, or that are stipulated in grant awards. There are no unorthodox strategies for mental health care under these funding guidelines.

But mental health exceeds therapeutic intervention, psychoanalytic approaches, or pseudo-shrink talk, or federal "solution" guidelines.

People are paranoid today because of the put-down strategies of society, because they are conscious of being manipulated for the system's benefit, and there doesn't seem to be a thing they can do about it. Perhaps mental health should be re-interpreted today to teach man survival strategies, instead of telling him that it's all in his head. And survival techniques are not delivered in mental health services now.

Instead of letting a system examine you, and find you wanting, examine it and start screaming. That's a beginning.

Karen McCarthy

COMMUNITY MENTAL HEALTH SERVICES IN VERMONT

Address	Phone number (area code 802)
United Counseling Service Dewey Street Bennington, Vermont 05201	442–5429
Windham County Mental Health Service, Inc. 67 Main Street Brattleboro, Vermont 05301	254–6028
Rutland Mental Health Service Box 222 Rutland, Vermont 05701	775–2381
Windsor County Mental Health Service P.O. Box 6 Springfield, Vermont 05156 also 32 Pleasant Street Woodstock, Vermont 05091	885–2766 885–2719 457–1208
Counseling Service of Addison County Municipal Building Middlebury, Vermont 05753	388–7641
Howard Mental Health Service 260 College Street Burlington, Vermont 05401	862–6514 862–1714
Washington County Mental Health Service 100 E. State Street Montpelier, Vermont 05602	223–6277 223–6303
Franklin–N. Grand Isle M.H. Service, Inc. 8 Ferris Street St. Albans, Vermont 05478	524–6554
Northeast Kingdom Mental Health Service 90 Main Street Newport, Vermont 05855 also 28 Pearl Street St. Johnsbury, Vermont 05819	334–7951 748–2346

MENTAL HEALTH CLINICS IN VERMONT

Address	Phone number (area code 802)
Lamoille County Mental Health Service Copley Hospital Morrisville, Vermont 05661	888–4635
Orange County Mental Health Service 5 Maple Street Randolph, Vermont 05060	728–3230 728–9011
also Bradford, Vermont 05033	222–4477
also Wells River, Vermont 05081	757–2197

Rev. 6/19/72

NOTES

PSYCHOLOGICAL PROBLEMS

Psychological problems involve the relationship of a person with some important other person. This "other person" is not necessarily present or alive, and may even be imaginary. In general, our society reacts to psychological problems by ignoring them, or, when they become too blatant, punishing them. This is not the most effective way to approach the problem. The approach of most communes to psychological problems is to deal with these problems in a non-assertive, accepting manner. This method is more likely to be beneficial, but it is not always effective, and may occasionally be harmful to the individual or community involved. A common approach to the treatment of persons behaving in ways harmful to themselves or others is based on the thought that such behavior results from societal problems. Left alone for a long enough period of time, treated with kindness, love and respect, these people will give up their "symptoms" and again become part of the community of man. Even if we accept the first assumption—that is, that destructive behavior is a function of society rather than of the individual—we must carefully consider our approach to treatment.

In general, persons in psychological distress are people with relatively poor reality judgment or perception. The inner turmoil which they are experiencing causes them to behave in certain ways which are probably most comfortable for them but which, at the same time, are generally found to be inappropriate to the situation they are responding to and to the people they must live with. Thus the community is probably more quickly aware of the difficulties someone is experiencing than he, himself, is. To ignore these difficulties is to do both the person and the community a great disservice.

People generally have the need to belong, to feel that they are important to someone else. One of the major premises underlying the idea of "psychological first aid" is that this feeling of belonging or esteem can be generated in the relationship of one person with another where troubles and feelings can be talked out. If a community is working under the model that everyone should be allowed to "do his own thing," this may prevent meaningful communication between people for fear of imposing or interfering. When this happens, first-line psychological aid within the community is almost impossible.

Should attempts to allow the expression of internal turmoil appear to fail, then the response must be to turn outward for assistance. No one person can be an expert on everything, and when you are dealing with the life and health of another individual for whom you claim some feeling, it is important to get assistance as soon as possible.

Just as individuals may be victimized and made to suffer by the destructive behavior of another individual, so communities may be harmed by the destructive behavior of another person. Such people may take advantage of a community given the opportunity to do so. When the community's response is to say, "We will turn the other cheek," then the community is explicity

PSYCHOLOGICAL PROBLEMS

denying its own responsibility to help to teach the destructive individual the logical consequences of his own behavior. This is what growth is really all about. If the community refuses to point out to the individual the effect of his behavior and to respond to this behavior, the community may be destroyed as an effective working and living unit by the behavior of only one person. There must be some rules to existence, and it is up to each community to make them explicit.

A final, and important, problem faced in many communities is the problem of suicide. There are times when a person may feel that his existence has become so painful and unrewarding that the only answer is suicide. This is not generally something that is arrived at as a logical response to a difficult situation. It generally occurs in one of three situations. The first situation is that of the child who is saying "after I'm gone they will be sorry that they treated me this way." This approach is characteristic of a person who feels that he is not appreciated and whose feelings of esteem for self are quite low. People in this situation who attempt suicide often feel that after death they will be able to look down upon the sorrowing people who did not appreciate them in their own life.

The second general group of people who attempt suicide tend to be highly impulsive and, if they do succeed in taking their own lives, it is more of a tragic accident than anything else. Finally, there is a third group of people, though it be small, whose choice of suicide as a termination to existence is a logical solution based upon the problem they are confronted with. Such people generally take great care to set their affairs in order and are generally quite successful in their attempt upon their own lives.

We generally grow suspicious and concerned about a person's designs upon himself in the presence of certain personality changes, disastrous emotional situations, etc. This is especially true when we know that the person we are dealing with has always been impulsive and tended to act before thinking out any of the consequences of his own behavior. At this point the answer is to get help. While the feeling that I alone saved someone else's life is a warm and good one, nothing will be lost by sharing that feeling with a number of other people. Never hesitate in situations such as these to ask the opinion of somebody else. A potential suicide presents you with a "one time only" situation. You cannot afford to guess incorrectly.

Some of the things to do if you are afraid that someone may be thinking of suicide are the following:

1. Ask them if they are thinking of hurting themselves. Most people will tell you if they have considered suicide.
2. If they have thought of harming themselves, ask them how they planned to do this. If they have made definite plans, you should be even more concerned about the possibility of suicide.
3. If they or any member of their family have made previous suicide attempts, you should be more concerned about the possibility of suicide.
4. If you are concerned about the possibility of suicide, attempt to keep someone with them as much as possible.
5. Never hesitate to ask for outside help if you are concerned that someone may try to commit suicide.

Steve Goldstein

NOTES

WOMEN'S HEALTH

ANATOMY

The purpose of this section is to explain the anatomy of our reproductive organs so that as women we can have an understanding and control over our bodies. It is important to become familiar with our anatomy in order to understand our menstrual cycle, pregnancy, birth control, and gynecological problems.

Use the diagram while we explain the different parts. Externally the *vulva* is the collective name for the female sexual parts. The two outer lips of the vagina are called *labia majora*. These protect the more delicate inner structures. The *labia minora* are seen when the labia majora are separated. The labia minora extend from the *clitoris* back to the sides of the vaginal opening. One part passes above the clitoris to meet the lip on the other side, forming the *clitoral hood*. The other part passes beneath the clitoris and attaches to its undersurface forming the base of the clitoris. To best understand get a mirror out and examine yourself. The clitoris itself is the primary organ of sexual excitment in the female. It has functions of erection and orgasm. Erection occurs when blood flows into the hollow areas of the organ causing it to stiffen. The clitoris is composed of a shaft and *glans clitoridis,* which is the tip of the clitoris. The shaft is hidden under the hood (formed by the labia minora), but the glans protrudes. If you are not sure of the location of your clitoris, feel your outer genitals until you hit upon the most sensitive spot. This will more than likely be the clitoris. The clitoris is richly supplied with nerves.

The area between the minor lips and behind the glans clitoridis is called the *vestibule*. This contains the urinary orifice (urethra) and vaginal opening. The urinary opening is just between the clitoris and vagina. The vaginal opening is beneath the urinary opening. Located around the vaginal opening are two glands (Bartholin's glands). Each opens by means of a duct; they secrete a mucus which contributes very little to lubrication during sexual excitement.

The *hymen* is a thin fold of membrane situated at the vaginal opening, usually seen in a virgin. When this membrane is torn, often people say "virginity has been lost." This is not always true; a tampax can be inserted while the membrane is still intact and menstrual fluid is shed through the opening. The hymen may be entirely absent even in a virgin and when present may assume many shapes and degrees of thickness.

We will now briefly describe the internal female organs. See the section on physiology to understand how these organs function.

The *vagina* leads through the *cervix* to the *uterus* which is a heavily muscled organ, about the size of your fist, where a child may develop. When a woman isn't pregnant she sheds the uterine lining once a month during her menstrual period. On either side of the uterus is an *ovary*.

164   THE HOME HEALTH HANDBOOK

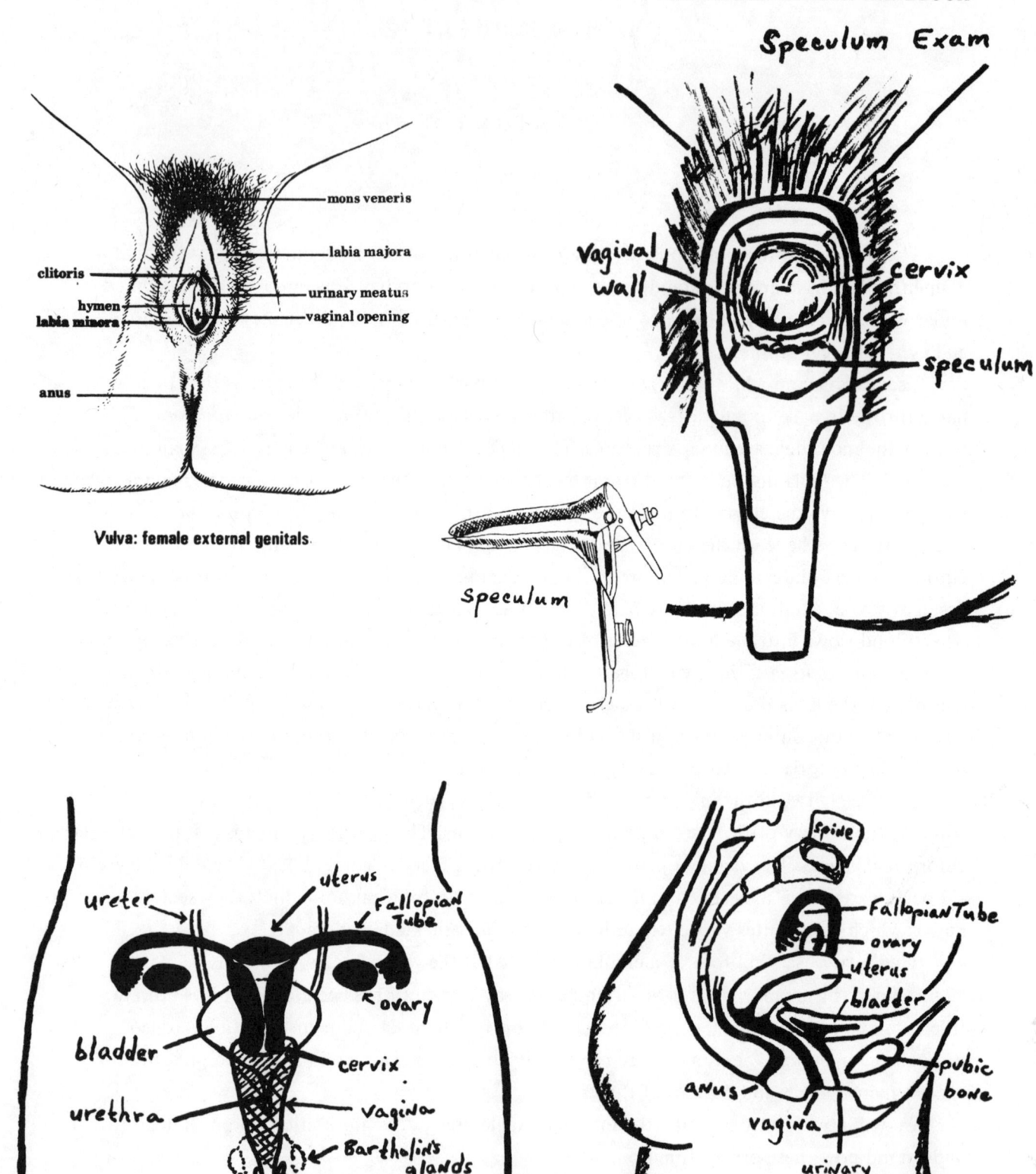

Vulva: female external genitals.

Speculum Exam

speculum

Female Pelvic Organs

An ovary is about the size and shape of an unshelled almond. Ovaries produce the ovarian follicle which produces the ovum or egg. Ovulation is the process of releasing eggs from our ovaries. The *fallopian* tubes extend toward the side of the ovaries from the uterus. When ovulation occurs, the egg travels down a fallopian tube to the uterus. A good reference is *Our Bodies—Our Selves* by Boston Women's Health Course Collective.

EXAMINATION OF A WOMAN'S ORGANS

PELVIC EXAMS. Most pelvic exams are done by doctors. But more and more of us are learning about our bodies and about how to do pelvics on ourselves and each other. With mirrors, plastic speculums and diagrams, we can examine ourselves.

The following is a description of a pelvic exam. The exam is more comfortable if you urinate first. You lie on the examining table with your feet in the stirrups. It's important to try to relax so that the examination is more comfortable.

Examination of outer genitals. The examiner should look at the vulva and anus checking for signs of infections (such as inflammation, swelling, or sores) and for infected glands and for growths (such as warts, cysts, tumors, or polyps) and also for signs of damage.

Speculum exam. The speculum is an instrument that holds the wall of the vagina open so the examiner can see the walls of the vagina and the cervix. She or he looks at the color of the mucous membrane lining the vagina and to see whether there's a discharge, signs of infection, damage or growths. At this point the examiner may perform some tests: a pap test for cancer of the cervix and uterus, tests for infection, and tests for gonorrhea. These are described later in the article.

Bimanual exam. The examiner places two fingers against the cervix and with the other hand feels the top of the uterus through the abdomen wall. She or he notes the size of the uterus, whether it's soft and whether it can move easily and if there are any obvious lumps or pain. Then the examiner feels the ovaries and tubes, checking for signs of lumps or infection and inflammation.

BREAST EXAMS. More than one-fifth of cancer in adult women is cancer of the breast and in most cases it can be cured if its treated early. You should examine your breasts every month, about one week after each menstrual period. Be sure to continue these checkups after menopause. The chances of getting breast cancer increase if you are over thirty.

There are slightly different methods of examination you might have learned. The important thing is to learn one and to become familiar with your own breasts—so that any changes can be noted.

If you find a lump or thickening, leave it alone until you go to a clinic or doctor. Don't be frightened. Most breast lumps or changes are not cancer, but they should be checked.

BREAST SELF-EXAMINATION

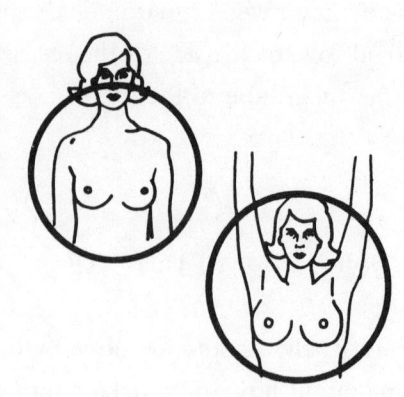

1

Sit or stand in front of your mirror, arms relaxed at your sides, and look for any changes in size, shape and contour. Also look for puckering or dimpling of the skin and changes on the surface of the nipples. Gently press each nipple to see if any discharge occurs.

2

Raise both arms over your head, and look for exactly the same things. Note differences since you last examined your breasts.

3

From here on you will be trying to find a lump or thickening. Lie down on your bed, put a pillow or a bath towel under your left shoulder, and your left hand under your head. With the fingers of your right hand held together flat, press gently against the breast with small circular motions to feel the inner, upper portion of your left breast, starting at your breastbone and going outward toward the nipple line. Also feel the area around the nipple.

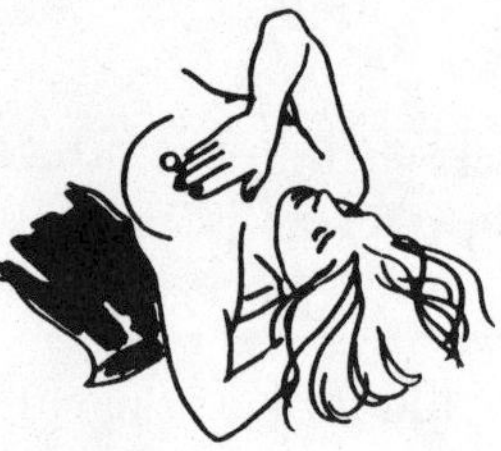

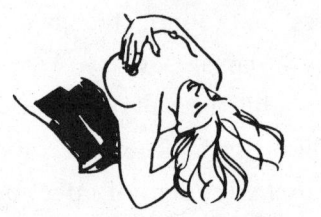

4

With the same gentle pressure, feel the low inner part of your breast. Incidentally, in this area you will feel a ridge of firm tissue. Don't be alarmed. This is normal.

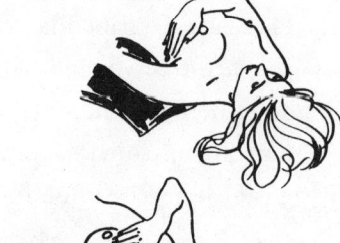

5

Now bring your left arm down to your side and, still using the flat part of the fingers of your right hand, feel under your left armpit.

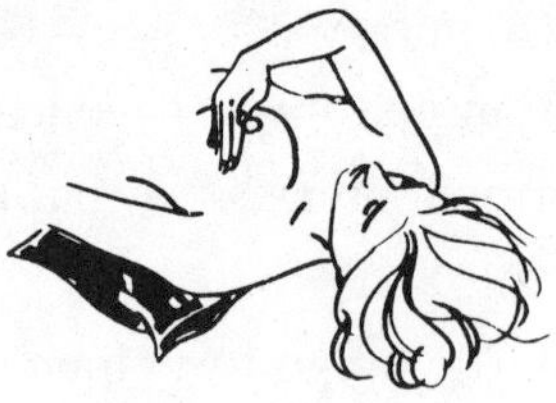

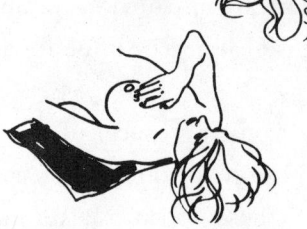

6

Use the same gentle pressure to feel the upper, outer portion of your left breast from the nipple line to where your arm is resting.

7

And finally, feel the lower outer portion of your breast, going from the outer part to the nipple.

8

Repeat the entire procedure, as described, on the right breast using the left hand for the examination.

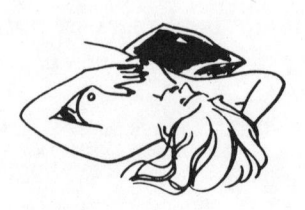

COMMON PROBLEMS OF WOMEN'S ORGANS

Normal condition of the vagina. In all women, glands in the cervix and the membranes that line the vagina secrete moisture and mucus. This discharge is transparent or slightly milky and may be somewhat slimy. When dry it may look yellow. This secretion increases in a woman who is sexually aroused. It is a normal discharge and causes no irritation or inflammation of the vagina or vulva. The cells of the cervix and vagina and the discharge are affected by the female sex hormones, estrogen and progesterone, which are involved in the menstrual cycle. Therefore the amount and consistency of a woman's discharge may vary during her menstrual cycle and may also depend on a woman's personal hormone balance.

Every woman normally has many different types of bacteria inside her vagina. These help keep the vagina acid and keep down some harmful germs. Constant douching or the use of vaginal sprays and deodorants can destroy these bacteria and upset the natural balance in your vagina, leaving it open to infection.

VAGINAL INFECTIONS. These infections are usually marked by soreness, irritation, or itching accompanied by a discharge that's different from normal.

Yeast infections (also called *monilia* or *candida*). The discharge is white and usually curdy, though sometimes thin. It causes intense itching, inflammation, and sometimes chafing and soreness of the vulva. White patches may be seen on the vaginal or cervical mucous membrane.

Factors that favor the growth of yeast are abnormal pH of the vagina and an abundance of glycogen (sugar). So yeast infections are more prevalent in pregnancy, just before menstruation, in diabetes, and when a woman is taking birth-control pills. Antibiotics, too, make yeast infection more likely by cutting down the bacterial competition, allowing the yeast in the vagina to flourish.

Diagnosis can be made by seeing the threads or spores of the yeast under a microscope.

Treatment can be on several levels. Yogurt douche increases the bacterial population, which should help restore the bacterial-yeast balance. Eating yogurt returns important bacteria to the intestines after antibiotics. Vinegar and water douche makes the vagina more acid and helps relieve symptoms. Mycostatin prescribed for 10 days can clear up the infection (Mycostatin is usually used as a vaginal suppository, and sometimes is taken orally in tablet form).

Trichomoniasis. This is an infection by a protozoan. As with yeast, a woman may be very uncomfortable or she may harbor the organism and have no symptoms. The discharge is usually greenish-yellow and is foamy or slimy. There are often small red spots on the cervix and vaginal walls. Often the vulva is red and tender and burns.

Below-normal acidity of the vagina from cervical mucus or menstrual blood; estrogens; and bacterial flora predispose a woman to infections by trichomonis. Symptoms worsen just before, during, and right after menstruation.

Diagnosis is made by a microscopic demonstration of the trichomonads in a wet mount of the vaginal discharge with a drop of normal saline solution.

Treatment is usually a prescription of Flagyl tablets: 250 mg. by mouth 3 times a day for 10 days. When taking this drug, you shouldn't drink alcohol because it can lead to nausea and vomiting. Douching with vinegar may give relief from the symptoms. Use 1 tablespoon of vinegar per quart of water. Sometimes a woman is reinfected by her sexual partner. If this is the case, he should also be treated.

Non-specific vaginitis. A vaginal discharge with vaginal irritation and inflammation may be nonspecific vaginitis if trich and yeast are excluded. Most of these cases are due to Hemophilus vaginalis, a particular type of bacteria. The discharge is grayish white and smelly. Other cases are due to a mixture of organisms including normal flora plus various strains of bacteria (strep, staph, or colon bacillus). Diagnosis is made by gram stain. Treatment for non-specific vaginitis is usually a sulfa drug, Triple Sulfa cream or AVC cream.

Prevention. There are a couple of things you can do to help prevent vaginal infection. Wiping yourself from front to back keeps bacteria from the anus from being spread to the vagina and urinary opening. Wearing cotton underpants is helpful in absorbing moisture and cutting down irritation.

CERVICAL EROSION. This is a term for a red and raw-looking cervix. Sometimes it is caused by a vaginal or cervical infection and it clears up when the infection does. The cervix of a woman taking birth-control pills sometimes looks eroded because the pills can make the uterine lining grow out over part of the cervix. When the woman stops taking pills, this goes away. Sometimes a woman has chronic cervical erosion with no known reason. If it causes no pain or soreness or bleeding, there is no reason to do anything except get it checked every six months so a pap test can be done and the cervix looked at. If a woman has erosion with tenderness or bleeding or other complications, she is often advised to have her cervix cauterized. This is a simple process in which the surface of the cervix is electrically burned. It is done to make the cervix less sensitive which cuts down on the irritation and inflammation.

VENEREAL DISEASE. (See the article on VD for symptoms, diagnosis, and treatment.)

Gonorrhea is an especially serious problem for women. Since most of us experience very slight or no symptoms at first, we don't know that we have it (unless someone who we've had sexual contact with tells us). If we don't know, we don't get treated. In its later stages, gonorrhea infects the inner pelvic lining of the fallopian tubes often causing pregnancy complications or sterility.

It is extremely important for her own health that every woman who has had sexual relations be routinely tested for gonorrhea by means of a pelvic exam and cervical and anal cultures.

A routine blood test for syphilis should be done too.

CANCER. Cancer is a scary idea for many of us. It's important to realize that there are simple, routine tests that can be done to see if we are developing cancer. Most cancer discovered and treated early enough can be cured.

A discussion of breast cancer and *self-examination* of breasts appears earlier in this article.

A *pap test* is a test for detection of cancer of the cervix or uterus. It can be easily and painlessly done during a pelvic exam. Using a Q-tip or wooden spatula, the examiner removes some of the cells from the cervix and vaginal wall. These are sent to a lab and studied to see if there are any signs of cancer developing. There are some differences of opinion as to how often a woman should have a pap test. Most people agree that a woman over 30 be tested once a year. Women 20–30 need one less often: once a year to once every 2 or 3 years. If she is taking birth-control pills, a woman should get a pap test every 6 months to once a year.

Chris Allen
Ginny Lyman

NOTES

PHYSIOLOGY

The effects of hormones on women are great. There is a great need to understand their function and how they effect women. In order to truly understand birth control, especially the birth control pill, this is true. This section will concern itself with the explanation of hormonal effects on the ovaries, uterus and cervix.

The hormones that effect the menstrual cycle originate from the ovaries and the pituitary gland. The pituitary sends a hormone FSH (follicle-stimulating hormone) that stimulates the ovaries to produce follicles and therefore estrogen.

Follicles are usually called the egg when female physiology is talked about. Actually the growth of the follicles produces the egg. This occurs as the follicle responds to the pituitary hormones, such as FSH, as mentioned above. These hormones cause the follicle to release estrogen into the blood stream until the egg is released. At this point the follicle begins to form the corpus luteum which produces and releases estrogen and progesterone. At the end of each menstrual cycle, the corpus luteum (once the follicle) degenerates and the production of estrogen and progesterone stops. This decline stimulates the pituitary gland and the cycle begins again. To help you understand this better I will explain how the pituitary hormones affect the follicle.

As the estrogen level rises it causes a decrease in the FSH. As the estrogen level continues to rise it also causes the pituitary to secrete two other hormones: LH (Luteinizing hormones) and LTH (Luteotrophic hormones). LH is responsible for ovulation and LTH is necessary for a layer of the follicle which produces progesterone. Progesterone leads to the decrease of LH and LTH. When these levels decrease this leads to estrogen and progesterone decline and a decline of follicle. Estrogen decline leads to an FSH rise and therefore a new cycle begins.

During this time the hormones have been effecting change in the uterus. Estrogen causes the uterine lining to grow, thicken, and secrete hormones which would nourish an embryo. It also maintains the lining. Progesterone is the hormone that makes the uterus expel the nourishing lining. During this time, when the egg is being ovulated and is moving from the fallopian tubes to the uterus, the hormones are changing, i.e., progesterone is preparing the lining of the uterus for the implant of the fertilized egg.

The hormones also affect the cervix. The cervical mucus changes characteristics because of each hormone. Estrogen causes the mucus to become thinner and wetter and progesterone causes it to become thicker and dryer. There also appears to be a sharp peak in calcium and sodium concentrations at the time of ovulation, which is apparently very beneficial to the sperm as it seeks union with the egg.

Therefore menstruation is really a result of hormonal withdrawal. Because of this withdrawal the uterine lining cannot be maintained and it is shed.

Menopause begins when a woman runs out of follicles that will ripen, with a resulting estrogen deficiency. The symptoms are caused when FSH goes to very high levels because of no controlling hormones. Symptoms often include irregular monthly flow, hot flushes, dizziness, weakness, nervousness, and insommia, and the eventual cessation of menstruation. The menopause is not a complete change of life as some authorities would have us believe. The normal sex desire remains, and often women enjoy better health than they have for years.

INFERTILITY. Often this subject is left uncovered in this day of population control. Actually this is a very real problem to women—a problem which is often hard to handle emotionally because of intense training to place value on ourselves only as mothers and procreators. Women are also subjected to constant questioning as to when they will have children and why they aren't pregnant. This constant social pressure manages to make this medical problem a very overwhelming problem object in women's lives.

First of all, both men and women should be examined, since the problem could arise in either person. The man should be examined first, since tests for the woman are more expensive and time consuming.

In the woman, the organs of reproduction and the glands must be evaluated to find the problem. There are many factors which might cause infertility; among these are endocrine disorders, congenital anomalies (bummers you're born with), gynecologic infections, psychic factors, or general physical condition.

Diagnosis can be made by several basic tests. The *Huhner test* gives an estimation of the number of sperm alive and their ability to survive in the vagina several hours after intercourse. A *Rubin test* is essential to determine whether the fallopian tubes are open: this is done by introducing carbon dioxide through a tube into the uterus and the fallopian tubes, then measuring the resulting pressure in the uterus and other parts of the body. A *basal body temperature test* is also quite helpful to determine frequency and time of ovulation. (Refer to Birth Control section for further explanation)

If no problem is found in the female after these tests, quite often the male may have more intensive testing done. The treatment of infertility is a difficult matter because it may involve a number of and any combination of different factors. Each woman must decide how long and expensive testing procedures she wishes to endure, in order to find the problem. There seems to be a lack of treatment which will "cure" infertility. Often social, psychological, and general health are to blame. If this is the case, remedies can be found in examining feelings of sexuality and social roles which often make a person feel uptight about life.

—Ginny Lyman

NOTES

A WOMAN'S EXPERIENCE OF PREGNANCY AND CHILDBIRTH

This is a time to know yourself like never before. Think about why you are pregnant, why you want a child, what this means to you as a free being. Think about how you feel. Next, learn everything you can learn about your body. How pregnancy will affect it; how to help yourself through pregnancy; how to pick your medical care; how you want to experience labor and delivery; and if you want to breast feed. Read everything you can get your hands on. Here is a list of things to start with (all in paperback—see pp. 179-180 for authors and publishers of these and other works):

> Our Bodies—Our Selves
> Commonsense Childbirth
> Childbirth Without Fear
> Awake & Aware

Talk to other women about being pregnant. Share your feelings—you will soon find out that they are normal and shared. Most of all, remember who you are. Keep your own life going and active. You have your own life, as the baby will have its own life.

First off is the process of detecting pregnancy. This usually means seeing a doctor. He or she will ask for a urine specimen, which should be collected in the morning, and kept cool until the test can be done. This test checks the urine for a hormone which is secreted when a woman is more than 40 days pregnant. This means a woman must be 10 days over her last missed menstrual period, for the test to be accurate.

The doctor may do a pelvic examination. The following things will be checked for, indicating pregnancy:

> 1) Feel if the tip of cervix has softened.
> 2) Cervix will have changed color from pale pink to a blush red.
> 3) Uterus will feel softer.
> 4) The shape of uterus will change by having a bulge where the embryo is attached to the wall of the uterus.

Next you should find a doctor to do prenatal care and deliver you. This is a very important step. Find someone you can talk to easily, figure out if you want educated childbirth (natural), if you want to have a home delivery, or pick the hospital that best fits your needs—and remember, cost and philosophy are both important!

Now start your hunt for a doctor. Know what you want before you start. If having the baby in a hospital, find out the list of doctors who deliver there. You may want to consider location; remember, you will see the doctor once a month until seventh month, then twice a month, and every week in the ninth month. Next, phone doctors to find out which ones are enthusiastic about the methods you want. Ask the nurse if the doctor practices family-centered childbirth. If the answer is yes, leave your number. When the doctor is on the phone, explain that you are looking for someone who practices natural childbirth, and you would like to know how he or she feels about family-centered obstetrics. Now listen very carefully and decide if he or she is enthusiastic about this philosophy.

If money is a problem and you can't afford a private doctor, go to a clinic at a hospital. Medical supervision is very important during your pregnancy. Most women are healthy with few problems, but some have problems which could be helped or prevented by seeing a doctor. If you go to a clinic, remember that you have a right to know and understand what is being done to you. Ask questions and demand answers. The doctor may not want to take time with you, but ask your questions anyway. In between visits it is a good idea to make a list of questions you may have or things you are worried about.

Pregnancy is a time of great change in a woman's body. It helps a lot if we know what is happening to cause these changes.

The pregnancy is usually divided into 3 trimesters. First trimester is the first three months, second trimester 4, 5, 6 and third trimester 7, 8, 9 months. I will describe the trimesters and what is going on. There are many books and pamphlets which can give more detail. This will give the basic changes occuring in the uterus; then we can move on to how this affects the mother.

THE FIRST TRIMESTER: THE FETUS

End of four weeks: ¾ inches long—heart pulsating and pumping blood—backbone and spinal canal forming—no eyes, nose, or external ears—digestive system beginning to develop.

End of eight weeks: 1-1/8 inches long—1/30 ounce—face and features forming—eyelids fused—limbs show distinct divisions—unbilical cord formed—tail-like process disappears.

End of twelve weeks: 3 inches long—1 ounce—arms, hands, legs, feet, toes are fully formed—external ears present—nails begin to grow—tooth sockets and buds forming in the jawbones—heartbeat can be detected with special instruments—eyelids close for the first time—sex can be distinguished—small amount of urine is produced—movements may occur but are too weak to be felt by the mother.

THE SECOND TRIMESTER: THE FETUS

End of 16 weeks: 6½ to 7 inches long—4 ounces—strong heart beat—fair digestion—active muscles—skin covered with fine down-like hair—skeleton hardens.

End of 20 weeks: 10 to 12 inches long—½ to 1 pound—hair starts to grow on head—eyelashes and eyebrows begin—heartbeat can be heard externally—movement can be felt—sleeps and wakes like newborn.

End of 24 weeks: 11 to 14 inches long—1¼ to 1½ pounds—fingernails extend to end of fingers—hair on head grows long—fetus can and does suck thumb—umbilical cord reaches maximum length.

THE THIRD TRIMESTER: THE FETUS

End of 28th week: 16 inches long—3 pounds—fetus is "legally viable"—is fatter—has smoother skin.

End of 32nd week: 17 inches long—4½ pounds—resembles a little old man—bones of head are soft and flexible—will gain 2 to 2½ pounds this month. If born now has a better chance of survival than does the 7th-month fetus, although there is a popular fallacy to the contrary.

End of 36th week: 19 inches long—6 pounds—skin coated with creamy coating—fine downy hair disappeared—fingernails protrude beyond ends of the fingers—due to weight gain body is less wrinkled and red.

36 to 40 weeks: 20 inches long—7 to 7½ pounds—full term now reached.

Now we will explain what is happening to you while all this is going on in your uterus.

FIRST TRIMESTER: THE MOTHER

1. No menstrual periods.
2. Nausea, vomiting, "morning sickness"—this is caused by increased acid in the mother's stomach. It can be relieved by eating crackers on first arising in the morning. This absorbs the excess acid.
3. Frequency of urinating—caused by increased pressure on bladder from growing uterus—giving the sensation of being full of urine.
4. Breasts will begin to get larger firmer and more tender. The nipple and areola will begin to get darker in color. The areola, the area around the nipple, will become puffy and will gradually increase in size.
5. Fatigue—mother may feel very tired and drowsy. This will be relieved by lying down each afternoon and relaxing. You may be unable to sleep. This usually only lasts for the first couple of months.

THE SECOND TRIMESTER: THE MOTHER

This time period is usually very good for the mother. Your body has made the necessary adjustments for the pregnancy.

You won't feel as tired as you have been. The frequency of urinating will have stopped because the uterus has grown out of pelvis and doesn't exert pressure on the bladder any longer. The nausea and vomiting will have dissappeared now, with your body adapting to the new state of pregnancy. For the first time you will feel the movements of the baby. They can best be described as like a butterfly. This will occur about the middle of the fourth month. The doctor will usually be able to detect the heart beat at 18–22 weeks if the child is in a position favorable for sending the sound through your abdominal wall. Weight gain may be a problem, but it may help to remember that your greatest weight gains will occur in the fifth and sixth months. This occurs so that you will have the weight for the child to gain in the last three months. Weight gain is often blown out of proportion. The reason doctors are so concerned about too much weight gain is because of the toxemia of pregnancy. This is a condition which only occurs in pregnancy that is accompanied by a rapid weight gain consisting of fluid retention. This means swollen ankles, hands and face. This condition is rare and often this is what concerns the obstetrician about your weight gain. Remember, the important part of weight gain is what you eat. Eat well, try to eat high-protein foods, greens, vegetables, milk and fruits in moderate amounts. Your diet is very important for both you and your baby.

THE THIRD TRIMESTER: THE MOTHER

It is marked by the increase in size. Your body must adapt to the growing baby. Remember to stand up straight, as this will help prevent backaches. Wear good shoes to give your feet support. You may have problems with heartburn during the last months. If you do, don't eat real spicy food, eat slowly, and if you still have problems, try lemon juice and water ½ & ½, about 2 tablespoons of lemon juice.

You may find yourself short of breath during the last weeks of pregnancy. This occurs because of pressure on the lower part of the lung. Cramps in the legs may also occur. These also occur because of pressure by the enlarged uterus on the nerves supplying the lower extremities. These can be avoided to some degree by an exercise done daily. Sit with your legs straight in front of you on the floor. Rotate your feet in circles—go clockwise for 2 minutes, go counter clockwise for 2 minutes.

Swelling of the ankles and lower legs may be a problem. This can be relieved by resting frequently during the day. Elevating the feet or taking the right-angle position against a wall often gives relief.

Vaginal discharge will greatly increase; it should not itch or be yellow in color, or be thick like cottage cheese. If you have any discharge with these symptoms, see your doctor. This may indicate that you have a vaginal infection and it should be treated immediately before your due date is very close.

Frequent urination is also very common in the last weeks. This is caused from pressure on the bladder from the uterus. Don't reduce your water and fluid intake, which should not be less than 6 or 8 glasses a day.

Remember, pregnancy doesn't last forever and if these things get on your nerves, they will be over fairly soon.

While writing this section on pregnancy I have been nine months pregnant myself and battling the various problems involved. I think many things can be said about the basic facts of pregnancy, but the personal exchange is the most important. I have found talking to other women to be most helpful in dealing with the changes in my life while pregnant.

Most facts about pregnancy can be obtained easily or with a little effort. I would now like to give my own reaction to pregnancy with the problems and solutions I have found.

First off, I found problems dealing with people's reaction to my pregnancy. People will either be elated telling the joys of pregnancy and motherhood, or else they have you a complete invalid needing constant help. As women we must know that pregnancy is a normal state of being for us; we are not sick. People may be convinced we are. Often I had to firmly insist on carrying things, and doing certain activities. I found that exercise *every day* was very important. Use your muscles. Take walks, or walk where you need to go. You will feel better. Keep yourself as active as possible. Now, I don't mean running constantly for 12–14 hours; I mean doing the things you like to do, going places, and seeing people. Keep your own personal interests going. You and everyone will be concerned about the baby—getting ready for the child—but remember, the baby isn't *you.* You have your own self to remember. The baby is only sharing your body for a short time; the child isn't taking your life over. I feel this is extremely important to remember while pregnant.

Since you are going to keep busy on your own projects while pregnant, rest will be important.

Start taking a nap, or at least lying down each day. I found an hour before the evening meal was an excellent time. Read, or doze with your feet up. Don't think about anything except yourself during this time. Please try to get into a habit of this. I found it a life saver on many days. It is also important once the baby arrives that you sleep for short periods of time, as I am finding out!

Another thing I think played a large part in my healthy pregnancy and labor was nutrition. Eat three meals a day, drink *lots* of water. Eat as many vegetables and fruits as you can get a hold of. High protein foods are important also. A supplementary vitamin capsule may fill in, if you can't get the foods you need. I know good nutritious foods are expensive.

The next important thing in my pregnancy was my knowledge of what was happening to my body. I read everything I could find on pregnancy, labor and delivery. Start with your doctor. See if he has any pamphlets. Next try your library. Some drug stores carry paperbacks on natural childbirth, which give lots of information. I felt having this information month to month was important because I could read what was happening. Often the change in the child's development had a direct influence on how I felt.

In the last 3 months I would occasionally have heartburn; this is caused by the baby placing pressure on the stomach. I found this out through reading the various pamphlets I had collected. If we know what is happening in our bodies, I feel we are better able to adapt to the changes. From this idea I decided the natural childbirth would be the only way for me to go through labor. Natural childbirth or LaMaze Training I feel is a logical extension of knowing and having control over your body. I got more books on the theories and started with my husband to practice breathing and relaxation. I practiced relaxation everywhere—whenever I felt really tense. I think this is a great way to learn this technique. If you decide to use LaMaze Training in labor, the first thing you should do is find a coach. A coach is a *very* important aspect of the training and success. My husband coached me, but anyone that you can work with is fine. The important thing to remember is that it is a team effort; you must listen carefully to your coach, and your coach must listen carefully to you. Talk about the things which you think will be important to you. For me touch was very important. I wanted him next to me and actually touching me all the time. Each woman has something which will be important for the coach to know. Very close communication is essential for the team work. I felt that this communication was the key factor in making my labor a short, productive and beautiful event. So pick your coach carefully and then put both your energies into a fantastic delivery. Practice very hard. Learn the breathing so that it is an automatic response.

I wanted to have my child at home, but I soon discovered I could not find a doctor to attend the delivery. This is my first child so I decided on having this child in a hospital. Hospitals and LaMaze Training don't mix too well in this country. Hospitals are for sick people. We know we are not sick, but the hospital doesn't.

I found several ways to deal with the hospital. First of all remember *you* are having the baby, and you are in control of yourself and nothing is going to interfere with that. Next, try to ignore the bullshit that people may give, such as calling contractions pains, or riding in the wheelchair even though you can walk. Don't listen and get upset, only concern yourself with your breathing. Try to get your doctor not to order an enema and a prep, but if he does, explain your breathing to the nurse. Explain that she should stop while you are breathing with a contraction. Insist firmly and do your breathing. The word will spread quickly that a natural childbirth labor is happening. A number of nurses may stream in and out to watch. Again either ignore this or have your coach assure the nurses that if you need anything he/she will let them know.

Now settle down and have your coach get things organized for the later stages. I found a radio very comforting during labor; it made the labor room more friendly. Also remember to go to the bathroom every couple of hours. Finally the time will come for you to go to the delivery room. Don't panic—stay relaxed. Your coach will have to put on a gown, cap, and mask, but don't worry; the coach is still there—just slightly hidden. I panicked slightly when wheeled into the delivery room. The change of environment really affects you at this point, but keep cool. I concentrated very hard on my husband, using his face as a focus point. Which reminds me. I found a focus point very important through the entire labor—it gives a sense of reality to the situation.

When you are transferred to the delivery table, get the table up so that you are at an angle. Don't forget to ask for the mirror if you want to watch. I saw some, but I was very busy pushing and missed the actual delivery of the baby. I was getting discouraged and found having the mirror very encouraging. I could see the baby's head move down my vagina with each of my pushes. This was very exciting to realize your "labor" was really producing something.

Another important thing to know is that labor is hard work. That may sound very obvious, but often women are not prepared for this fact. Because it is hard work you may completely lose your concern over your surroundings. By this I mean you will be aware of your surroundings, but be only concerned about yourself. The hard work will cause you to grunt, hoot, and maybe give a whoop once in awhile. Don't worry, this is to be expected. Don't get uptight about it. Hard work always causes the human being to make noises.

Now, before you know it, your child is ready to be born. The doc gives the o.k. to push the head through and then the body. Now you hear the scream, and quickly you see the baby, lying there on your abdomen! A real baby—I really can't describe in words the emotions you will feel at this point. There are so many and they are so intense. My heart still quickens while I write this, remembering those emotions.

The baby will be bundled up and taken away to the other side of the room to be suctioned (removal of mucus) and to have ointment put in his eyes to prevent infection. The baby will be brought over to you after your episiotomy is finished. At this point you want to try to breast feed. This was my immediate reaction. This violates routine, but I recommend just doing it if you desire. Take the doctor and nurses by surprise. This usually works.

You will now be transferred back into a bed and wheeled either to a "recovery" room or to your own room. I recommend getting out of bed as soon as you want to. I was up in about 2 hours to the bathroom—taking it slowly, though. The more I moved around, the better I felt. If you must stay in the hospital for several days, take something to read. Plan each day—like when you are going to take a shower. It makes the time go faster. Next, if you are breast feeding, try to ignore the nurses if they hassle you. Again remember, once you are home, you and your baby can work out any problems. Nurses may make you feel ignorant and awkward with your baby. Again remember, motherhood is *learned*—it is not a natural inborn knowledge. Motherhood is an art in the truest sense of the word; it takes lots of time and patience to master it.

You will survive the hospital and go home. Home will really look great to you. At the same time you will now be confronted with the responsibility of this new little being. First, remember to get as much sleep as you can. At first this may mean sleeping every time the baby does. Next, remember your nutrition—please eat well. This is so important in helping your body adjust to the abrupt change and the awkward hours which you will be keeping.

Each day may bring a new problem to solve. Relax, you will find the solution. It may take some time, but remember you are learning. Feel free to call the pediatrician and ask questions. Call friends and talk to other women about how you feel. I have found this an immense help. Taking care of a baby is a big responsibility and adjusting one's life style can be very trying. It helps if you can express how you feel and realize other women have the same feelings and thoroughly understand.

The choice to have children in this society is a big decision. To become pregnant, deliver the baby, and raise it in a healthy manner is an act of revolution in this society.

This act of revolution occurs when we *demand* to know what is happening to our bodies and our children. Because with this knowledge we have control over our lives. Our decision and our ability to control having children in a healthy, human way is a commitment to the problems of women and children because we must now deal with those problems in a very real way. Women must share those problems together because only as a strong collective group can we change the process which women are subjected to during pregnancy, childbirth and child rearing.

BIBLIOGRAPHY

Our Bodies Our Selves. Boston Women's Health Course Collective. New England Free Press, 791 Tremont Street, Boston, Mass. 02118. April, 1971.

Birth Control Handbook. Students Society of McGill University, 3480 McTavish Street, Montreal. 1969.

Maternity Nursing. E. Fitzpatrick, N. Eastman, S. Reeder. J. B. Lippincott Company, Philadelphia, Toronto. 1966, Eleventh edition.

Pregnancy (pamphlet). Carnation Company, Medical Dept., 5045 Wilshire Boulevard, Los Angeles, California 90036. 1969.

Structure and Function in Man. S. Jacob, C. Francone. W. B. Saunders Company, Philadelphia. 1968.

Six Practical Lessons for an Easier Childbirth. Elisabeth Bing. Bantam Books, 51 Madison Avenue,

New York. June, 1969.

Commonsense Childbirth. Lester Hazell. Tower Publications, 185 Madison Avenue, New York, New York 10016.

Awake and Aware. Irwin Chabon. Dell Publishing Co., 750 Third Avenue, New York, New York 10017. Dec., 1970.

Childbirth Without Fear. Grantly Dick - Read. Har/Row Books, Harper and Row Publishers, 49 East 33rd Street, New York, New York 10016. 1970.

Having a Right-On Baby (pamphlet). Faith H. Liebert. Radical Education Project, Box 561-A, Detroit, Michigan 48232. 15 cents.

The Womanly Art of Breast-Feeding. LaLeche League, 9616 Minneapolis Ave., Franklin Park, Illinois.

Thank you Dr. Lamaze: A Mother's Experience in Painless Childbirth. Marjory Karmel. Doubleday Dolphin Books, Garden City, N.Y. 11530. 1959.

Please Breast Feed Your Baby. Alice Gerard. Signet Classics, The New American Library, Inc., 1301 Avenue of the Americas, New York, New York 10019. Feb., 1971.

Ginny Lyman

NOTES

PREGNANCY AND CHILDBIRTH

Having a baby is a beautiful thing. Delivering a baby is a beautiful thing. They are not, and should not be, the impersonal procedures that they too often are. Under the wrong circumstances, however, both having and delivering a baby can be a painful and frightening procedure. Until you've delivered a baby's head and discovered that you can't get the shoulders out, or delivered a baby and not been able to stop the mother's bleeding, it's hard to appreciate why anyone who has delivered many babies approaches each delivery with a sense of joyous expectation, but also with a little ball of fear in the pit of his stomach.

It is the right of a doctor to practice medicine only in situations where the ball of fear is small enough for him to manage. On the other hand, it is clearly the right of the parents to decide just what risks they want, or are willing to take.

Right now in many cases there is a gap between the risks a lot of people are willing to take, and the conditions the physician is willing to practice under. Hopefully things are improving, for gradually some of us are learning again that medicine can be practiced in other places than a fancy medical center, while many of our friends are gradually coming to realize that orthodox medicine, despite occasional spiritual deficiencies, does have valuable insights into the basic workings and needs of the human body, and that this information can be accepted and built upon, rather than thrown out with some of the unfortunate bureaucracy that often surrounds it.

In the United States at present, home deliveries carry a greater physical risk to both the mother and the child than hospital deliveries. In this section I hope to do four things. First, to point out the importance during pregnancy of regular examinations and good eating habits in reducing the risk of having a baby, whether at home or in the hospital. Second, to talk about the risks of having a baby at home so that you can make an informed decision about where and how you want to have your baby. Third, to list some of the essential things that should be done during your pregnancy and in delivering a baby if you find yourself in a place where no medical care is available. Fourth, to provide a list of references that should be consulted by anyone considering having a baby at home.

PRENATAL EXAMINATIONS. Data on patients in England has shown that patients receiving no prenatal care have a mortality rate five times the national average, and in a recent study in California it was found that 21% of maternal mortality could have been prevented by prenatal examinations. Prenatal examinations are obviously important, no matter how far you have to go to get them. If it is not possible to go for regular exams because of the distance you must travel, it is important to have at least two prenatal examinations by an MD or other qualified person, supplemented by regular exams at home performed by husband, friend, or midwife.

If you are only able to have two prenatal exams by an MD, the first should be early in pregnancy and include the following:

WOMEN'S HEALTH: PREGNANCY AND CHILDBIRTH

   a. General examination of the heart, lungs, abdomen, breasts and nipples.
   b. Measurement and evaluation of pelvic size.
   c. Pelvic examination and Pap Smear (a routine test for cervical cancer).
   d. Blood pressure.
   e. Blood tests, including test for syphilis (VORL), hematocrit (test for anemia), blood group (A, B, or O) and Rh (positive or negative) status of both mother and father.
   f. Weight
   g. Urine (clean midstream specimen) for protein, sugar, sediment and cells.

The second should be 36 to 37 weeks after your last menstrual period and should include:
   a. Repeat hematocrit
   b. Blood pressure
   c. Urinalysis
   d. Abdominal examination to evaluate the size and position of the baby
   e. Weight
   f. Repeat evaluation of heart, lungs and breasts

If there are any abnormalities found on either exam, or if there is a possibility of Rh incompatibility, additional examinations by an obstetrician may be important.

The other examinations, by a doctor or someone else with adequate equipment, should be done
   1 each month for months 1–6.
   2 each month for months 7 & 8.
   1 each week for month 9.

These exams should gather and record the following data:
   a. General condition
   b. Blood pressure
   c. Weight
   d. Urine specimen for protein, sugar, sediment (since the sediment exam requires a microscope, it may not be practical at home; but the test for sugar and protein can be done with a dipstick—Combistix, cost $13.50/100—and should be checked at every examination).
   e. Check ankles, wrists, hands for any swelling.
   f. *A vaginal exam should never be done by an untrained person during pregnancy because of the danger of infection, hermorrhage from a placenta previa, or premature rupture of the membranes.*
   g. Record when the mother first feels the movements of the baby.

Prenatal examinations are important to spot problems or signs of problems to come so that adequate treatment or delivery precautions can be carried out. Danger signs are as follows—if any of these appear during the course of pregnancy, contact a doctor, nurse, or clinic:
   1. Increase of blood pressure diastolic by more than 10mm. of mercury
   2. Excessive weight gain (3 lbs. in 1 month or 30 lbs. during the pregnancy)

3. Appearance of protein or sugar in the urine
4. Swelling of feet, ankles, hands, or face
5. Passage of decreased amounts of urine or of bloody urine
6. Blurring of vision
7. Severe continuous headaches
8. Bleeding from the vagina
9. Passage of fluid from the vagina
10. Occurrence of pain
11. Occurrence of fever or chills
12. Change in vaginal discharge
13. Pain or burning on voiding

PRENATAL INFLUENCES, ESPECIALLY DIET. It is gradually becoming clear that many things happening during pregnancy influence the development of the infant. As a result, during pregnancy it is important for the mother to remain healthy (see chapter on communal diseases) and to avoid all drugs including our socially acceptable ones such as tobacco, coffee and alcohol. No medicines with the possible exception of iron and vitamins should be taken without care and medical advice.

Many studies have shown that malnutrition during pregnancy is associated with increased complications of both pregnancy and delivery. In addition, recent studies have indicated that malnutrition during pregnancy may cause mental retardation in the children.

This does not mean you should eat large amounts during pregnancy. Most obstetricians recommend an intake of approximately 2,500 calories per day with a daily intake of 85 grams of protein and 150 to 200 grams of carbohydrate. Fats should be eaten sparingly. Important vitamins and minerals, their importance, and their sources are listed as follows:

Calcium and Phosphorus	Required for building the infant's skeleton, teeth	milk (1 pint to 1 quart per day)
Iron	Required to make additional blood; necessary to infant and mother	egg yolk, oysters, meat, liver, fruit, leafy vegs. (spinach and broccoli)
Iodine	Required for normal thyroid activity	ocean fish or iodized table salt
Vitamin A	promotes growth of the infant; deficiency may lead to miscarriage; helps prevent infection in the mother	whole milk, butter, eggs, green leafy veg., yellow veg., fish, liver, oils and coarse cereals
Vitamin B Vitamin B–complex	prevents beri-beri	whole grain, bread cereals, lean meat, fruits, vegetables, beans, peas, lentils

Vitamin C	prevents scurvy	citrus fruits, raw vegetables, tomatoes
Vitamin D	important in building bone	fish, liver, oil, milk, egg yolk
Vitamin E	deficiency may lead to miscarriage	wheat germ, oil
Vitamin K	prevents bleeding	may be given to mother before or during labor—or to infant after labor

While it is important to have an adequate intake of these various vitamins, it is important to remember that an excess of some vitamins is as harmful as a deficiency.

A basic diet providing adequate amounts of the various nutrients is as follows:
1) Whole grain bread—two slices a day
2) Coarse whole grain cereal—one moderate serving a day
3) Cheese, one ounce a day
4) Eggs, one a day
5) Milk (low fat), one pint a day
6) Leafy vegetables, twice a day
7) Butter or margarine, one tablespoon a day
8) Meat or chicken, moderate serving twice a day (may be replaced with whole soy beans)
9) Potato—one per day
10) One orange, or one-half grapefruit, or six ounces of tomato juice a day
11) Liver—once a week
12) Fish—once a week.

Many obstetricians also recommend supplemental iron and a prenatal vitamin and mineral supplement.

RISKS OF CHILD DELIVERY. It is the parents' decision about how they wish to have their baby. Before making any decisions about home birth, however, they should be aware of the risks involved in giving birth at home.

Much of the information on the risks of having children at home comes from England, but it is important to remember that in England provision is made for routine home deliveries. As a result, (1) home deliveries are done by highly skilled midwives equipped with sterile instruments and with medicines to help stop uterine bleeding after the delivery; (2) patients planning home deliveries all have regular prenatal examinations; and (3) a "Flying Squad" equipped with blood and an obstetrician is on call at all times to rush to the aid of the midwife during difficult deliveries. A typical flying squad reported in *Lancet* in 1964 that in their 25 years of operation they had administered 180 gallons of blood to hemorrhaging patients, and were averaging 120 calls a year. Forty-five percent of these calls were for bleeding after delivery, twenty-five percent were for retention of the placenta, and twenty percent were for excessive bleeding before delivery. There are no flying squads in the U.S.

Even with the above provisions, there are several conditions which in England are absolute indications for delivery in hospitals, because of the greater risk of both maternal and infant complications. In 1926 in England, one out of every 250 births resulted in the death of the mother. Now fewer than one out of 5,000 births result in the death of the mother. This improvement in maternal mortality may be attributed largely to three changes: the provision of dietary supplements to ensure adequate nutrition for the mother; the provision of regular prenatal care for mothers; and the identification of high-risk mothers for whom delivery at home would be dangerous, but who can have their baby safely in a hospital where blood transfusions, operating rooms for performing cesarean sections, and highly trained medical personnel are all immediately available.

WHEN HOSPITAL DELIVERY IS INDICATED. The following are the medical and obstetrical indications for delivering in a hospital under the care of a specialist in obstetrics:

1) Pregnancy four or more times before
    Risks: Rupture of the uterus
            Excessive bleeding after delivery
            Anemia
            Abnormal positioning of the baby in the uterus
            Excessive bleeding before delivery
2) History of previous postpartum hemorrhage
    Risk: Excessive bleeding after delivery
3) Any major medical disease (heart disease, kidney disease, diabetes, thyroid disease, anemia, etc.)
4) Twins or triplets
    Risk: Excessive bleeding after delivery
            Abnormal position of baby in uterus
            Anemia
            Prematurity
            Eclampsia (high blood pressure and convulsions)
5) Abnormal position of baby in uterus
    Risks: Rupture of uterus
            Risk to baby of birth damage
6) History of previous stillbirths, premature infants, premature labor
    Risks: Of the same problems, with death of the child if oxygen and other equipment is not available

7) Baby too large for birth canal
   Risks: If a cesarean section is not performed, the baby may die from continued labor, and the uterus may rupture with consequent hemorrhage and death of the mother.
8) Previous cesarean section
   Risks: Ruptured uterus, death of the mother
9) High Blood Pressure
   Risks: Kidney damage, convulsions, excessive bleeding
   Excessive bleeding before delivery
10) Rh negative mother
    Risks: If the baby is Rh+ and antibodies to the Rh factor are present, the baby may need a transfusion or other special treatment to prevent complications. Two test tubes of blood from the placenta should be collected from all babies with Rh-mothers and Rh+ fathers.

    This blood should be tested the day of delivery, for if it is Rh+, and the mother's blood shows no Rh antibodies, a special preparation (Rhogam) can be given to the mother to prevent her next child from developing Rh problems.
11) History of any previous gynecologic surgery
    Risks: Tearing of cervix or vaginal vault
12) First pregnancy in mother over 30 years of age
    Risks: Difficulties in delivery
13) History of infertility
    Risks: The baby may need oxygen or other special care immediately following delivery.
14) Gross obesity
    Risks: Bleeding after delivery
    High blood pressure
15) Age over 35 years
    Risks: Difficulty in delivery
    Postpartum hemorrhage
16) Patient on hard drugs
    Risks: Withdrawal symptoms in newborn baby

This list is *not* presented to frighten everyone into having babies in the hospital. It is presented to show what the risks are if the mother shows any of the above indications, so that the parents can decide in an informed manner whether to have the baby delivered at home or in a hospital. The risks are the same regardless of where the baby is born. The chances of overcoming those risks are better in a hospital. John Starr's article (immediately following) has more to say about the risks and the benefits. He also describes complications that may arise in the course of labor itself.

LABOR. Approximately 280 days after the first day of your last menstrual period (if you should happen to know for sure when that was and that it was a normal period), you should note the first signs of labor. If you have not had your baby by two weeks after the due date, you should consult with some qualified person.

The three indications of true labor are:

1) "Show"—the passage of the small blood-tinged plug of mucus that has blocked the entrance to the uterus.
2) Labor pains—regular, painful contractions, at first occuring approximately every 15 minutes, but gradually becoming more frequent until they are occurring every 2 to 3 minutes. These contractions last from 30 to 90 seconds.
3) Rupture of the bag of waters with passage of water from the vagina usually occurs after several hours of labor, but it may occur before labor has begun, or may not occur until after the baby has been born.

If it does occur before labor has begun, you should contact your obstetrician. Often labor will start soon after the breaking of the bag of waters; if it does not, however, it may be necessary to induce labor to prevent infection from developing.

The average labor for the first baby takes 14 hours, but may take as long as 30. For a second baby the average is 8 hours, but 20 hours is still considered normal. Prolonged labor occurs in roughly 1 out of 20 births and suggests that the baby may be too big for the birth canal or may be in an abnormal position.

DELIVERY IN AN EMERGENCY. As I stated earlier, the delivery should be done by a trained person. Like any other manual skill, it can't be learned by reading books.

If you suddenly find yourself having a baby, and can't get to the hospital, the thing to do is to relax, avoid panic, and do nothing. If there is time, put up two pieces of string and scissor in a pressure cooker for 20 minutes at maximum pressure (see p. 199), and get a clean piece of cloth or some fresh newspaper with some towels under it to lie on when you have the baby. If there is anyone there to help you, make sure they wash their hands thoroughly, and then make sure they don't do anything. In most cases the baby and the placenta will come out by themselves. In those few cases where they don't, unskilled manipulation is more likely to do harm than good. An untrained person should *NOT* pull on the baby, the cord, or the placenta. The placenta should be delivered within an hour after the birth.

If you were on your way to the hospital when the baby was born, or if your transportation arrives too late, it would still be wise to proceed to the hospital so the mother may be checked over, and the cord may be clamped and cut under sterile conditions. Otherwise, wearing sterile surgical gloves, tie the cord tightly with two pressure-cooked rubber bands or pieces of string and cut between them with the pressure-cooked scissors. Cut the cord 4 to 6 inches from the baby's navel, and be sure to keep it clean and dry to avoid infection. Usually some antiseptic is applied to the baby's cord stump after it is cut.

The baby should begin breathing with crying really soon, 30 seconds or so after birth.

Probably the breathing will begin without any help at all. There are a few simple things that might help the baby begin to breathe if it appears to be having trouble. Hold the baby with its head lower than its feet so any secretions in the airway can drain via gravity to the baby's mouth. Open the baby's mouth and extend its head so the airway will be maximally open. In the hospital the baby's mouth and throat will be carefully suctioned with a rubber tube. Suctioning of the nose and throat can also be done with a bulb syringe if it is done very carefully.

By tapping the feet sharply but gently, by rubbing the child's body vigorously, you can stimulate breathing. Everything done to the baby should be done very gently, taking care not to hurt the child.

The baby should always be kept warm.

After one minute, the hospital workers would compute an APGAR score for the baby. This is an estimation of a baby's condition based on its movement, respiration, heart rate, color, muscle tone. You should attend to these vital signs in a newborn. Breathing should be relatively clear and regular. Movement should be vigorous, muscle tone good. Heart rate should be 80–120 counts per minute, and not less than 60. Color should be pink, not blue.

If a child doesn't begin breathing within two minutes, it may require resuscitation. Place your mouth over the baby's mouth and nose. Blow gently into the baby every five seconds, just enough to inflate the lungs.

If the mother is Rh negative and the father is Rh positive, it is important to collect *two test tubes of blood* (20 cc or roughly 1 fluid ounce) *from the placental end of the cord* and bring it to the hospital for Rh testing, for if the mother is planning to have other babies it may be necessary for her to receive an injection of Rh antibodies within 72 hours to protect future children from incompatibility reactions. In addition it is worthwhile having the placenta examined by a physician, since this may give an indication of some difficulties the baby may develop.

POSTPARTUM (AFTER THE DELIVERY). After you have had your baby, it usually takes 6 to 8 weeks before your body returns to normal.

Your uterus gradually returns to normal size, and by two weeks after delivery usually cannot be felt in the abdomen.

During the first three days after delivery, the vaginal discharge consists of moderate amounts of reddish fluid. There should be no frank (quick, overt, overabundant) bleeding, and if any occurs you should be sure to contact your obstetrician. From day 4 to day 9 there will be less discharge and it will be pinkish brown in color. From day 10 to day 15 the discharge should gradually lessen in amount and become white in color. If the discharge continues to be red, it is again important to contact your obstetrician.

Because of the strain of the delivery, you may have difficulty urinating or having a bowel movement in the first few days after delivery. If this occurs, it may be necessary for your physician to catheterize you to release your urine or give a laxative or an enema until your bladder and bowels again begin to work. If you have a baby at home and don't urinate within

8 hours, you should see a physician or midwife.

During the early postpartum period it is important to prevent infection in the mother. The uterus is a wound where the placenta tore away, and is also undergoing the stress of shrinkage. There are many torn and open blood vessels which heal very rapidly but which do provide excellent environment for growth of other organisms until the healing is well begun. To prevent infection there are some precautions that can be taken, especially trying to keep those other organisms (bacteria) from reaching the mother. Keep the linens around the mother as clean as possible, and prevent people with runny noses, sore throats, fevers or infections of any other variety from coming too near.

Keep watch on the mother's pulse and temperature for the first 72 hours after birth as changes in these vital signs may be the first indications of infection. The pulse should be strong and steady (below 90 counts per minute), not light and rapid. If the temperature rises above 38 degrees C or 100 degrees F and remains there for several hours, there is cause for concern and a doctor should be consulted.

One other important problem which might follow delivery is emotional depression, sometimes accompanied by confusion, disorientation, or paranoia. Some physicians feel that this depression is due to sudden hormonal changes occurring at the time of delivery, but certainly in many cases, anxiety over ability to take care of the new baby plays a part in this depression.

This is a time when it is important for the mother to be with someone she really loves and trusts, someone who can reassure her about herself and her ability to care for the baby. She should get plenty of rest, sleep and good food. The best thing to be done for postpartum depression is to prevent it by being attuned to the mother, to who she is and what she needs and by seeing that she gets those needed things. If the depression does occur and becomes severe or complicated by confusion and disorientation, the people close to the mother might want to contact trusted professional help.

Short, mild pains similar to labor contraction feelings are common during the early postpartum period. However, for persistent or severe pain you should contact a doctor or other qualified person. Most doctors also feel that a routine postpartum examination six weeks after delivery is advisable.

Most obstetricians recommend abstinence from sexual intercourse for six weeks after delivery, to allow the uterus and vagina to regain health and normalcy. And with resumption of sexual activity, thoughts should be given to birth control, yes or no, and what method to use. Nursing the baby is a birth control method 80% effective, but if a woman wants closer to 100%, she should consider other methods (see section on birth control).

REFERENCES. There is still some conflict in the medical profession about just how much patients should know about what is happening or what could happen.

Doctors, who know the most about their own diseases, are far and away the worst possible patients. There are two dangers of too much reading: the first is the confusion of book knowledge with judgment or manual skills. You can't learn to ride a bicycle by reading books, and delivering a baby is the same kind of skill. The second is what has been called "the parade of imaginary horribles." Obstetrics textbooks list everything that can go wrong, no matter how infrequently it occurs. Reading a standard textbook may do nothing but terrify you.

For those interested in textbooks, I have listed some with brief summaries and evaluations. My personal recommendations for expectant parents are below:

1) *Prenatal Care* by Children's Bureau, Department of Health, Education and Welfare—20 cents

    A cheap, thorough, and generally complete presentation of information about pregnancy and childbirth, covering everything from intrauterine development to natural childbirth.

2) *Husband-Coached Childbirth* by Robert A. Bradley—$5.10

    An excellent book by an obstetrician who allows fathers to help their wives during childbirth.

3) *Childbirth, A Manual for Pregnancy and Delivery* by John S. Miller—$4.07

    Another book by an obstetrician who believes in working with couples.

4) *The First Nine Months of Life* by Geraldine L. Flanagan—$3.95 hardback; 75 cents paperback

    The story of the baby's development from conception to birth.

5) *A Baby is Born* by Maternity Center Association—$3.95

    Prenatal development and birth.

6) *A Child is Born* by Nilsson, Ingelman and Sundberg—$9.95

    Superb photographs of prenatal development and birth. If you can afford it, buy it.

7) *Emergency Childbirth* by Gregory J. White—$3.00

    Especially valuable if you live in the woods and your car won't start.

8) *Preparation for Childbearing* by Maternity Center Association—$1.00

    A small book of exercises, advice on posture, lifting, etc., during and after pregnancy.

9) *The New Childbirth* by Erma Wright

    A well-written guide to natural childbirth, highly recommended by several friends. Available from: American Society for Psychophylaxis in Obstetrics, Inc., 164 West 79th Street, New York, New York 10024.

10) *Natural Health and Pregnancy* by J. I. Rodale

    A book by a leading proponent of organic food. It contains much good information but occasional misinformation. His emphasis on sound nutrition and a healthful way of living are to be commended but at times his uncritical acceptance of uncontrolled studies is disturbing.

GOOD SOURCES OF INFORMATION AND PUBLICATIONS ARE:

1) Maternity Center Association
   48 East 92nd Street
   New York, New York 10028

    For books numbers 5 and 8, and other publications.

2) Boston Association for Childbirth Education
Box 29
Newtonville, Massachusetts 02160

For information and publications on childbirth.

3) International Childbirth Education Association
208 Ditty Building
Bellevue, Washington 98004

For all books listed other than numbers 1, 5, 8.

4) Superintendent of Documents
U.S. Government Printing Office
Washington, D.C. 20402

For *Prenatal Care* (number 1) and other publications.

5) Ross Laboratories
Columbus, Ohio 43216

For publications on pregnancy and childbirth (free).

6) Mead, Johnson & Company
Evansville, Indiana 47421

For publications on pregnancy and childbirth (free).

7) Ortho Pharmaceutical Company
Raritan, New Jersey 08869

For *Rapid Post Natal Figure Recovery* (free).

As I said earlier, I do not recommend reading an obstetrics textbook. If you insist on reading one, however, my personal preference is McLennan—inexpensive, thorough, and concise—or perhaps Taylor (*Beck's Obstetrical Practice*). There are also several midwives' texts available; again not recommended because of gory details. My preference here would be Myles. *The Manual for Rural Midwives* is the cheapest, but it seems willing to accept a much higher prenatal and maternal death rate than Myles or the other British Midwives' Handbooks, and I personally feel that several of its recommendations (such as delivering multigravida breeches at home) are contraindicated. *The Manual for Rural Midwives* is obtainable from the *Whole Earth Catalog.* The American texts can be obtained from the publishers, or from any medical bookstore, and the British Midwives' textbooks should be obtainable from Blackwell's.

TEXTS

Prenatal Influences by M. F. Ashley Montagu

　A superb book on prenatal development and the factors that influence it.

Pregnancy, Childbirth and the Newborn—A Manual for Rural Midwives by Leo Eloesser, Edith Galt and Isabel Hemingway (1959)

　Written for people without access to hospitals. A good guide if you're sure you're willing to take the risks.

Obstetrics by J. P. Greenhill (1965)

　Big, complete, and expensive.

Textbook for Midwives by Margaret F. Myles, E. S. Livingstone, Ltd., Edinburgh and London (1968)

　Far and away the best of the books on midwifery—the British midwife's bible.

WOMEN'S HEALTH: PREGNANCY AND CHILDBIRTH

Williams Obstetrics by N. J. Eastman and L. M. Hellman (1966)
> Big, complete and, again, expensive.

Mayes' Handbook of Midwifery by V. DaCruz, London, Baillier, Tindall, and Cassell (1967)

Synopsis of Obstetrics by Charles E. McLennan (1970)
> Complete, concise, and inexpensive.

Human Labor & Birth by H. Oxorn, W. R. Foote, New York, Appleton-Century Crafts (1968)
> Outline form with lots of pictures.

Beck's Obstetrical Practice by E. Stewart Taylor, Baltimore, (1966), Williams & Wilkins Company
> Detailed, complete, and dear—well illustrated.

ADDRESSES:

Whole Earth Catalog
558 Santa Cruz
Menlo Park, California 94025

Blackwell's
Broad Street
Oxford, England

Stuart Copans

NOTES

HOME DELIVERY OF BABIES*
Rewards vs. Risks

As recently as 1935, 65% of all babies born in the United States were delivered at home. At present, slightly less than 5% of this country's mothers deliver at home. Maternal deaths, during the same time interval, were cut from 60 per 10,000 to 5 per 10,000 and—as might be expected—the medical profession generally seems to feel that there's a direct correlation between the two sets of figures.

Some of us are not so easily persuaded by that reasoning, however. We know that much of this reduction in risk to a mother is due to the discovery of antibiotics and the widespread adoption of prenatal checkups (which detect and ward off complications of pregnancy before the actual delivery).

We also know that few medical people are apt to seek out and publicize the ways in which home deliveries actually *reduce* the risks involved in childbirth. For example, a mother at home will usually be watched and attended far more faithfully than she would if she were in a hospital; she will be less anxious in many cases; she will be much less likely to receive drugs that might poison the baby; her delivery will not be rushed by an obstetrician who is anxious to get on to something else; the baby will not be exposed to the virulent staphylococcus germs which breed in hospital nurseries.

On the other hand, serious complications can develop during any birth, and such complications can definitely represent a larger danger to both mother and child in a wilderness cabin than when encountered in a hospital. If you decide to have your baby at home (after having gone through properly-supervised prenatal care) with an experienced nurse, midwife, or M.D. in attendance, the odds are about one in 50 that something will happen during labor and delivery to send you to a hospital. Once in every 200 home deliveries, that "something" will be potentially life-threatening.

Yes, this is entirely "natural." Even wild animals occasionally have trouble delivering and any farmer can tell you of complications he's had delivering a cow of her calf. It is pointless to deny—no matter how good your "vibes"—that problems can occur. It's much better if you know about these potential complications *before* rather than *after* they happen and the following description of some of the worst is not meant to scare, but to inform.

TWINS, TRIPLETS, ETC. One in every 89 deliveries results in twins, and only 60% of twin pregnancies are recognized as such prior to the actual birth—so they can be quite a surprise.

*Reprinted with the permission of THE MOTHER EARTH NEWS, P.O. Box 38, Madison, Ohio 44057.

A mother may suspect that she's carrying twins if her abdomen is much bigger than seems normal. If you have sensitive hands you can sometimes distinguish two hard, round baby heads instead of one when you touch the mother's abdomen. If you want to make a more professional check for twins, get a stethoscope at any physician's supply house and listen for the rapid tic-tac of the unborn baby's heart. If you hear two heart beats at different points over the abdomen (and particularly if there's more than 10 beats a minute difference in the pulse count) you can practically assume you have twins coming. The diagnosis can be confirmed by X-ray if there's any doubt.

Now, twins, triplets, and other multiple births are great to have in the family once they're delivered, but, unfortunately, they frequently are born hind end first (breech birth) and that's a difficult form of delivery. They're also smaller in size (hence weaker for a time) and are more apt to get sick following delivery.

Twins could be delivered at home and everything might go OK, but, if I was called upon to supervise the delivery, I would be jumpy until both babies were out and doing well. Any twin (any baby, in fact) weighing under four pounds would have a better chance if taken to a hospital nursery.

MOTHER'S PELVIS TOO SMALL. In about 1%–2% of hospital deliveries, the mother's pelvis is too small for the baby to be born. This is usually caused by rickets (vitamin D deficiency) which resulted in a misshapen pelvis as the mother's bone structure was being developed.

A doctor or midwife generally suspects this complication (called cephalopelvic disproportion) early in pregnancy and can advise against home delivery. In some cases, however, the condition is not noticed until labor has persisted longer than normal with no progress of the baby's head through the birth passageway.

The usual duration of labor for a first baby is about 12–14 hours. Labor lasts about 6–8 hours for subsequent children, and, if a mother has already had one child, you can generally assume that her pelvis is of adequate size for a later pregnancy.

In the event that a mother's pelvis is too small (or the baby's head is too large), labor will simply continue for days and a *Caesarian section* (the operation which removes a baby through a surgical incision into the abdomen) will have to be performed. A hospital is definitely the best place for such an operation.

ABNORMAL PRESENTATIONS. When a part of the baby other than its head comes out first, the birth is known as an abnormal presentation, and most knowledgeable people worry a great deal about delivering an abnormally presenting baby at home. The odds of such a birth are [reported to be] about one in 20 hospital deliveries. Get your M.D., nurse or midwife to show you how to feel the baby's head and wiggle it just above the pubic bone to make sure your baby is presenting its head first.

BLEEDING FROM A MISPLACED PLACENTA. This complication occurs in about one of every

200 hospital deliveries. Instead of growing on the side of the uterus where it should, the placenta grows over the mouth of the uterus, interfering with the passage of the baby. The symptom to watch for is continuous bleeding from the vagina either before labor or after labor begins. A "mucous plug" which is passed with a small amount of blood (called a "bloody show") early in labor is normal and should not cause alarm.

Misplaced placenta (placenta previa) is a very serious complication because of the rapid and severe bleeding which occurs. It is usually necessary to do a C-section to avoid catastrophe in the event of a misplaced placenta, and if bleeding occurs during labor, you've got some hard thinking to do in a hurry.

BLEEDING AFTER DELIVERY. At the time the placenta is expelled from the uterus, what seems like an amazing amount of blood is also expelled. This is normal, but it's a good idea to have someone on hand who knows how much bleeding is OK and how much is too much.

Sometimes a fragment of placenta is retained in the uterus following delivery. When this happens, the uterus does not flex its muscles to stop bleeding and you will notice that instead of feeling like a firm orange when you massage it below the belly button, the uterus is large and flabby. Blood loss from this condition can be rapid.

If this complication develops, the baby should be placed at the mother's breast and her blood pressure checked frequently. If the bleeding continues, if the mother's pulse becomes rapid and weak, or if her blood pressure starts to fall, you've got a problem. The mother needs qualified help immediately to evacuate the retained placental fragment and start a blood transfusion—and that means a hospital.

The average amount of blood lost during a normal delivery is about a cupful. Loss of over two cupfuls is worrisome and occurs in about one in 20 hospital deliveries.

PREMATURE LABOR. If labor begins a month or more before the baby is due to arrive, it can be predicted that the child will be small and weak (a premature infant). Such deliveries are tricky and should not be conducted at home. Certainly, any baby that weighs less than four pounds at birth is much more apt to get seriously sick in the days following delivery than is a baby of average weight. Low birth-weight babies also chill rapidly and should be put in a warm place as soon after birth as possible.

COMPRESSION OF THE UMBILICAL CORD. If the umbilical cord (which carries blood to the baby) slips past the baby's head and into the vagina, the cord will be compressed during the passage of the baby. This causes a shutting off of the baby's blood supply. This complication is estimated to occur about once in every 300 hospital deliveries.

Although cord compression does not threaten the mother, it will frequently result in a dead baby unless a rapid delivery of the child (usually by C-section) can be performed.

A trained person would feel the cord by doing a vaginal examination, would place the mother in the knees-to-chest position (have nurse, midwife or M.D. show you how) to reduce pressure on the cord and would rush the mother to the hospital.

Compression of the umbilical cord is much more apt to occur during breech deliveries; less likely when the baby's head is presenting. This complication is one of several conditions which may make the baby's heart rate (listened to over the abdomen) drop below 100-per-minute and which may cause the passage of watery and greenish baby stool from the mother's vagina during labor. Another possible cause of such symptoms is medication which a doctor sometimes gives the mother for pain.

INFECTION OF BABY AFTER DELIVERY. If you run a test on any 100 women, 5 will probably have gonorrhea germs even though they have no symptoms. If a baby is infected with gonorrhea during delivery, that infection can cause blindness. This is prevented by putting either silver nitrate drops or penicillin drops in the baby's eyes immediately after birth. You should obtain these drops at the prenatal clinic and always apply them following a delivery at home.

In those instances where the bag of water breaks before labor pains begin (dry labor) there is increased risk of fever and infection in both the mother and baby. This particularly true if the bag breaks and no labor pains begin for 24 hours or more (premature rupture of the membranes). In such cases (estimated to occur in about one in 80 hospital deliveries) the mother may develop a fever and the baby may be born covered with foul-smelling amniotic fluid. Such a baby must be watched carefully by experienced persons, since it may develop a life-threatening infection during the first week of life.

CHILDBED FEVER AND KIDNEY INFECTIONS. Both childbed fever and kidney infections can occur in the mother at any time during the eight days following delivery.

The symptoms of childbed fever are a high temperature, smelly vaginal discharge and abdominal pain. The condition is caused by germs getting into the uterus during or after delivery. Usually these germs are introduced into the vagina by the person doing the delivery. Always use sterile gloves (available from a physician's supply house)! Kidney infections are identified by a high fever and pain on one side of the mother's back.

In general, if significant fever occurs in the post-delivery period, you have reason to consult an M.D.

OTHER COMPLICATIONS. Almost all other possible childbirth complications—including blood incompatibility, anemia, swelling of the feet, blood pressure elevation, diabetes and syphilis—can be detected by prenatal checkups. Some of the complications I've mentioned—twins, small pelvic size and abnormal presentation—are also frequently detected in such examinations. Additionally, problems such as a bad heart or bad kidneys in the mother would probably be noted and home delivery properly discouraged.

I'm sold on regular prenatal examinations, in other words...don't wait until the last moment to sign up.

In England, where high-risk deliveries are handled in hospitals and normal deliveries are performed either at home or in the hospital, a 1968 study done in the city of Wolverhampton produced this interesting comparison: Of 7,133 home deliveries under midwife supervision, there were 54 stillbirths (babies born dead) and no maternal deaths. Among 12,163 hospital deliveries, there were 369 stillbirths and four maternal deaths.

Although it would be unfair to take these figures as evidence of the greater safety of home deliveries—since, admittedly, the higher risk deliveries *are* shunted to the hospital—they do indicate that home delivery following adequate prenatal care and attended by experienced people is not as risky as our medical profession would have us believe.

ADDENDUM

Note: Contrary to popular belief, boiling is *not* a guaranteed effective way of killing germs on either scissors or the material used to tie an umbilical cord. Heat resistant tetanus and hepatitis germs can be killed only by pressure cooking the objects to be sterilized at maximum pressure setting for at least 20 minutes.

Surgical gloves (sterile and disposable, size 7 or 8) should be worn when tying baby's cord or whenever touching any area of mother injured in birth.

Tetanus (in the baby) and childbed fever (in the mother) can result from improper sterilizing techniques and from not using gloves and masks to perform the delivery. Surgical masks and gloves are available from a physician's supply house (see the yellow pages).

John Starr

NOTES

HOME EXPERIENCE OF CHILDBIRTH

Kerosene lamp yellows the room where in one corner a woman is in childbirth labor, lying on a pallet of folded newspapers and a clean sheet. We enter, carrying with us a cloud of snow flakes into the drama of birth. Her friends standing or sitting around the pallet, someone at her head to breathe with her the controlled breathing of practiced childbirth, the mother flashes a welcome between contractions. She is completely absorbed in her work. Her whole being is strained and concentrating on pushing out the baby she has carried for nine months. She is the focus of all energy in the room. Several of the participants have had their own babies at home and know quite a lot about the course of labor, the control by breathing and proper pushing, and are able to help when needed.

The minutes tick on. The woman waits, then breathes more rapidly into a contraction, then relaxes, waits some more. The contractions come closer and closer together. Then, "I want to push."

"Then push!"

Everyone gathers closer, pushing and breathing together to bring about this birth. Push—the head shows a little. Push—shows a little more. Push—you can see a little dark hair. Push, push, push—

Then, "Don't push now! Let it come out slowly so you don't tear." The perineum stretches more and more as the mother exerts all effort not to push and the baby still keeps coming. Then, out pops the head. The medic with sterile gloved hands clears the baby's head of the membrane, checks around the neck to see if the cord is strangling the baby, clears the baby's mouth gently.

Another push, and the baby spills onto the sheets. A hush for a long moment, then a choked gasp, then a cry, tentative and growing stronger.

The room bursts with the glow and the joy into smiling, laughing, hugging people.

"She's a girl!"

"Let me hold her," cries the mother.

"Nurse her if you want. It's good for contracting the uterus," advises a helper.

More waiting now for the next series of contractions which will deliver the afterbirth. This is an anticlimactic period but soon over. The placenta pops out in a gush of blood. The medic puts it in a pan and checks it over carefully to try to ascertain if any is left in the mother. This done, the placenta is held slightly higher than the baby so the blood will drain into the child. Then the cord is tied and cut.

The baby is cleaned off gently with a damp cloth, wrapped in new blankets and handed to the mother who is glowing but tired. She puts the baby beside her and cuddles around her.

We wait around, checking on the size of the mother's fundus, her blood pressure, temperature and pulse for an hour or so. Then after instructing the family what danger signs to watch for, we pack up and go back into the snow and our car.

We're high from the courage of the people who, knowing the dangers of home delivery, accept the risk and the challenge to do it themselves. This was my third birth attendance outside a hospital—none of those labors have been longer than seven hours—each has been controlled, the baby born healthy and responsive. The experiences have been beautiful and affirming.

There are dangers. That's why we go, a team of three poorly trained and equipped women. We know we're insufficient, but people beg us to come, because we know a little more and are a little better equipped than they.

We've learned and gained a lot from the people we've met who've birthed at home. They add to our courage and strength and belief in the power and spirit of the people.

But why do women give birth at home? In large part for the wholeness of the experience just described with the participation of loved ones in familiar surroundings. But there are other reasons.

The hospitals and doctors available in an area may leave a good deal to be desired. Child delivery in hospitals is expensive and the process is pretty much out of the mother's control. Many women want to feel themselves giving birth, to be strong and controlled and without fear and beautiful. For someone who wants that experience, a hospital is at best neutral and at worst a real opponent, unless it is a hospital where controlled childbirth and rooming-in of the baby are an integral part of the hospital's practice and philosophy. Hospitals are generally sterile and unattractive environments, although efficient, and one must be very aggressive about one's needs to have them met.

Hospitals may not be so good for the baby. The hospital may not encourage nursing, may separate mother and baby by not having rooming in or other facilities which make it possible for mother and child to be together, or by having facilities that are prohibitively expensive. The baby may run more risk of contracting serious infection in a hospital because of exposure to antibiotic-resistant strains of bacteria which would not be found in the home.

The mother or parents-to-be may feel little choice but to do the birth themselves because of the failure of the medical establishment to provide the kind of care they want. Until those institutions become responsive to what people want and need, there will be some who will take control themselves, against frightening odds. Let us hope that those odds go down by our efforts to change our health care system.

Barbara McIntosh

RECORDING A BIRTH

Vermont law requires that a baby's birth be recorded within ten days of the birth. Each state has its own laws concerning this. Hospitals record births routinely. If you want to record a birth in Vermont:

1) Obtain a birth certificate from the Department of Health. This certificate must be signed by someone who attended the birth besides the mother—midwife, doctor, or other responsible party.
2) Within ten days of the birth, the certificate must be filed with the town clerk of the town where the baby was born.

BREASTFEEDING

Human milk is Nature's perfect food for babies. If your baby is healthy and full-term, your milk will provide complete nourishment for your baby for the first four to six months of life. In addition, your milk contains immunity factors which will help your baby resist infections and disease. If your baby has nothing but breast milk for the early months of his life, he will be less likely to develop allergies later.

Breastfeeding is healthy for you, too. When you nurse your baby, your uterus contracts, resulting in less bleeding and a quicker return to normal size after childbirth. Some experts think that breastfeeding greatly reduces your chances of developing breast cancer. If you do not give your baby any solid foods or bottles of formula for the first six months or so, you probably will not ovulate or menstruate for eight months or more. Thus, complete breastfeeding is a good—though not foolproof: it is about 80% effective—method of spacing babies.

Besides the physical advantages, successful breastfeeding promotes a close mother-child relationship. You need each other—baby needs you for food, you need baby to relieve the fullness of your breasts. The close physical contact is good for your baby's psychological development. Even after your baby stops nursing, the habit of observing your child's needs, necessary for successful breastfeeding, will help you be a good mother in the years to come.

Nursing a baby is a simple, natural act which nearly all women can do well if they know the right techniques. The basic thing to remember is that the more your baby nurses, the more milk you will have. The breast operates on a supply-and-demand system. The more your baby demands, the more you will supply. If your baby is not getting enough, he will want to nurse more often. This increased nursing will cause you to produce more milk, satisfying your baby's hunger.

A. HOW TO BEGIN. Nature helps prepare your breasts for nursing when you are pregnant. There are a few things you can do, too, to help the early weeks be more comfortable for you. The most important thing is to avoid using soap on your nipples during your pregnancy and for the entire time you are breastfeeding. Soap removes natural skin oils and this can cause dry, cracked nipples. Just wash your breasts with water every day and keep your bra or clothing clean. You may also do the "nipple pull" daily during the last month or two of pregnancy. Wash your hands and gently pull the nipple out until it begins to be uncomfortable; do not hurt yourself. Follow with a light application of lanolin or other mild lubricating cream. You should also practice hand-expression of colostrum. Just cup the breast in your washed hand, with your thumb and forefinger at the edge of the dark area (thumb on top, forefinger below). Then press thumb and forefinger together. In a while you may see some clear, yellowish fluid (colostrum). Do this for a few minutes occasionally in the last months of pregnancy. Knowing the technique of hand-expression can be valuable when you need to relieve fullness after your baby arrives.

When your baby is born, try to nurse as soon as possible after delivery, even before the cord is cut, if you can. Nursing causes the uterus to contract, thus reducing bleeding. Your baby's sucking instinct is strong in the first hour after delivery, if you have not had any drugs during labor. The colostrum in your breasts is rich in protein and vitamins and many immunizing substances. Early and frequent nursing after delivery will provide the fluid your baby needs and help prevent excessive weight loss (though all newborns lose weight—this is normal). Also, your milk will come in sooner if you nurse more often. To get your baby started, stroke his cheek on the side toward the breast. He will automatically turn toward the breast and open his mouth. Then put your nipple in his mouth, being sure to get as much of the dark skin in as possible. Never let your baby chew or suck on the nipple itself. This can damage the nipple. After five minutes or so the first day, take the baby off by pressing your breast away from the corner of your baby's mouth to release the suction. When milk comes in a few days, your breasts may feel swollen. This is called engorgement. To relieve it, nurse the baby often, take hot showers or apply hot washcloths to your breasts, and express your milk until the fullness is relieved. In a few days, engorgement will pass, but you will still have a good milk supply for your baby. If you are very full and your breasts are very firm when the time comes to nurse, the baby may not be able to grasp the dark area around the nipple properly. Hand-expressing a small amount of milk first helps this.

B. NURSING YOUR BABY. Breastfed babies usually like to nurse every 2 or 3 hours. Just feed your baby when he is hungry and you will have enough milk. Don't worry about schedules; but if you have a baby who regularly sleeps several hours between feedings, wake him to nurse if he sleeps longer than 3 hours. Wash your hands, and nurse for ten minutes or so on one side, then take time for a burp, diaper change, and a bit of play, and then nurse for as long as your baby likes on the other side. Start with this side at the next feeding, and use the same procedure. Sometimes your baby will have a growth spurt and will want to nurse more often. Go along with his demands, and in a day or two, he will probably go back to fewer feedings as your milk supply is built up. Your baby does not need water, formula or other foods. If you are feeding him nothing but breast milk (no water), and he has six or more wet diapers every day, you can be sure he is getting enough. Also check for good bowel movements. The normal breastfed baby's stool is very liquid, usually yellow or gold, and may come with every feeding or sometimes not for several days, but in that case it will be abundant when it comes. (For a few days after birth, your baby will excrete a tar-like substance called meconium). A weight gain of about a pound a month is generally considered adequate. If your baby is not gaining this much, try nursing more often. If your baby fails to gain weight despite more frequent nursing, you should have him checked by a doctor.

C. THINGS TO REMEMBER. Be sure to eat an adequate diet while you are nursing. High-protein foods, fruits and vegetables, and fluids are most important. If you do not eat right, you will feel tired and will not have enough energy. There are no foods which you must eat or avoid. A good, balanced diet will insure that your milk has all the vitamins your baby needs. Since drugs you take appear in the milk and some can be harmful to the baby, be very careful about anything you take and do not use drugs or medicine except on the advice of your doctor. If he prescribes any drugs, be sure to tell him you are nursing. Do not take birth-control pills while you are nursing. Above all, remember that your baby needs *you*. Do not be afraid of "spoiling" him. Your baby needs the comfort of your presence as much as he needs your milk. Try to keep him with you when he is awake.

D. SOME COMMON PROBLEMS. Many women have no problems at all with breastfeeding. But you should know what to do in case of difficulty. Some women are bothered by sore nipples. If this happens to you, be sure to avoid soap and dry the nipples thoroughly after each nursing by exposing them to the air. Do not use any bras with plastic-lined cups or plastic-backed nursing pads. A little pure lanolin applied to your nipples will be soothing and help them heal. Don't let your baby get too hungry, or he will suck very hard and cause pain. Nurse on the less sore side first, or express some milk to get the flow started. You do not need to wean your baby because of sore nipples. Keep nursing; the soreness will soon pass.

If your breast gets sore or red, you may have a plugged duct or be developing a breast infection. Apply heat to the sore breast (hot wash cloths, heating pads, or hot water bottle), but be careful not to burn yourself. Get lots of rest, preferably bed rest. Keep the sore breast empty, by nursing more often on that side and hand-expressing, if necessary. If you have a fever or if the soreness does not improve in a day, you must get in touch with a doctor. Be sure to tell him you want to keep on nursing. If he prescribes medication, be sure he knows you are nursing so he will give you a drug which will not harm your baby. If you do not contact a doctor, a breast infection can develop into a breast abscess, which may require hospitalization. However, the infection usually disappears promptly with proper treatment.

Most breastfed babies are happy and contented. Occasionally, though, a baby seems to cry a lot, even with the best of care. If your baby cries, first rule out hunger by nursing more often for a few days. If the crying continues, overfeeding could be the problem. The overfed baby usually gains weight well, is an eager eater, and seems to spit up a lot. He may nurse for a long time and fall asleep, but wakes up in 20 minutes or so acting as if his tummy hurts. If you suspect overfeeding, offer just one breast at a feeding and do not nurse more than every three hours. To satisfy your baby's sucking needs, you can let him suck on the empty breast or use a pacifier while you hold him in your arms. Eventually, your baby's stomach capacity will increase and you can again nurse on both sides at each feeding. If neither underfeeding or overfeeding is the problem, and your baby still cries a lot, and the doctor says he is healthy, he may have "colic," which is just a name for unexplained crying in the early weeks. Hold your baby and do whatever you can to make him comfortable, and remember that nearly all crying disappears by the time your baby is three months old.

E. SOLID FOODS. After four to six months, the supply of iron your baby was born with begins to run out. Then he needs iron-rich foods, in addition to your milk. If your four-month or older baby demands to be fed more often and keeps it up for several days despite more frequent nursings, you may assume he needs to start solids. Mashed ripe banana thinned with breast milk or a little water (boiled if you're not sure it's pure) is good to begin with. Put a little on the tip of a spoon and feed the baby slowly. Give him time to get used to this new way of eating. Strained or pureed meat can be added next. Nurse the baby first, before feeding solids, for a few months. This will keep up your milk supply. You can start juice and cow's milk from a cup and will not need to use bottles at all. Give one new food at a time, observing your baby for allergy or upsets.

F. WEANING. The easiest way is to let your baby wean himself. He will gradually lose interest in nursing, one feeding at a time. If he seems uninterested, eliminate the nursing, unless he asks for it. Proceed slowly and be flexible about it. Some babies quit around nine months, and others may nurse until they are three. Just remember, your baby will eventually quit. If you let him satisfy his dependent needs until he is ready to give them up, he will be more independent in his future life.

SUGGESTED READING:

The Womanly Art of Breastfeeding (La Leche League: 9616 Minneapolis Ave., Franklin Park, Ill. 60131). This is a practical, non-technical book written by mothers for mothers. Most nursing situations are covered. The League can also send you the name of someone you can contact for encouragement or breastfeeding help.

Nursing Your Baby, Karen Pryer (Harper & Row, New York).

The Family Book of Child Care, Niles Newton (Harper & Row). This book covers the whole gamut of family living. Particularly fine on breastfeeding, family nutrition, and household management.

Please Breastfeed Your Baby, Alice Gerard (Hawthorne, New York).

Abreast of the Times, R. M. Applebaum, M.D. (available from La Leche League). This author is, alas, a male chauvinist. He says some nasty things about women who choose not to nurse their babies and has a very traditional view of the role of women. Nevertheless, he does give a lot of solid information on breastfeeding, based on his pediatric practice with over 90% successful nursing mothers.

Judith Miner

NOTES

BIRTH CONTROL

Couples usually want to make love a lot, but want to make a baby only a very few times. Every couple should be able to decide when and how many children to have. At present many obstacles stand in the way of this: inadequate contraceptives, inadequate access to contraceptives due to lack of knowledge or money, real and imagined legal barriers, and doctors' attitudes and lack of knowledge. In Vermont there is probably a Planned Parenthood not too far from you where prices are based on what you can afford to pay. In other states it is often necessary to travel long distances to find low-cost care. The Supreme Court recently ruled it unconstitutional to deny birth control to women just because they aren't married, but single and young women still often have trouble getting contraceptives. We can all help each other by searching out relatively good doctors and clinics and passing the word on. We can also try to educate doctors about birth control and improve their attitudes toward women. But the biggest problem remains.

Contrary to a popular myth (current especially among population "experts"), *there is no adequate method of birth control:* all methods have drawbacks, whether these be lack of effectiveness, hassles in use, side-effects or limited acceptability. With that in mind I'm going to talk about those methods that can be considered relatively effective. They are male or female sterilization, diaphragm with spermicide, foam and condoms together, IUD's (intra-uterine devices), and the birth control pill. I refuse to play the game of not stepping on religious toes by pretending that rhythm is a reasonable method of contraception (see appendix). In this paper I'm walking a tightrope. I don't want to discourage you, but I want to tell you the situation as best as I understand it. What I say is based on my experience and reading, but that does not mean that it is the Truth. Don't trust any one source—and that goes for doctors and "experts." Use your own head. Read critically.

PERMANENT METHODS

Sterilization is the most effective method of birth control, but it can only be used when you are sure that you don't want to bring any more children into this world. Although sometimes sterilization can be reversed and research is being done on this, it must be considered irreversible at the present time.

MALE STERILIZATION: If you are a monogamous couple who want no more children and you, the man, are not freaked out by being sterile, male sterilization is the best method for you because it is so much safer and cheaper than female sterilization. The operation, called a vasectomy, is safe, simple, relatively cheap and can be done with a local anaesthetic in a clinic or doctor's office in about 20 minutes. Planned Parenthood has a vasectomy clinic in Burlington where the cost ranges from $5–55. A private doctor runs about $150. If you are under 25, single or childless, you'll have some self-convincing to do. The operation won't make you impotent or unmanly and you will still ejaculate. All the doctor does is remove a small section of the vas deferens. The sole purpose of the vas deferens is to transport sperm. Sexual desire and secondary sex characteristics (low voice, slim hips, etc.) depend on the hormone testosterone, which is produced in the testicles and circulated through the body in the blood. A vasectomy does not affect this. You probably won't notice any difference in the amount of ejaculate because sperm is only 5–10% of the semen. You are not immediately sterile after the operation because there will be sperm hanging around in the ampulla, seminal vesicles, and cowper's glands. The doctor will ask you to come back for a sperm count to determine when you are sterile.

FEMALE STERILIZATION: If you, a woman, decide that you don't want to bear any more children, you may want to consider getting sterilized. If you are married, even if you are separated from your husband, Vermont law says you must have signed consent from him. (Note that a man does not need his wife's consent.) Just as for a man, sterilization will not unsex you. You will still be a woman, still have a uterus, periods and normal hormonal cycles. There are two operations done in this country. The old tubal ligation requires major surgery and a long and expensive hospital stay. The newer laparascopic tubal ligation, nicknamed band-aid surgery, is a vast improvement, but you may have to travel quite a ways to find a hospital that has the equipment. Also, be prepared to do some fighting to get the operation. A lot of doctors and hospitals think that it is their business to decide whether or not you should get sterilized. Generally, though, rules are becoming less restrictive because concern with overpopulation is growing. The surgery itself can be done on an out-patient basis with a local anaesthetic, but right now most places require at least a one-night stay and use a general anaesthetic. The abdomen is inflated slightly with carbon dioxide gas (your shoulder joints will probably ache that evening from this), and two small incisions are made just below your belly button. Through one the doctor inserts a laparascope (same idea as a periscope) and through the other he inserts a forceps with which he electrically cauterizes the tubes. A friend of mine had this procedure done at the Hitchcock Clinic in Hanover, N.H. She paid $800, had a general anaesthetic and stayed two nights. A McCall's article (July 1971) said $300 is the average price.

TEMPORARY METHODS

O.K. What if you just want to wait awhile before you have a kid? There are four possible methods: two, diaphragm with spermicide, and foam and condoms can involve both partners and only involve a physical risk for the woman when they fail, and two, the IUD and the pill, are the woman's responsibility alone and involve a physical risk for her in and of themselves. If it is absolutely imperative that you not get pregnant—that is, if it would be too difficult to have a baby or to get a safe abortion—the pill is the most effective method.

BIRTH CONTROL

DIAPHRAGM WITH SPERMICIDE: The diaphragm is a rubber cup with a rubber-covered, flexible metal rim. It is used with a spermicidal jelly or cream and is placed in the vagina before intercourse. Statistics on effectiveness are quite variable. I've read claims that range from an effectiveness equal to that of the pill (99.5%) down to 15 pregnancies out of 100 women in a year (85%). You will have to judge for yourself if you think it will be effective for you. Here are some reasons why the failure statistics are so high and why it might fail for you: You don't trust it or don't like it (too messy, a hassle, etc.) and so you "forget" it sometimes. You go to a doctor who is incompetent and so fails to fit it properly, gives you inadequate or wrong instructions, or gives you a low-effectiveness spermicide. You are afraid of having a doctor stick his fingers up inside you, so you don't go for a checkup to see that it still fits. (Some doctors do hurt. Others don't. If your doctor is hurting you, it makes sense to find one who doesn't.) You take poor care of it and it develops a leak. If you can stay on top of these potential problems, the diaphragm will probably be highly effective for you. One thing to keep in mind is that there are no hazardous side effects with this method. In terms of mortality statistics it is safer to use a diaphragm with the vacuum aspirator abortion as a back-up than to use the pill. (However, carrying a pregnancy to term carries a higher death risk than using the pill.)

Instructions for use: Since diaphragms vary in size from about 2–4 inches, a doctor or paraprofessional must find out what size you need by inserting increasingly larger diaphragms into your vagina until he/she finds the biggest one that will fit. You will need to have the fit checked every year and after first intercourse (if you are a virgin), after a pregnancy, or after gaining or losing more than 10 pounds. You should get yearly pap smears anyhow so you could get the diaphragm checked at the same time. The doctor should give you instructions for using it, ask you to insert it, and check to see that you got it in properly.

(One nice way to use the diaphragm is for the man to learn to prepare and insert it as part of foreplay. I know some couples who do that and are really happy about it. Or simply insert it every day just before the time you usually make love (like before going to bed). It can be inserted up to an hour before intercourse, but the fresher the spermicide the more effective it is. Another possibility is for you, the woman, to become the main initiator of love-making and so prepare yourself before you start. If none of these things works for you, you will probably have to interrupt foreplay to put in your diaphragm. Worse than that, you will be worrying about whether or not you should put it in (are you making love or only making out?) and when you should stop to put it in instead of enjoying yourself and getting turned on. There is a strong possibility that if the woman is responsible for all of this, she will become resentful.)

OK, back to the mechanics. Put about a tablespoon of spermicide (you'll have to experiment to find out what kind of cream or jelly you like best) in the bowl of the diaphragm and some more around the rim and on the underside. Press the opposite sides of the diaphragm together so the rim forms kind of a figure eight and insert in into the vagina, cup side down. I found that I had to use two hands and that if I didn't keep the lower edge in contact with my vulva while I was sliding it in, I lost a mess of the spermicide on the outside. Push the diaphragm into the vagina until you feel the bottom edge slip up over the protrusion caused by the pelvic bone. The diaphragm should rest on this ledge. Then feel through the diaphragm for the cervix (see p. 164). This last step pushes the spermicide up onto the cervix, thus protecting you from sperm that get past the diaphragm. It may seem hard at first, but practice will make it easy. Inserters are available. The diaphragm must be left in place for at least 6 hours to give the spermicide plenty of time to get all the sperm, and you can't douche during that time. If you want to make love again before the 6 hours have passed, insert an applicator full of your spermicide into the vagina and don't remove the diaphragm for another 6 hours. If it is fitted properly, you won't feel it. It can be left in place for 24 hours or more. An added advantage is that it will hold quite a bit of menstrual blood so you won't make a mess if you make love during your period. When you remove it, wash it with lukewarm water, pat dry, and powder with corn starch. Never use petroleum products like vaseline because they will destroy the rubber. Check for cracks and holes every so often by holding it up to a bright light or filling the dome with water. When it isn't in your body, keep it in a closed container because air doesn't help the rubber either. Talcum powder or baby powder used to be recommended but aren't now. I've been told that they harm the rubber and cause cancer of the cervix. I don't know, but corn starch is certainly easy to use.

The Margaret Sanger Research Bureau in New York City has done test-tube tests on the sperm-killing abilities of different spermicides. Of the creams and jellies designed for use with the diaphragm, the following are the most effective (spermicides listed under the same number have the same strength): 1. Certane Creme, Contra Creme. 2. Creemoz Creme, Lactikol Jelly. 3. Ortho-Gynol Jelly. 4. Koromex Jelly, Marvosan Jelly, Verithol Jelly. Some creams and jellies were designed for use without a diaphragm, but they are less effective.

Myth: "Putting spermicide around the rim will make the diaphragm slip out of place or destroy the slight suction seal that develops." The amount of suction I feel removing the diaphragm is the same whether I've put spermicide around the rim or not. The walls of the vagina lubricate profusely while a woman is excited so there is plenty of slippery stuff present anyhow. Suction cups require moisture to work.

Myth: "When a woman is excited, her vagina expands so much that the diaphragm is free-floating and so doesn't really act as a barrier to sperm." When a woman is excited, her uterus rises so that the cervix is out of the way of the thrusting penis. When a man ejaculates, most of the semen forms a pool on the bottom or back side of the vagina. After a woman has an orgasm or is no longer excited, the vagina collapses to its normal size and the uterus lowers into its normal position bringing the cervix into contact with the seminal pool. The diaphragm is an effective barrier now because it is between the cervix and the seminal pool, and the seal that I was just talking about forms. It is during the time that the woman is excited that the spermicide is most important. From this you can see that the diaphragm is neither effective by itself nor merely a platform for the spermicide. If the man withdraws his penis during intercourse, make sure it is not reinserted so that the penis is between the cervix and diaphragm.

FOAM AND CONDOMS: This is another method that makes contraception a joint responsibility and does not involve hazardous side effects for the woman. As with the diaphragm, the mortality

BIRTH CONTROL

rate for using foam and condoms with vacuum aspirator abortion as a back-up method is lower than that for using the pill. Foam and condoms are non-prescription items available in most drugstores, so you can always rely on them in a pinch. Effectiveness, of course, is highly disputed. Claims range from 85% to over 95%, which means that out of 100 women, anywhere from less than 5 to 15 will get pregnant in a year. The more recent figures seem to be the lowest. Obviously, effectiveness depends on proper use. Either foam or condoms used alone is less effective.

Instructions for use—Foam: Foam comes in an aerosol canister with a plunger-type applicator. Be sure to get the kit with the applicator the first time. Fill the applicator, insert it into the vagina as far as it will go, withdraw it about half an inch, and push the plunger. This will deposit the foam just about at the opening of the cervix (see p. 164). You can use double the amount for added protection. Foam can be inserted up to 30 minutes before intercourse. (Some manufacturers claim up to two hours, but the fresher it is the safer you will be.) A new applicator full should be inserted every time you make love even if you do it again right away. If the woman gets up from bed before intercourse, the foam will fall away from the cervix, so another applicator full should be inserted. Do not douche for at least 6 hours after intercourse, but you can get up. If you do all this stuff yourself, it could well be a drag. If the guy does it, it can be fun and part of lovemaking. Foam is kind of like shaving cream in consistency. Delfen and Emco are equally effective according to the Margaret Sanger Research Bureau. You may want to try both to see which one you like best. Use a tampax if you drip too much afterwards.

Instructions for use—Condom: Condoms are thin latex rubber (0.0025 inches thick) or lamb membrane (skins) sheaths which cover the penis during intercourse. They come lubricated or not, with or without a teat at the end, and rolled or not. Condoms without teats should be worn so there is about a half an inch free at the end to catch and hold the semen. Unroll it onto the penis squeezing the air out of the space at the bottom. Be sure to put it on before penetration, preferrably as soon as the penis is erect, because secretions present before ejaculation contain sperm. This could be a bothersome interruption, but it could be an enjoyable part of foreplay if you have your partner put it on for you. If you need extra lubrication besides the foam and the woman's fluids to make intercourse comfortable for the woman or to protect the condom from tearing, saliva or K-Y Jelly are fine. If you plan to use the condom again, don't use vaseline because it will destroy the rubber. Apply the lubricant to the outside of the condom after you've put it on. Be sure to hold on to it when you withdraw. If you should discover that the condom has broken or if it slips off, insert another applicator full of foam and consider getting the morning-after pills.* A 1958 FDA report said about 1 in 350 condoms is defective, but oftentimes the defect is obvious when you put it on. High quality condoms can be reused 5 or 6 times if you take care of them. When you remove a condom that is to be reused drop it into some water. Later, dry and powder a rubber condom with corn starch and wash a skin condom and put it in a mild solution of household boric acid and water. Before you use it again you should check to make

---

*Morning-after pills are a very high dosage of the natural estrogen stilbesterol—25 mg. for five days. Try to get anti-nausea pills too. This is a pretty extreme thing to do to your body and so should only be done a few times during your whole life. Check with Planned Parenthood to find out where to get them.

sure there are no holes by blowing it up like a balloon. Don't store condoms in your wallet because perspiration and heat will disintegrate the rubber. Be sure to buy good quality ones, not the ones in vending machines. Skin condoms are supposed to transmit heat better and so are more sensitive; however, since they are packaged in water, glycerine, and a preservative, they are cold when you first put them on. Don't use any older than 2 years.

Now we're down to the methods of contraception that are entirely the woman's responsibility, are not connected with intercourse and tend to be the most frightening because they have side effects.

IUD. The most common IUD's (intrauterine devices) are the Saf-T-Coil, Lippes Loop and Dalkon Shield. Statistics on effectiveness of all IUD's vary from 91–99% which means that in one year 1–9 women out of 100 will get pregnant. Effectiveness varies with the size and shape of the specific device. Many women who try the IUD cannot use it, either because it is expelled by the uterus (10–12% of insertions) or it is removed because of pain and bleeding (8–10%). All of these figures are higher for nulliparous women (women who have never been pregnant). The shield, developed specifically for nulliparous women, is an exception. The expulsion rate is lower, but the failure rate is higher than for the other two. To be effective the shield must remain at the top of the uterus where the Fallopian tubes enter. The doctor may place it improperly or it may be pushed into the cervical canal by uterine contractions (see p. 164). These IUD's are made of flexible plastic. The coil and loop have a core of metal salts so that they can be seen on an X-ray. The shield has copper embedded in it to make it pliable and also for X-ray visibility. It is unknown whether any of this copper gets into your blood. (Large quantities of copper in the bloodstream can be harmful. The Food and Drug Administration recalled a newly developed device called the "copper 7" because part of its contraceptive action involved releasing copper.) There is no theoretical time limit on how long the coil or loop can remain in the uterus, but some clinics want to replace them every five years. The shield must be replaced about every two years. Calcium deposits build up and reduce its pliability, and this can lead to a reoccurrence of the pain and bleeding experienced during the first few cycles after insertion. Removing the old shield and inserting a new one relieves these problems. Of course, if insertion really hurts, this is a drawback.

Instructions for use: You must first get a medical exam to see if there are any anatomical abnormalities that would interfere with the insertion of the IUD, any vaginal or uterine infections or anemia. If you have had a lot of uterine (not vaginal) infections, be sure to tell the doctor. You must wait for your period before you can actually get the IUD inserted because it is easier for them and less painful for you at this time, since your cervix is slightly dilated. Also they'll be reasonably sure that you aren't pregnant. After examining you again briefly, the doctor or paraprofessional will pass a probe through your cervix to see that your cervix and uterus are not obstructed and what size device will fit. This probably will hurt but it is usually fast. Next he/she will grasp your cervix with a tenaculum (like a long tweezers) to hold it steady for the insertion. This may feel like a pin prick, or it may hurt. The sensation dies away quickly, though. The coil and loop are then straightened out by being pulled into a plunger-type inserter. This is passed into

BIRTH CONTROL

the uterus, where the IUD is expelled when the plunger is slowly pressed. The IUD then returns to its original shape. The shield is put on the end of an inserter which is passed into the uterus. The inserter is then removed leaving the shield in place. The time it takes to insert this device is much less than for the other two. All three of these devices have nylon strings which hang down into your vagina. Contraceptive action begins as soon as the IUD is in place. You may feel pain or cramping for a while because the uterus is contracting trying to get rid of the foreign object. It should taper off fairly rapidly although you may have some discomfort for several days. If this is extreme—which means more pain than you can or want to stand—get the IUD removed. Your first period after insertion may come early or it may be delayed and is likely to be heavier and involve more cramping than usual. This should taper off in a few months to a year.

If you have trouble with one device you may want to try another because expulsions, pregnancies and removals vary with the device. If you expel the IUD, you can have another inserted, but sources vary as to whether your chances of expelling the second one are increased or not. Some expulsions are accompanied by pain, some aren't. Since most expulsions occur during your period, you should always check the surface of your napkins or tampax and you should feel for the strings after your period is over. Usually a doctor asks you to come in after your first period so he/she can check to make sure the strings are still there. After that you're on your own.

Pain: If you are nulliparous, getting an IUD is likely to be painful. If you have had children and to a lesser extent if you've had an abortion or miscarriage, the opening in the cervix is slightly stretched. Consequently the doctor doesn't have to force it to open as much as he does for a nulliparous woman, and the pain will generally be less. Of course, each individual will have a different sensitivity. Some nulliparous women experience so much pain that the attempt at insertion has to be abandoned. Some barely feel pain. Some women who have had several babies have to be told that the IUD is in because they haven't felt it. This is especially true if the insertion is done immediately post partum or post abortion. (There is a very confused controversy about when an IUD should be inserted after a birth. In the absense of any convincing evidence, each doctor makes his/her own decision.) If you think the insertion is going to be difficult for you, learn deep breathing exercises and try to get a pain killer, muscle relaxant, or tranquilizer.

Method of Action: Unknown. There are about ten theories. Here are a few: The egg is hurried through the Fallopian tubes so that it doesn't have time to be fertilized or if fertilized is not mature enough to implant by the time it reaches the uterus. The lining of the uterus is chemically or physically inhospitable so the fertilized egg can't implant. White blood cells try to eat up what they think is a germ (the IUD) and failing that they attack the egg, sperm, or fertilized egg. (Pregnancy is not considered to have started until after implantation.)

Side effects: The long-range side effects are unknown including the posibility that the IUD might cause cancer. An incompetent doctor may perforate the uterus during insertion. Sometimes uterine contractions later will push the IUD through the uterus. If a coil, loop or shield goes all the way through, nothing needs to be done. It will float freely in the abdominal cavity and should cause you no trouble. If it only goes part way through it will have to be removed. Both of these are fairly rare. Perforation happens about once in 2000 insertions. The uterus may heal itself or it may require medical treatment. If you bleed much heavier than a normal period (more than one tampax an hour), seek medical attention. Slight infection probably occurs in the uterus immediately after insertions but clears up quickly. However, in about 2 to 4% of women, it doesn't. Some infections are treated with the IUD in place, but sometimes it has to be removed. If you get pregnant you have a slightly higher chance of miscarrying than if you didn't have an IUD. If you want to carry the pregnancy to term generally the IUD is left in place and is delivered with the baby. The baby is not harmed because the IUD remains outside of the liquid and tissues that surround the fetus.

BIRTH CONTROL PILL: This is the most controversial of the methods of birth control. I would recommend reading the *Birth Control Handbook,* Cherniak and Feingold, as a follow-up to this article because I can do no more than scratch the surface. Birth control pills contain a synthetic version of the hormones estrogen and progesterone which normally occur in women's bodies (see p. 170). There are two main kinds of pills—combination and sequential. Sequentials contain estrogen for the first part of the month and estrogen and progesterone for the last part. They were originally thought to be better, but now it is known that they are less effective and more dangerous. Combination pills contain estrogen and progesterone in every tablet. Of the combination pills, you should get low-dose estrogen ones: like Demulen 1, Demulen .5, Norlestin 1, Norlestrin 2.5, Norynyl 1, Ortho-Novum 1/50 and Ovral. (Norlestrin 2.5 is only for people who have suffered from estrogen excess symptoms.) Low dose means that there is .05 mg. of estrogen. Pills with more estrogen than this are no longer on the market in England because of the increased danger associated with them. If your doctor is giving you pills with more than .05 mg. of estrogen, make him give you a good reason why or switch doctors. If you have progesterone-excess symptoms, ask for a pill with less progesterone, not more estrogen.

Instructions for use: Pills require a doctor's prescription. Your medical history will help her/him determine how dangerous it is for you to take the pill and what kind would be best for you. All good doctors require at least a yearly pap smear so they will only give you a 12-month prescription at a time. Some put the limit at 6 months. A month of pills is 20, 21, or 28 tablets one a day. Specific instructions will come with the pills, but be prepared to wait until your next period to start taking them. Although contraceptive action begins right away, failure is much more possible during the first month, so it is a good idea to use foam too for that time. Follow the same precaution if you switch brands. It is best to take the pills at the same time every day and on a full stomach.

How they work: Some questions remain, but the pills are believed to produce a hormonal pseudo-pregnancy. The estrogen and progesterone in the combination pills seem to prevent the mid-cycle rise of LH so that no egg is released (see p. 170).

Side effects: Most side effects are caused by estrogen excess, so if your pill has a low estrogen content (.05), you shouldn't have much trouble. Nuisance side effects caused by estrogen excess include nausea accompanied sometimes by vomiting (combat this by taking the pill after a meal or by eating when you feel nauseous), fluid retention, breast tenderness, chloasma (giant freckles on your face, a rare side effect) and a heavy discharge. Estrogen excess also makes you more susceptible to vaginitis, especially yeast infections. Progesterone-excess side effects can include mood changes, including depression and changes in sexual desire, increased appetite and weight gain, decrease in amount and duration of your menstrual flow, oily scalp and skin, changes in facial or body hair distribution and breast enlargement. Break-through bleeding (spotting in the middle of the month) is usually associated with too little progesterone, while a missed period is associated with too much. If either of these happens several months in a row, consult your doctor. While the estrogen-related side effects disappear after a few months, those related to progesterone remain constant or worsen.

The biochemical activities which keep you alive are called metabolism. The pill causes many undesirable changes in these metabolic processes. Low-dosage estrogen (.05) significantly reduces these changes. The most serious side effect presently known is blood clotting: an unnecessary blood clot forms in a blood vessel, obstructing the flow of blood and starving body tissues (thromboembolism). The death rate from thromboembolism attributed to the pill is 1.3 per 100,000 women ages 20–34 and 3.4 per 100,000 women ages 35–44. This is lower for women taking low-dose estrogen or having type O blood. It is highest for women taking sequentials and high-dose estrogen. No conclusive evidence has yet been found showing that the pill does or does not cause cancer. In susceptible women it does cause an increase in blood pressure, which could cause stroke (a rupture of a blood vessel leading to the brain), but the risk is considered to be small.

If you get migraine headaches, blurred vision, dizziness, or sharp pain in your legs, call your doctor immediately and stop taking the pill. These can be symptoms of the dangerous side effects.

APPENDIX

RHYTHM: If you are Catholic and don't mind a few contraceptive failures—an estimated 15 to 30 out of 100 women get pregnant each year using this method—or if you want to increase the effectiveness of another method you are using by adding rhythm to it, here is the simplest way to do it. A woman ovulates 14–16 days before her period. Generally the egg must be fertilized within 24 hours of ovulation. Sperm usually live for 48 hours (although I've been told that they sometimes live as long as eight days). For the calendar method, keep a record of your cycle for at least 8 months. The cycle is measured from the first day of one period to the first day of the next. Forget this method if there is more than eight days difference between the length of your shortest and longest cycle because your ovulation will be too irregular.

The arithmetic—divide the number of days in your longest cycle in half and add 3 days. The shortest cycle is halved and 3 days are subtracted. Abstain between these two days. *Example:* Say your shortest cycle is 26 days and your longest is 34. $34 \div 2 + 3 = 20$. $26 \div 2 - 3 = 10$. In this case, abstain from day 10 through day 20. You may make love from the first day of your period to day 9 and again from day 21 until your next period, at which time you refigure. Drop the first cycle and add the one just completed to maintain your eight-cycle record. After a pregnancy, allow several months to build up a new chart.

If you are using rhythm just to increase the effectiveness of your other method, use your own discretion about when to refrain. For the temperature method, get a basal temperature thermometer and take your temperature every morning as soon as you wake up. A graph of your daily temperature should show a dip followed by a rise about mid-cycle. This is when you ovulate. Abstain from day 1 until 24 hours after your temperature rises. This can be combined with the calendar method so that you only abstain from 3 days before your earliest ovulation until 24 hours after your temperature rises. Your earliest ovulation probably occurred 14 days before the end of your shortest cycle.

Lleni Jeffrey

NOTES

ABORTION

Abortion is often a back-up birth control method, because as we know all too well, none of the methods are 100% effective. Abortion is often used as a primary method of birth control.

Repeated abortions, no matter what method, are a strain on the woman's body. Abortion should not be used as a primary method of birth control over and over again. There is a significant risk that the uterus may be damaged, especially with a D & C (see below). The uterus heals quickly, but a slight scar may remain, making it difficult for a fertilized egg to implant. Women who want to have children should avoid repeated abortions because the cervix is dilated (the muscle is forced open against its natural state) and if this happens too often the cervix may not go back to its original size; this could make it difficult to physically carry a child.

Often women who are desperate or poor turn a self-induced abortion. These methods are usually very harmful. At the end of this article is a list of places to receive help when you want an abortion. If you need an abortion, *please* try these places; don't attempt a self-induced abortion.

If you know of anyone who has tried the following methods, get her to medical help; they can lead to extreme pain, injury, permanent disability, infection, and death.

UNSAFE PROCEDURES

ORAL MEANS
ergot compounds—overdose is poison; can cause fatal kidney damage
quinine sulphate—can cause deformities in the fetus or death to the mother
birth control pills—often taken in large quantities; this actually supports the pregnancy if there is
    one; are suspected of causing genital deformities in the fetus. Taken as prescribed by a doctor
    will bring on the woman's period if she is not pregnant and just has a delayed period.
castor oil—useless

EXTERNAL MEANS: Women may try hot baths, severe or prolonged exercise, violence to lower abdomen, and sharp tools of self-mutilation. These methods only cause damage to the woman, usually not to the fetus. Douching will not work; it will only cause damage to the woman.

Solids inserted into uterus, such as knitting needles, coat hangers, pastes, catheters, gauze packing, paint brushes—all present the danger of perforation of the uterus and bladder; all may cause death from infection or hemmorrhage.

Almost any type of fluid—such as soap suds, alcohol or lye—can be inserted into the uterus; these solutions usually cause severe burning of the tissues, hemmorrhage, shock, and death.

Air pumped into the uterus causes an air embolism (bubble) in the bloodstream and sudden and violent death.

Various other means such as falling down stairs will cause severe injury to the woman but no abortion.

SAFE PROCEDURES

If you are pregnant and need an abortion, try to contact some one to help find a legal abortion. Even if you don't have money for the abortion, still contact these places. Often the fee may be covered by Medicaid, health insurance, or the people who run various clinics may have their own policies. Don't let the price deter you from seeking abortion counseling, because the counselor may have some ideas about where to get money.

The earlier the abortion is done, the safer it is for the woman. Many states or doctors place a cut-off point at twenty weeks from the last menstrual period. This varies from place to place but speed is always important. The first step is to find out for sure if you are pregnant. Get in contact with either Planned Parenthood, Clergy Consultation Service, or Women's Liberation; also check the list at the end of this article. The pregnancy test may have a cost.

It is important for a woman to know the whole range of abortion methods, so she will know what she is talking about to her doctor and so that she may protect herself against the illegal abortionist.

There are only four safe medical abortion procedures. The first two—dilatation and curettage (D and C) and vacuum aspiration—are used until the 12th or 13th week of pregnancy; after this time the saline technique or hysterotomy are used, both of which usually require a hospital stay. This points out how important time is in saving a woman both money and emotional trauma.

A. DILATATION AND CURETTAGE—up to 12 weeks from last menstrual period ($150–200)

This is the most standard in the U.S. This procedure involves dilation of the cervix and scraping the uterus with a curette. The cervix is dilated by means of graduated dilators. The curette is a metal loop on the end of a long thin handle. The patient quite often receives a local anesthetic called the paracervical block. This means the patient is conscious during the operation. This local blocks sensation in the uterus and the cervix. The entire operation takes about 10–15 minutes.

B. VACUUM ASPIRATION—up to 12 weeks from last menstrual period (about $150)

Preparation for this method is the same as for the D and C, including the paracervical block and the cervical dilation. Once the cervix is dilated, the doctor inserts a hollow tube called the vacurette. The vacurette is connected to a collection bottle. The vacuum pressure is turned on for 20–40 seconds. When the uterus is emptied, the doctor will go over the uterus lining with a curette to insure that no placental tissue is left. Recuperation from this method is almost immediate. Some women experience cramps similar to menstrual cramps. A woman will have menstrual-like bleeding for a day to a week after an abortion. Her period may resume from three to six weeks after the abortion. She should consider herself fertile and begin birth control immediately upon

ABORTION

resuming sex, which should be delayed for 4 weeks after the abortion procedure.

C. SALINE INJECTION—after 16th week ($150–250 plus hospital costs)

A long needle is passed through the locally anaesthetized abdomen and withdraws some of the amniotic fluid surrounding the fetus. This fluid is then replaced with an equal amount of a concentrated salt solution. This solution kills the fetus and induces labor and miscarriage in 20 to 24 hours. This method is useful only at 16 weeks because the amniotic sac must be big enough to find. Although this method is more painful and emotionally harrowing, it is cheaper and less time-consuming than the hysterotomy. This procedure must be done with extreme caution and precision because it is dangerous.

D. HYSTEROTOMY—after 16th week ($700–900 total cost)

This operation is similar to the cesarean section done in childbirth. This operation shouldn't be confused with hysterectomy, which is the removal of the uterus. In the hysterotomy the fetus is removed through a small abdominal incision, usually below the pubic hair line. This procedure must be done in the hospital and the woman must be hospitalized for a week afterwards.

It is well known that risks involved with incorrectly performed abortions are very high. Infection can lead to permanent disablement, sterility, or death. On the other hand, an abortion performed by a competent gynecologist after a three-months or shorter pregnancy involve little danger at all.

The dangers from hysterotomy are slightly higher. This is because danger always increases with abdominal surgery. Reports from communist countries where abortion is performed legally on demand reveal that early abortion (before 3 months) is at least 10–20 times safer than actually having the baby (*Birth Control Handbook*, p 3).

IF YOU ARE PREGNANT AND DON'T WANT TO BE

Women's centers and women's groups often have abortion information and counselling. Wherever you are, try to contact a local women's group. If they don't have specific information, they will probably be able to refer you to someone who does.

The Clergy Consultation Service is located in most larger cities. It's sometimes listed in the phone book under "clergyman's council." These services generally counsel only women from their particular states. But new services are being formed. If no service is listed for your state, call National Clergy Consultation on Abortion 9 AM–12, Monday–Friday, 212-254-6230.

Planned Parenthood in your city is also a good, reliable service. Check your phone book. If none are listed, call the Central Abortion Information Service at 212–541–7800, weekdays from 9 AM to 7 PM. They will refer you to a counsellor in your area or help you to set up arrangements for an abortion in New York state.

In Burlington, you can have a pregnancy test done at the People's Free Clinic or the Elizabeth Lund Home.

Probably the best place to go in Vermont for pregnancy tests, however, is the Vermont Women's Health Center located in Colchester, Vermont. Hours are 8–4, Monday through Saturday. The phone there is (802) 655–1600. The center offers pregnancy testing, pregnancy counseling, voluntary termination of pregnancy under 12 weeks, birth control devices and counseling, VD testing, and pap smears. Fees are on a sliding scale according to individual income.

Ginny Lyman

NOTES

A WORD ABOUT ROUTINE PEDIATRIC CARE

Children naturally grow and thrive and are able to tolerate wide variations in emotional and nutritional input. Personal preferences or needs in such matters as feedings (breast or formula) and type of family (one or many children) are important, but it must be admitted that one can see children doing well in widely different situations.

Many guides for child rearing are available and parents or a community should have one available for immediate or casual reference. Dr. Spock is excellent and a classic.

In addition, periodic checks on growth and development should be made. These are more important during infancy when children change seemingly overnight. Visits to a doctor or nurse-practioner on a periodic basis are advisable. In many areas the public health nurse or visiting nurse association can direct people to clinics that exist for well-child care.

Preventive medicine means more than checks on growth and development. A program of immunizations protects adults and children from numerous diseases. Children, and especially small children, benefit the most from immunization. There is no reason why such diseases as polio, measles, tetanus, and diphtheria need to be of risk to individual children or population groups. Once again the public health and visiting nurses can direct one to clinics available for children.

Certain information is valuable to doctors and others responsible for child care. Parents or responsible parties for children should keep a record of the following:

—birth weight and some general record of subsequent growth and development such as weight, age when first walking, etc.
—immunizations
—medications used regularly
—injuries, operations or allergies

The following pages discuss some of the more common pediatric problems.

DIARRHEA is usually too many and too loose stools. Color and odor may change. It may accompany other signs and symptoms. Remember the frequency and type.

The greatest dangers are:
1. dehydration. Children, especially infants, have less reserve of fluid and get into trouble faster than adults.
2. The underlying cause, such as infection, allergy, etc.

What to do:

See a doctor if:
—you are not sure the child is handling the diarrhea without excessive risk
—if any evidence of excessive fluid loss is present, such as weight loss, sunken eyes or fontanelle (the membrane between sections of the skull in very young children), loss of urine output

—blood or pus in stools
—the child is "out of it"
—diarrhea continues longer than 48–72 hours

If the child is less than 18 months: Remember again, fluids are more important the younger the child. Young children and infants have less proportionate body reserve than older children and adults.

1. Stop solid foods but maintain liquids
   —if breast feeding, continue
   —if bottle feeding, initially give just formula. Formula or milk may be diluted ½ strength for short periods if better tolerated
2. When diarrhea is stable and stool frequency is decreasing, and if stool is becoming less liquid, then:
   —return to full strength formula or milk
   —after 12–24 hours, begin solids again but slowly. Start with one food per day initially, such as cereal or junket. Add fruits last.

If the child is over 18 months: Fluids ad lib with soft solids such as gelatin, junket; discontinue fruits.

SEVERE DIARRHEA. Treatment of fluid loss to be used: until child seen by doctor; when doctor not available (do not continue longer than 24 hours without improvement or without seeing doctor):

Glucose-Saline Solution
8 oz. boiled water with 1 level teaspoon cane-sugar and ¼ level teaspoon salt.
Less than 18 months—give 1–4 oz. every 2–3 hours
Over 18 months—use as tolerated in moderate amounts only.

When improvement begins, advance slowly through liquids, to liquids plus bland soft solids, to regular diet, taking 3–4 days until back to normal.

VOMITING—WITH OR WITHOUT DIARRHEA—is forceful ejection of stomach contents. (It is *not* regurgitation)

The greatest dangers are:
—the same as for diarrhea

What to do:

See a doctor if:
—same as under diarrhea
—child vomits blood
—vomiting seems to be getting more frequent and more forceful (projectile).

If the child is less than 18 months:
—nothing by mouth for 1–3 hours.
—then give flat, room-temperature coke or ginger ale in frequent, small amounts (as

A WORD ABOUT ROUTINE PEDIATRIC CARE

0–6 months ½ tablespoon every ½ hour.)
—gradually increase amount if tolerated; *then* may change to other bland, warm liquids.
If the child is over 18 months:
—nothing by mouth for 4–6 hours
—then give flat room-temperature coke or ginger ale and then advance diet slowly.

CONSTIPATION is infrequent stools that are often hard and perhaps painful.

It is not the normal variation in frequency that can occur. Children and adults may have stools several times a day or less than once a day.

Temporary Constipation occurs with illness especially with fever and dehydration. This will usually clear naturally.

The greatest dangers are relatively uncommon. Excessive concern over bowel movements, which are a natural function, can cause problems.

What to do:
See a doctor if:
—blood appears on stools
—stools are black and tarry
—persistent pain with movement leads to avoidance

For infants: more sugar or a change from white to dark granulated sugar or syrup will loosen stools; fruits or juices—especially prunes—will loosen stools.

For older children: increase liquids and fruits and vegetables.

WHAT NOT TO DO: Don't use suppositories or laxatives repeatedly and/or over a long period of time unless under a doctor's instructions.

FEVER is any body temperature above the normal (98.6 F)

An elevated temperature is a normal body defense mechanism which is accentuated in children. Small children in particular can have rapid appearance of fever.

Thus, fever to reasonable levels (103–104 F) is frequent and by itself is not a severe hazard.

The greatest dangers are:
—not being concerned about the underlying cause of fever.
—persistent fever beyond the usual 48–72 hours.
—dehydration
—febrile convulsions from high temperatures in small children.

What to do: if a temperature is greater than 104 degrees:
—do not dress warmly: remove clothes and remember body heat must escape through the skin. For example, if transporting a febrile child to a doctor, protect him from the Vermont winter but do not raise his temperature further by excessive bundling.
—tepid water (not cool or cold) sponging should be used to bring temperature down to 103 degree range. Place your child right in a basin or tub with 2–3 inches of water.

—Aspirin, ½ child aspirin per year of age up to 5 is helpful. Use only every 4—6 hours and not more than 3 times without consulting a physician.

Seizures with Fever are to be avoided, if possible, but often occur before one is aware the child has a temperature. If a child has had a previous seizure he is more susceptible when future fever occurs.

When a seizure occurs:

—don't panic; a seizure is usually self-limiting.

—follow the basic principles of maintaining a passage for breathing outlined elsewhere in this manual (see pp. 31-32).

—do not restrain the child's activity but protect from injury.

—turn the child on his side so he won't inhale vomitus

Seizures occur most often in small children with fever but other causes exist.

ANY SEIZURE WITH OR WITHOUT FEVER MEANS A DOCTOR SHOULD BE CONSULTED.

SORE THROAT is any symptomatic discomfort in the throat, especially if accompanied by pain on swallowing. It can be caused by virus or bacterial infection.

The greatest danger is prolonged untreated strep (bacterial) sore throat. Streptococcal disease can sometimes cause severe heart, kidney, joint, or other systemic disease.

What to do: If the sore throat is mild with temperature less than 102 degrees and little other evidence of disease:

—force fluids

—warm diluted saline gargles frequently give relief.

See a doctor if:

—fever is over 102 degrees

—illness persists past 48—72 hours

—the throat is fiery red and/or develops white spots or patches.

George Little

NOTES

COMMUNAL DISEASES

In our living situations we must deal with stress, close quarters, and sometimes improper sanitation facilities. Because of this, disease spreads quickly and comes often. A few things to remember when you or a member of your family is sick are 1) keep the patient as isolated as is feasible; 2) rest and quiet work wonders; 3) the patient should be kept out of the kitchen; 4) patient's eating utensils should be washed separately and should be his or her own for the duration. Another thing to remember is that you're not doing your brothers and sisters a favor by going to meetings or meeting other responsibilities in situations where you may infect them.

The following are some common diseases that visit us frequently:

URINARY TRACT INFECTIONS. Urinary tract infections are fairly common in women. They can occur in the bladder, ureters, and less commonly, the kidneys.

Symptoms: Pain and burning on urination and the feeling that you have to pee often but nothing comes, are common symptoms. There may be pus and/or blood in the urine. There is usually a fever, muscle aches and a run-down feeling. A urinalysis is needed for a positive diagnosis.

Treatment: Sulfa drugs are used for treatment, usually gantricin. The full prescription, usually 10 to 12 days, should be used because many times you'll feel better after 3 or 4 days, but the infection is only suppressed and will keep cropping up. A second urinalysis will tell you if the infection is gone.

MONONUCLEOSIS.

Symptoms: Loss of appetite, lethargy or irritability, change in bowel habits, usually constipation, nausea and vomiting, fever, chills or chills and sweating, sore throat, enlarged glands in the neck and sometimes a slight rash. A blood test is needed to be sure that you have the disease.

Treatment: Treatment in most cases is just making the patient comfortable and relieving the symptoms. How it is passed from person to person is not known, but it is infectious and the patient should be isolated to protect those around and to protect him or her from getting a secondary infection. Gargling with salt and warm water will relieve the sore throat and a cold pack will help the swollen glands. Aspirin and alcohol rubs will reduce the fever. Plenty of rest is essential. Although loss of appetite may make it difficult, it is important to drink a lot of fluids. Prune and apple juice is good.

LICE. There are several types of lice: head, body, and crabs. Infestation usually comes through direct contact but can be acquired from toilet seats, bedding, clothing and furniture. Head lice, more common among kids, is usually passed when kids sleep together or use the same brushes, combs, or hats.

COMMUNAL DISEASES

Symptoms: With head lice, there is itching and where the lice have fed several bumps appear. The nape of the neck is usually affected first. Small eggs can be seen in tiny clusters at the base of the hairs. The eggs range in color from white to dark brown. Crab lice usually occur in the pubic hairs, and that includes the beard. It starts with persistent itching and may go unsuspected until you see the eggs on the hairs. Sometimes spots appear on the inner thighs or abdomen and will go away when the lice are gone. Body lice are fairly common where heavy clothing is worn. At first, small red points will appear and then they will swell, similar to mosquito bites.

Treatment: Benzyl-benzoate is the cheapest and must be ordered from a drug company. It is therefore sometimes difficult to obtain. If you are unable to get it, there are two other kinds of treatment, kerosene and lindane. Pyrinade A-200 and Cuprex are both kerosene-based, and I would not recommend them for people who are around an open flame very often. Kwell is a lindane-based treatment, but lindane is a chlorinated hydrocarbon which is a long-lasting toxin similar to DDT, so it must be used with care and washed out thoroughly. All of these treatments are used about the same way. Wash the affected areas with it, leave it on about 30 minutes, and wash it out thoroughly. Use it once a day for about 3 days and that usually does it. Lice in clothing can be killed by putting the clothes in a commercial dryer on the hottest setting.

PINWORMS. Pinworms are small round worms that live and breed in the intestine. At night, the female crawls outside the body and lays eggs around the anal opening. The eggs are light enough to be carried through the air and can infect bed linen and the hands through scratching. This is why it is important to wash hands after going to the bathroom and before meals. Cleaning the fingernails is also important.

Symptoms: Though there may be no symptoms, itching, especially at night, usually occurs.

Treatment: Everyone in the house should be treated because you probably all have it. Piperozine is the medicine usually prescribed. Getting rid of them entirely is impossible in our situation, but keeping their numbers down is desirable. They usually do not affect your health much unless they are in very large numbers. Soaking bed linen in a solution of 2 cups ammonia to 10 gallons of water before washing will help. Normal laundering will not kill the eggs. It is important to wear your own clothes and keep your hands and nails as clean as possible.

GASTROENTERITIS. Gastroenteritis is commonly referred to as stomach virus.

Symptoms: The symptoms include nausea, vomiting and/or diarrhia, loss of appetite, and severe stomach cramps which may be mistaken for appendicitis. Other symptoms which may occur are chills, moderate fever, and dizziness.

Treatment: Kaopectate or Donagel will control the diarrhea. A doctor can prescribe Thorazine or Compazine to control the vomiting. The important thing to remember is that your body is losing a lot of fluid and it must be replaced. When the vomiting subsides, drink lots of water, juice, and clear soup which is room-temperature or possibly warmer. Again, the patient should be isolated.

ATHLETES FOOT. Athletes foot is a fungal infection that can sometimes be prevented by keeping the feet dry. The best and cheapest preparation is Desenex ointment or powder. If that does not work, you should be able to get a prescription for Tinactin from a physician. Athlete's foot is contagious, so do not walk around in your bare feet. Try to wear white sox and keep your feet dry. Powder helps a lot.

Sherry Oake

NOTES

VENEREAL DISEASE

Venereal Disease is the most widespread communicable disease in the country. It infects about one American in every 100; the young and poor are the largest groups infected.

VD is a complicated problem because it is a disease spread by sexual contact. Public attitudes toward the disease are intermixed with attitudes about sex. In this country, sex is treated very moralistically—it is considered sinful, dirty, and something to be hidden. So information about sex, even sexual disease, is often hidden, hard to get, hard to admit that you need or want. Instead of treating the epidemic, some authorities tell people not to have sex. If you run into these attitudes when you go for testing and treatment, you are made to feel ashamed.

The VD problem is further complicated by society's attitudes toward women. Women frequently have no recognizable symptoms of gonorrhea, though the men they contact do. So the simplest way for a woman to learn she has gonorrhea and get it treated is to be told by the man or men with whom she is in contact. Because women are often thought of as commodities to be exploited, to be used and discarded, especially if associated with disease, all to frequently the warning does not get to them.

Controlling venereal disease needs a widespread national effort. We need education about the disease as it now exists and research to find a control for it quickly. For this effort we need the cooperation of the government, schools, drug companies, and the medical establishment. We need to strengthen our sense of responsibility to each other to talk freely of symptoms and treatment. We also need to talk about why VD is so hard to curb, so that people will begin to change their attitudes about it.

Chris Allen
Barbara McIntosh

SYMPTOMS, DIAGNOSIS, AND TREATMENT OF VD

Venereal diseases are transmitted by intimate physical and sexual contact. The two most common and dangerous types of VD are syphilis and gonorrhea. Gonorrhea is more common and less likely to be fatal than syphilis. VD germs live only in a warm, moist environment. Since they are killed by exposure to air, drying, soaps, and disinfectants, VD is not spread by towels, dishes, toilet seats, etc.

GONORRHEA is acquired through intimate, body-to-body contact with the body exits of an infected person; the penis, vagina, anus, or mouth. The infection attacks the linings of the genital-urinary organs, causing symptoms to appear in 3–14 days. The symptoms occur much more often and are usually far more obvious in a man. He will notice a thick, whitish-yellow pussy discharge from the end of the penis and feel discomfort or burning while urinating. He will probably urinate more often and feel more of an urgency to do so. The pus is very infectious and may be carelessly transferred to the eyes, possibly causing blindness. If untreated in men, the disease may cause narrowing of the urethra due to scarring, as well as scarring in the tubes through which sperm pass. If the scarring is severe, it can cause sterility.

In a woman the first organs infected by gonorrhea are the urethra and the cervical canal (entrance to uterus). She might feel a little discomfort when urinating or she might have vaginal discharge. These symptoms may not be very noticeable, or there may not be any symptoms at all. But if the disease goes untreated, various complications can arise. The glands in the genital area may be swollen and tender. The infection can spread up the urethra into the bladder causing cystitis. (Urination will be more frequent and painful.) Or it may spread to the rectum. Most serious of all is the spread of the infection to the woman's fallopian tubes (tubes through which eggs move on their way from ovaries to the uterus) and to the tissues lining the pelvic area. This may be manifested as chills, fever, fatique, muscle pains, loss of appetite, nausea, vomiting, irregular menstrual periods, and lower abdominal pain. If it still goes untreated, a lot of scar tissue will form in the fallopian tubes; often so much that the eggs can't pass through them. This will cause pregnancy complications and/or sterility.

If a pregnant woman has gonorrhea and doesn't get treatment before her child is born, the disease can infect her child's eyes during birth, possibly causing blindness. Silver nitrate, often put in newborn babies' eyes, kills gonorrhea germs.

Untreated, the disease may also cause arthritis and endocarditis (inflammation of the inner lining of the heart and its valves) in both men and women.

To diagnose gonorrhea in a man, some discharge is looked at under a microscope. Usually there are so many germs they can be seen and identified right away. In women it is more difficult, since the germs spread out in her body more. So with women a culture is taken. (Some of the secretions from her cervix are put into a culture medium and allowed to multiply and are examined a couple of days later.) The culture is not totally reliable, so it is good to be retested and maybe treated on the basis of positive contacts.

SYPHILIS is caught by intimate body-to-body contact with an infected person. The disease germs may enter the body through the mouth, genitals, anus, or break in the skin.

The first symptoms of syphilis appear within 10–90 days, usually in about 3 weeks. A sore called a *chancre* usually appears where the syphilis germs entered the body. This looks like a blister or open sore. It's pussy and looks as if it should hurt a lot; it doesn't. The chancre may appear on the penis, in the vagina or vulva, on the fingers, breasts, or in the mouth. If it's inside the penis or vagina, it will probably not be noticed. This sore disappears even without treatment, but the disease does not.

After the chancre disappears, about 1–6 months after a person has caught the disease, other symptoms show up which may include: rash, sores in the mouth, sore throat, swollen glands, head-

VENEREAL DISEASES

ache, fever, sore and swollen joints, sore bones, patchy hair loss. As these symptoms are not very specific, they may be mistaken for any of several other illnesses. For this reason syphilis has been called the "great deceiver."

During the third stage of the disease, the syphilis infection becomes general throughout the body. The germs may be invading inner organs like the heart or the brain. There are no outwardly visible signs of the disease. The infectiousness of the disease fades out. This systemic infection begins about 5 years after the disease was contracted and lasts usually 10–20 years.

The last stage is when the serious effects appear. Depending on which organs the syphilis germs have attacked during the latent phase, a person may have serious heart disease, crippling, blindness, mental incapacity, paralysis, and maybe death.

A pregnant woman with syphilis will probably give the disease to the unborn child. The child may be born deformed or diseased or dead. But if the woman's syphilis is treated before the 18th week of pregnancy, the fetus probably won't be infected at all. Therefore it is very important that every pregnant woman get tested for syphilis as soon as she knows she's pregnant. So if she has the disease, she can be treated for it before giving it to her child.

The test for syphilis is a special blood test called a VDRL. The germs show up in the blood within 1–3 weeks after the sore appears. It's usually best to have 2 tests several weeks apart, even if the first one was negative, because sometimes the results are not reliable.

Both syphilis and gonorrhea can be cured quickly and cheaply by large doses of penicillin or other antibiotics. It is vital to have correct treatment; for inadequate treatment may cause recurrence of the disease or a resistant strain. Herbal remedies do not work. With both syphilis and gonorrhea the disappearance of symptoms usually does not mean a cure unless there has been proper medical treatment. Treatment stops the disease but cannot repair the damage that has already been done.

Whenever you get penicillin treatment, it is best not to drink any alcoholic beverages for 48 hours afterwards. Alcohol deactivates the white blood cells, which are the agents that kill the disease. Penicillin will stop the growth of new germs in that time, but the treatment will not be as effective if the white blood cells are inactive.

There is no such thing as immunity to VD. You can have both syphilis and gonorrhea over and over again and you can have them both at once.

If you think you have VD, either by a positive contact or by experiencing any of the symptoms, get it checked out. You can be tested and treated for VD by people's clinics, planned parenthood clinics, hospital emergency rooms, or private physicians. In Burlington, Vt., you can go to the People's Free Clinic or the VD clinic at the Medical Center Hospital. Don't rely on just one test. If the first test for gonorrhea or syphilis doesn't show anything, have another one just to be sure.

If you find out you have VD, don't have sexual relations with anyone until you are well (condoms help, but aren't totally reliable). If you had sex with someone when you had VD, you should tell that person right away so she or he can be treated. It's especially important for men to tell women that they might be infected with gonorrhea, because the woman probably won't notice any symptoms in herself until the disease has already done a lot of damage. Also make sure you get rechecked to be certain the treatment was adequate.

Possible symptoms	*Diagnosis*	*Complications*
SYPHILIS		
1st stage (9–90 days after infection): chancre	examination of pus from chancre	
2nd (few weeks–6 months later): rash, sores in mouth, sore throat, mild fever, sore bones, swollen joints, headache, patchy balding	examination of swollen lymph glands	
3rd stage (10–20 years): no outward symptoms	blood test (valid 1–3 weeks after appearance of chancre throughout duration)	Disease invading organs such as brain or heart
4th stage: systemic destruction becomes obvious depending on which organs the syphilis germs have attacked in the third stage		Heart disease, crippling, deafness, blindness, insanity, paralysis, death
GONORRHEA **In Women:**		
May be vaginal discharge, maybe some pain when urinating	Culture from cervix and anus	Infected cervical canal infected bladder infected rectum infected tubes scarring & pregnancy complications & sterility arthritis endocarditis blindness
Later: Lower abdominal pain, chills, fever, loss of appetite, nausea, vomiting, irregular menstrual periods		
In Men: Discharge from penis Burning during urination Urgency & frequency of urinations	examination of discharge under microscope	Infected bladder infected tubes sterility arthritis endocarditis blindness
Later: Maybe sore, swollen testicles		

Peter Marsh
Chris Allen

NOTES

HEPATITIS

The following article on hepatitis is not intended as a complete, in-depth treatise on the subject. It is rather intended to give the reader some understanding of the disease, its presentation as a clinical problem and an approach to its control. With some knowledge of the clinical problem, it is hoped that the reader can recognize the signs of hepatitis and refer patients to a physician for medical care. With a knowledge of how hepatitis is spread, it is hoped that some cases may be prevented.

In spite of the many startling and significant advances in our understanding and characterization of many of the known human viruses during the last two to three decades, viral hepatitis remains today, at least in the United States, the leading still-unconquered viral disease. During the last peak year, 1961, 73,000 cases of hepatitis were reported in the United States alone. Among the military, viral hepatitis still remains the leading single infectious disease causing the greatest loss of man hours from duty. In the United States, a clinical pattern of disease has been noted with disease peaks occurring approximately every 7 years. Peak years have been noted in 1954 and in 1961. During the late 1960's and early 1970's a gradual increase in the number of reported cases of hepatitis has been noted. During the last 20 years, cases have averaged between 30,000 and 70,000 per year.

SIGNS OF THE DISEASE: Hepatitis usually has the symptoms of influenza, with a feeling of weakness, fatigue, sweatiness, and frequent depression. There may be gastrointestinal upset with loss of appetite, nausea, and vomiting. Smokers notice a loss of taste for cigarettes. Patients may note increased irritability and general crabbiness, said to be more pronounced in women. Women may also note the appearance of abnormal menstrual periods. Acne-like rashes have also been described, these being confined chiefly to the face. Physical examination may be entirely negative. There may be simply be a tender liver which may or may not enlarge. When jaundice is present (characterized by yellow skin and deep yellow urine) this is the most prominent clinical feature of disease. When jaundice reaches its peak intensity in benign hepatitis, the patient usually begins to feel better. Jaundice will peak 2 weeks after the onset of the disease and then gradually recede over the next 2 to 6 weeks. Patients who follow an uncomplicated course will recover in 2 to 6 weeks but in approximately 15% of cases, relapse will occur. This is usually milder than the primary benign hepatitis and in most instances leads to complete recovery.

TREATMENT: The hallmark of treatment is rest. Careful attention should also be given to diet and an attempt made to increase calories. The patient with hepatitis may have a very finicky appetite and should be allowed to eat what foods he or she wishes at whatever hour of day is most comfortable for the patient. It is not infrequent for patients to prefer their largest meal in the morning rather than in the evening. It is extremely important that the patient have no alcoholic beverages during the course of his or her illness. It should also be emphasized that NO DRUGS be used for symptomatic relief of appetite loss, vomiting, irritability or tiredness. Almost all drugs are toxic to the liver, especially tranquilizers and drugs that suppress vomiting, and it is imperative that all unnecessary drugs be avoided. In cases of complications secondary to hepatitis, the patient should definitely be followed by a physician. This is particularly true in chronic progressive hepatitis.

PREVENTIVE TREATMENT: It has been well documented that the use of gamma globulin, 0.01 ml per pound body weight intramuscularly, is effective in preventing the clinical manifestations of short incubation (infectious) hepatitis. Some reports have indicated that it is also useful in the prevention of the manifestations of long incubation (serum) hepatitis. In case of intimate exposure to documented cases of hepatitis, gamma globulin should be used for prevention.

ROUTE OF INFECTION: It is terribly important for all to understand the basic principle of the spread and transmission of infectious hepatitis and serum hepatitis, because in understanding this one may prevent many cases. Although it was felt for a long time that infectious hepatitis was spread by contact with feces and serum hepatitis by infected injection equipment, it is now felt that although these are the usual routes of infection, infectious hepatitis may on occasion be acquired by infected needles and serum hepatitis may be acquired via the airborne route. The virus in both instances may be present in urine, feces, and blood and since it is not clear how long these materials remain infected, a person should be cautioned about the sanitary disposal of fecal and urine material and should follow precautions for at least 5 years after disease and perhaps for a lifetime.

Major epidemics of hepatitis have been caused by the eating of raw clams and oysters grown in fecally contaminated water. In this regard, improper steaming will not inactivate hepatitis virus. Waterborne epidemics of hepatitis have accounted for the largest epidemics reported. Chimpanzees and other primates imported from Africa may harbor the virus for periods of time after their arrival in the United States; and finally, man-to-man transmission of virus via feces, urine, and blood has been reported.

CONTROL: From the account presented above, it should be evident that isolation and quarantine of hepatitis cases is ineffective. Patients are infective both before and after the onset of the disease, and furthermore, most cases of infectious hepatitis are not diagnosed as such. The best one can do is to stress personal cleanliness and instruct those with the disease on the disposal of fecal and urine material. Use of disposable needles and syringes is also indicated. Water supplies should be carefully watched and allowed to settle and should be filtered and chlorinated according to public health standards. People should avoid eating raw shellfish or poorly steamed clams. More control of the use of blood products is also being instituted. Careful selection of blood donors should decrease the possibility of transmitting serum hepatitis to recipients. Finally, the use of gamma globulin in immediate or intimate contacts of patients who have diagnosed hepatitis can prevent secondary spread of the disease.

SUMMARY: Hepatitis remains a major problem in the United States today in spite of some recent advances. It is possible that within the next five to ten years an effective vaccine may be developed which can prevent the spread of hepatitis. In the meantime, care should be taken to recognize clinical cases and refer them to a physician for follow up, to dispose of waste products carefully, and to treat immediate contacts with gamma globulin. Careful attention to water supply, proper preparation of foods, particularly shellfish and clams, and use of disposable needles and syringes can help contribute to the control of this major infectious disease problem.

Charles Phillips

NOTES

SAFE USE OF FARM EQUIPMENT

For those of us new to the farming life in Vermont, the use of farm machinery is a new experience. It can be a very bad experience if people are not extremely careful. There are over 1200 reported tractor deaths a year in the United States; there are countless other serious farm accidents involving chain saws, balers, axes, and other farm equipment. Although some of these are accidents of inexperienced people, many happen to old hands around the farm.

There are some basic rules to remember whenever one uses farm equipment.

1) Never operate machinery without understanding how it works.
2) Make sure the equipment you use is in good working order.
3) Never operate any machinery after drinking any alcoholic beverages, smoking dope, or using any other drugs including drugs such as antihistimines, cold tablets or tranquilizers.
4) Never work when you are tired.
5) The old proverb "haste makes waste" is especially true in using farm machinery.
6) Never fix or change machinery while the machine is on.
7) Dress appropriately to the kind of work being done. Especially dangerous are bell-bottoms or similar loose-fitting clothes.
8) Long hair should always be tied back or braided, and the braid kept from dangling free.

TRACTORS. The tractor is the most common piece of farm equipment and can be one of the most dangerous. Tractors are like cars: they operate best when they are maintained well, and safest when they are driven carefully. Safe practices to remember when driving a tractor include the following:

1) Reduce speed when turning or applying the brakes.
2) A tractor will tip over at the speed of 8 mph if one of the wheels hits a hole.
3) Remember to turn the tractor off when you dismount.
4) When driving up and down a steep hill, you should drive at a diagonal to the top of the hill.
5) When plowing on a hill, you should plow downwards.

A great deal of farm equipment is attached to a tractor by a hitch to a draw bar, and often by a drive shaft to the power take-off. Any load hitched to the draw bar should be kept as low as possible. Be particularly careful on a sidehill. When pulling a loaded wagon downhill, it is important to remember the extra force behind the tractor. Start off in first or second, and stay in that gear until you reach level ground. Then pulling a plow or a harrow, the greatest danger is falling off the tractor and being run over. When pulling balers, rakes and other haying equipment, it is important to wear tight clothing and to be sure the power take-off has a shield over it.

WOOD-CUTTING TOOLS. Other machines and tools often found on the farm are to cut wood. The ax is a dangerous tool to a person who does not know how to use it. Learn from someone who knows. Make sure no part of your body is in line with the spot at which you are swinging the ax—this mostly applies to your legs and your head. (With a double-bitted ax, you run the risk of being hit on the backswing or on the follow-through.)

A chain saw is a great machine if you are careful. It can cut your work down considerably; however, it can also cut off a hand or a leg. Follow the safety rules list in the beginning of the article.

GUNS. Another common tool on the farm are guns. There are many good books on guns and many people who are knowledgeable about them. Consult with these people and books when you are learning to use a gun. Never leave a gun loaded if you are not going to shoot it immediately. Know the range of your ammunition and know what you are shooting at and what's beind and around it.

Finally, the extension agent is a source of valuable information, especially in providing booklets on farm equipment.

Below is a chart showing the different causes of accidents on the farm.

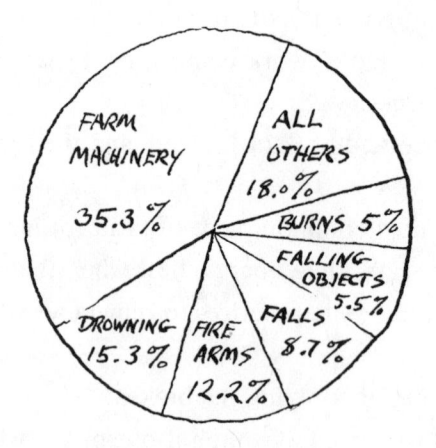

Living in the country is great, farming is fun, but safe farming is the healthiest.

Scott Lyman
assisted by Murray B. Hunt

NOTES

HOW TO MINIMIZE FIRE DANGER

House fires are a distinct health hazard for people who choose to live in heated wooden houses far away from fire plugs. Fortunately, few people were physically hurt by the many country fires that burned this last winter. But my experience was close enough to death to jar my awareness. The following checklist is based on the experiences/observations/suggestions of several people who built their homes and then watched them burn down. Many points can only be used when you are building or rebuilding; others involve minor alterations; the rest are things to be conscious of at anytime.

HOUSE CONSTRUCTION AND LAYOUT:
Avoid flues: put firebreaks between studs in walls; put doors at the bottom of stairways.
Connect rooms with closeable doors.
When possible use fire-retarding materials in walls and ceilings. Sheetrock is ugly, but you can panel over it with almost the same effect.
Provide useable exits to the outside on each floor—two if possible. An 18" x 24" window with a 10 foot drop won't do.
Build separate structures for fuel storage, workshops, barn. In Vermont you have to bundle up to get firewood no matter how close it is to the back door. Also fire insurance companies specify fifty feet between house and barn. They know how to save their money.

WOOD HEAT
One big stove is safer, more efficient than several small ones.
Store wood, tinder, trash away from stove.
Fireproof the stove area below, behind, and above to contain sparks. Asbestos is best, since it insulates as well. If another combination of materials is used, put metal sheet facing stove backed by unburnable insulating material.
Straight stove pipes stay cleaner than ones with elbows. In any case, clean pipes of soot and creosote once a month during the winter. These residues are still flammable; on a cold night with a hot stove they will ignite in the pipe.
Seal stoves and pipes. Cracks, holes, and loose fittings can allow sparks to escape, as well as causing poor draft and build-up of pipe residues.
Insulate pipes, especially near walls, ceilings. This (1) protects the walls and ceilings from getting hot, and (2) prevents flue gases from cooling enough in the pipe to inhibit draft and deposit more soot and creosote.
Check chimneys for crumbly mortar. Scrape lining annually. Line new chimneys with clay tile. Avoid venting more than one stove in each flue.

HOW TO MINIMIZE FIRE DANGER

Avoid burning trash, especially glossy magazines, in stoves, since trash creates much soot and fly-ash. Avoid burning the coniferous woods (pine, spruce, fir, cedar, hemlock, etc.), since they create excessive creosote.

GAS AND OIL APPLIANCES

Avoid unvented oil and gas heaters.

Do *not* use oil "pot burner" heaters. They can be deadly if not kept perfectly clean. Because they are illegal in many places, they are cheap heat in junk stores.

Protect oil and gas pipes from physical injury. Building codes require oil pipes to be buried.

Place gas ranges, heaters, and water heaters away from drafts that would blow out the pilot lights. Keep pilot burners and tubes clean.

Check gas smells immediately.

Know where oil and gas shut-off valves are at the tanks.

ELECTRIC WIRING AND FIXTURES

Wire installation details are important. Protect insulation from injury: run it along ceiling-wall corners when possible; don't set cable staples so hard that they break the outer cable jacket; run wire in accessible crawlspace, attic, cellar, rather than hidden in walls.

Over-estimate future circuit loads.

Frequently check motors in unattended equipment (furnaces, fans, compressors, pumps) for heating. As equipment gets older and less efficient, motors work harder. The greatest cause of electrical related fires is hot motors.

If lights blink or dim a lot, find out why. A poor connection or over-loaded wire can heat dangerously without blowing a fuse.

Install main switch near a fire exit or outside. In any case know where it is.

Avoid using extension cords and double plugs.

Use ground wire on tools and heavy appliances.

KEROSENE, GAS, AND GASOLINE LAMPS; CANDLES

Store kerosene and gasoline in vented, shaded containers *outside* of buildings.

Keep mantles in good condition; keep Coleman (and similar) lamp generators clean.

Do not use cracked globes.

Do not use wooden or unstable candle holders.

Avoid leaving lamps or candles unattended.

Try to make lamps kid-proof: fastened wall and ceiling lamps are better than easily knocked over table lamps.

BARNS

Decentralize: if possible, keep animals, hay, and equipment in separate, unconnected buildings.

Ventilate hay and grain storage areas. Wet organic matter can heat very quickly; therefore,

NEVER put anything but brittle-dry hay in the barn, and
Store manure in a separate shelter.
Keep wiring and fixtures high, protected from injury and moisture.

LIGHTNING

You should get protection if your house is in a precipitous or open place; if there are tall trees near your house, they should be wired to protect the house.

Check electric system, phone line for good ground connections. Antennas should have a lightning arrester and a good ground. A good ground is a copper or galvanized (not aluminum) pipe driven into *permanently* moist earth.

FIRE EXTINGUISHERS

Dry chemical is best over all, except in a barn where its use on a limited fire could poison feed; there a CO_2 extinguisher would be as effective and non-toxic.

Water is only good for wood, paper, grass fires. It tends to spread oil, chemical, or electrical fires.

Try to have one extinguisher near (but not behind) each stove, on each floor, and easily accessable to sleeping area.

HOUSEKEEPING CONSCIOUSNESS

Get rid of gasoline/kerosene/paint/oil soaked rags.

Keep solvents and household chemicals well covered. Lye, for example, heats rapidly when water drips into the can.

Don't store trash, tinder, or wood near stoves.

Store ashes in a fireproof container away from house.

A WORD ABOUT BONFIRES

A burning permit is free. It protects you from a fine, and assures you that the fire warden thinks that the day is still and damp enough for you to burn safely. It also lets the fire department know that you are burning, gives them a jump on location if your fire gets away, and gives them advance notice in case someone else (who doesn't know your plans) sees your smoke and reports a fire in your locality.

Start a small pile and add to it, rather than a large one.

Burn downwind from trees.

Make a moat of bare or damp ground around the fire.

Have water, broom, shovel, rake available.

Do not burn in even a slight breeze.

Do not burn alone.

WHAT TO DO IF A FIRE STARTS

Feel doors before opening—if a door is hot and you open it, you could be hit with a six-foot-high blowtorch. If you must use a warm door, open it slooooowly.

Close windows and doors behind you—that will slow the progress of the fire.

Use your judgment. If there is a chance that this is a major fire, make sure that everybody knows what is happening before you battle it.

Turn off power, gas, and oil at tanks.

For localized oil, gas, and electric fires, use dry chemical or CO_2 extinguishers, or anything (like blankets) that will smother the flames. Play extinguisher at *base* of flames.

Localized wood, paper, or fabric fires can be cooled with water. Anything dense, like stuffed chairs or books, should be thoroughly soaked.

Fat fires on ranges can be killed with a layer of sodium bicarbonate (baking soda).

There are a number of specific pamphlets available from the U.S. Dept. of Agriculture on house fireproofing, wiring, lightning protection, safe hay storage, and chimney construction. There are several good books on house construction and safe wiring listed in the *Last Whole Earth Catalogue*. I will try to prepare a bibliography for the next edition of this book.

Owen Lindsay

PREVENTION OF FIRE

A neat house seldom burns. Accumulated trash and general clutter often provides fuel for a fire that would not spread otherwise.

Heating equipment should also be kept clean and properly adjusted. Dirty oil burners account for many fires and much smoke damage.

While layers of newspapers can be effective insulation, unless the wall or ceiling has a fire-resistant finish (such as gypsum board) the fire hazard is extremely high. Walls, if insulated in this manner, should have fire stops (wood barriers at intervals to prevent "flue effect" in case a fire does start).

Electrical wiring can be a fire hazard if the insulation is worn, brittle, or frayed or if the wiring is overloaded. Never use pennies or extra-large fuses in place of the proper fuse size. The extra current produces heat which deteriorates the insulation. Never run extension cords over nails, etc., or under rugs. An extension cord should never be a permanent part of the wiring. When the insulation becomes worn or brittle, discard the extension cord.

Improper use of solvents or cleaning fluids causes many fires. Solvents should not be used in confined places. Gasoline, benzene, or other flammable fluids should not be used for any indoor cleaning such as clothing, furnishings, or floors.

Oily rags can ignite spontaneously in a very short period of time. They should be kept in a tightly closed metal container or disposed of by burying or burning.

PUTTING OUT FIRES THAT HAVE STARTED

Extinguishing a small blaze promptly can often prevent a major fire. A bucket of water kept handy can extinguish a fire in a wastebasket, etc., but many fires do not involve wood, paper or cloth alone, so water is not always suitable. If the fuel is oil, grease, paint, or varnish, water will probably only spread it. The best extinguisher for this type of fire would be a commercial extinguisher of the dry chemical type. It should have a capacity of at least 2½ pounds (U.L. rating of 4B, C). This type is also suitable where electrical equipment is involved.

Baking soda can be valuable for extinguishing fires involving grease, oil, paint or varnish. It can also work for wastebaskets, ash trays or unupholstered furniture. It is wise to keep a supply of at least one pound of baking soda available at all times.

A blanket or coat (wool is best) can often be used to smother a fire. This is especially useful to put out a clothing fire.

If a fire becomes large it is important to have an adequate supply of water. Ponds can often be constructed for this purpose. They have many other benefits also. Help in constructing a farm pond is available through the local Soil Conservation Service Division of the United States Department of Agriculture. Construction should include a frost-proof hydrant for a fire hose. The SCS or the local fire department should be able to help on this detail. In lieu of the frost-proof hydrant, a floating plug can be used to provide access through the ice in winter. A brine-filled barrel or plastic garbage can could provide a one-time access by merely smashing a hole through the bottom to insert a suction hose.

Milo Moore

NOTES

SIMPLE BURIAL

Death is a universal experience that few people really like to think about. The emotional impact of death on the survivors is always a crushing one, and it is usually made even more oppressive by the financial burden that death in the United States imposes. The cost of an average American funeral is between $1,500.00 and $2,000.00, and prices in the three to four thousand dollar range are not at all unusual.

There is no other area of purchased service in which the consumer has less real choice in selecting a product than in the funeral industry. Mark Twain put it neatly:

> There's one thing in this world which a person don't say: "I'll look around a little and if I can't do better I'll come back and take it." That's a coffin. And you take your poor man, and if you work him right, he'll bust himself on a single layout.

The idea is still held by many Americans that the more money that is spent on a person's funeral, the more loved and respected he was in life. Thus funeral directors are only too happy to encourage purchases of burial vaults, caskets with inner springs, and (in "funeralese") "restorative services for the creation of a lasting memory picture." There is no other country in the world where corpses are so commonly creamed, wired, and stuffed so that they may be viewed and their "life-like" appearance commented on.

THE ALTERNATIVES

I. MEMORIAL SERVICES. Fortunately there are some alternatives to these barbaric practices. Many people are realizing that there can be real meaning and comfort in a simple burial and memorial service where the physical remains are not dwelled upon. A gathering is held after the burial to emphasize the beautiful and joyful aspects of the person's life rather than to center on his death. Funeral directors do (when pushed) handle such services, but the overall costs will still run in the five to seven hundred dollar range, depending on the mood of the director.

II. MEMORIAL SOCIETIES. In some instances, collective pressure can help bring down the high cost of dying. Consumer-controlled organizations called "Memorial Societies" have become much more popular over the past few years, and well over 300,000 people in the United States hold membership in one of these groups.

Generally, a memorial society helps its members obtain simple, dignified and economical funeral arrangements through advance planning. Collective pressure is brought against funeral homes, and members contract with cooperating funeral directors to provide the desired services at death.

The usual one-time membership fee to join a society is $10.00. Further information on the philosophy and services of these citizens groups can be obtained from the following organizations in New England:

> A. Memorial Society of New England
> 25 Monmouth Street
> Brookline, Massachusetts 02146 (covers Vermont)
>
> B. Memorial Society of New Hampshire
> 274 Pleasant Street
> Concord, New Hampshire 03301
>
> C. Greater New Haven Memorial Society
> 60 Connolly Parkway
> Hamden, Connecticut 06514
>
> D. Memorial Society of Connecticut
> 10 Lyons Plains Road
> Westport, Connecticut 06882

For information on Memorial Societies in other parts of the country, write to:

> Funeral and Memorial Societies
> 59 E. Van Buren Street
> Chicago, Illinois 60605

III. HOME BURIAL. Under Vermont law, it is not necessary to embalm the body of a person who has died in Vermont if the body is to be buried in the state. (If the health officer determines that it is a threat to the public health, he can order it to be embalmed and/or immediately buried, entombed, or cremated.) But if the body is to be *taken across a state line* by *common carrier,* it may have to be embalmed. In addition, it is still possible under Vermont law for a person who is not a licensed funeral director to handle a burial and to bury a body in a place other than an already established public cemetery. These are the steps that must be taken:

> A. A plot of land, *owned by the family,* should be set aside for burial purposes. The Town health regulations should be reviewed, and it should be made certain that the burial site *will not cause a public health problem.* When in doubt, the Town health officer should be contacted.
>
> B. When a death occurs, *a death certificate must be signed by a physician within 24 hours.* It should be delivered to the family of the deceased person or to the person who has charge of the body within 36 hours.
>
> C. The *death certificate should be filed at once with the Town Clerk,* who will issue a "burial-transit or removal permit." This certificate serves as either a permission for burial (when the burial is to take place in the town where the death occurred), or a permission for removal and burial (if the body is to be moved and disposed of in some other place). In either case, such information as time, place, and manner of disposal must be stated on the permit.

D. The law says that at burial "the bottom of the outside coffin shall be at least five feet below the natural surface of the ground, excepting infants under four years . . . where the bottom of the coffin enclosing them shall be at least three and one half feet below the natural surface of the ground."*

E. During the first week of the month following the burial, the *burial-transit or removal permit must be delivered to the clerk of the Town* in which the burial takes place.

IV. CREMATION. Cremation is another alternative. In Vermont, this method may also be handled by the immediate family or friends. The procedure to obtain permission for cremation is as follows:

A. A *death certificate should be signed by a physician* and a *burial-transit or removal permit should be obtained from the Town Clerk.* (See section "B" and "C" under HOME BURIAL).

B. The person in charge of the body must obtain an "Examiner's Permit to Cremate a Dead Human Body" from the Chief Medical Examiner or Regional Medical Examiner serving his area. This person *must keep this permit in his possession for 3 years.*

C. Again, the *burial-transit or removal permit should be returned to the Town Clerk* after cremation.

There is only one crematorium in Vermont: Mount Pleasant in St. Johnsbury. They have a rule that the body must be enclosed in a wooden container. The total cost is $66.00 and the ashes are mailed to the family for disposal. Burial of the ashes may take place on land owned by the immediate family of the deceased.

There *are* other crematoriums that are close to Vermont. Montreal, Boston, and Albany all have such facilities; in these cities, however, cremation must be handled through a funeral director.

REFERENCES: *A Manual of Simple Burial* by Ernest Morgan, the Celo Press; Burnsville, North Carolina ($1.00).

This is an excellent little book that discusses the subject in more detail. A list of memorial societies is included as well as an extensive section on anatomical gifts.

The *Whole Earth Catalog* says: "As a part of the literature of funerals (this book) is like a living rosebud in a bouquet of plastic flowers."

David Osgood

*Vermont Title 18, Chapter 121, Section 5319 (b)

NOTES

BACK TO THE LAND: POINT

I don't speak for all farmer's wives, only for myself. I'd like to try to tell you how I feel about our lives, our similarities, and in a few cases, our resentments with young people who also have returned to the land.

The world I know, of nature and of people, is full of cycles. I feel that you've come full circle, around to some of what we are and what we've always been. You, of course, might think of us as being two steps behind you. Chances are we are more alike than we are different. At least we're more like you than many others you've known and have left.

We, too, have found our riches in the environment (human and natural) in which we live. We've willed ourselves to a standard of consumption less than many others. This has been a choice for us. For many others who farm there was no choice. They were stranded on the farm with no place else to go. We could have jobs in town but we'd have to give up too much.

We feel a real sense of accomplishment in our work here. We can see "progress" in the amount of milk a cow makes, the yield from a corn field we've raised, and in a calf that was sick and is now well. Our labors are meaningful and rewarding. Sometimes there are too many. It bothers us if someone thoughtlessly adds to our work by forgetting to close a gate or tramping down a field of hay.

We, too, get very concerned about the role of technology in our world, on our farm. As our tractors get bigger, we have a feeling we're selling out our way of life to technology. I remember my grandfather whose job on the farm was to carry milk in pails from the barn to the milkhouse and to wash the milk things. He had a meaningful job. Today both jobs are done automatically by a pipeline and a washing system. My grandfather wouldn't have a task on our farm he could do.

We know the farm is the best place to raise children. There still are opportunities here to teach them self-reliance, a kinship to their environment, a love for all living things and skills for expression in a cooperative venture. We don't really worry about where they'll fit in when they're grown. We think they'll fit into their world because they are in tune with nature and with man. The skills and knowledge we can share have meaning to them.

We don't have a great deal of time to worry about things off the farm. Our days are very long. If you think we're not concerned about social wrongs, it's because we simply don't see them.

We don't get excited about women's rights. We've long been partners with our husbands, making the major decisions together. In a way we feel we were liberated a long time ago, just as our husbands were.

We love our land and consider it our real wealth. We feel very protective of it and its inhabitants. We've gotten angry with people who have offended it: bow-and-arrow hunters who leave wounded animals, snowmobilers who run over little trees we've just planted to prevent erosion, and campers who litter or leave fires.

We have a lot of skills and knowledge you might find helpful. If you'll ask us, we will tell you, even if we chuckle a little over your not knowing. It's nice to have someone consider what we know to be valuable.

There is one thing we resent a little about you. Sometimes I think you're living off the land as a diversion. As soon as you tire of the hard work, the long hours, your husband's premature aging, you can and will cut out. I guess I'm saying I won't take you too seriously until you show us differently. But who knows? Maybe once you've tried it you will find you do like it. Maybe you'll feel the advantages are worth whatever your next diversion might have been.

Jeannie—a farmer's wife

BACK TO THE LAND: COUNTERPOINT

I take great issue with many of the statements in *Back to the Land: Point*, and with the overall somewhat questioning acceptance of persons who newly decide on a life style close to the land (is a way of life good only if one sticks to it for a long, long time; and only if it requires long hours of hard physical labor?).

I speak for myself, too—not as a wife, or mother, though these roles have been mine. I speak for myself: whole female.

I agree about the "cycles" of life, but not about the "back." Within these United States I hope there is no such thing as "going back." People have to grow and develop: i.e. move forward. The status-quo, if there is any such thing, and going back, are the death-knell to an alive democracy and to any individual who is part of it. Reformation and renaissance are necessarily constant phenomena—not just periods of history (my school teachers were wrong!). I'm very sure of this.

I do get excited about women's rights: about concrete objectives like equal wages for equal work, equal job opportunities, fair property legislation, and other matters where women have been subject to injustice over many centuries of history.

That's right: so many Americans "don't see" the "social wrongs" and, therefore, are not concerned. The real world frontiers are no longer geographical: they are social. Those who advance to the land do so, I think and hope, in the context of both seeing and coping with these frontiers: basically, the acceptance of all people (each person) as dignified and worthy of human justice.

Real wealth is not just land: it's more nearly defined (I think) as working for and having one's fair share of what the good earth can produce for everyone (fairly shared), having one's physical place in the sun and rain, and living out to the fullest all the positive feeling relationships one can have with fellow creatures.

Joan Babbott

VERMONT LAWS

INTRODUCTION. To the disappointment of some and the relief of many, the "hippie" invasion of Vermont of the summer of 1971 never materialized. The first edition of this article was designed to serve as a guideline for those summer visitors. Although that immediate need is no longer at hand, knowledge of the law and of one's rights is an invaluable tool.

Although many Vermonters adopt a live-and-let-live attitude, it is reasonable to expect that not all Vermonters will welcome visitors and newcomers with open arms—particularly those whose appearance typifies the new life style. The poor and the young are particularly vulnerable to police scrutiny. They are the ones least likely to know their rights, and least able to enforce them.

This article will focus on Vermont law. In an age of increasing use of uniform and model laws, Vermont statutes may resemble those of other states. But they are different, and the laws of each state must be examined individually.

Reference is sometimes made to United States Supreme Court decisions, and these, of course, have nation-wide applicability. Even this is deceptive, however, since a state may continue to enforce a law virtually identical to that of another state which has been held unconstitutional until specifically enjoined by a court.

This article is not an exhaustive survey of Vermont law. To the contrary, it will outline only certain areas of the law where young people may be expected to run afoul. The purpose is not to give any definitive legal advice on specific legal problems. It is rather to alert the newcomer to certain peculiarities of Vermont law so that he can guide his conduct accordingly.

Neither is this article a political tract—political in the broad sense. Few need be reminded that civil rights are not self-enforcing. It is self-evident that in any given situation an individual has to determine for himself whether to acquiesce in the command of a law enforcement officer (L.E.O.), or to attempt to enforce what he believes are his civil rights. However admirable fighting for the principle may be, the choice is often between fighting and enjoying one's liberty. Enforcement of one's rights takes time, energy, and often money.

For example, the United States Supreme Court recently declared unconstitutional a Cincinnati ordinance which made it a criminal offense for three or more persons to assemble on a sidewalk and there conduct themselves in a manner annoying to persons passing by. *Coates v. City of Cincinnati*, 402 U.S. 611 (1971). The Court said that the standard of "annoying" conduct was unconstitutionally vague; "men of ordinary intelligence must guess at its meaning." A Vermont statute forbids "unnecessary and offensive noise" between sunset and sunrise. Based on the *Coates* decision, the Vermont statutes may well be unconstitutional, but *Coates* will probably not deter a L.E.O. from making an arrest when he feels the statute is being violated, and final adjudication will take several months at least.

Finally, the article will cover only passive activity, that which is involved in day-to-day living. Specialized conduct, e.g. demonstrations, will not be covered. For any activity in which confrontation with the law is anticipated, prior consultation with an attorney is recommended.

(A) CAMPING. A Vermont statute, passed by last year's (1971) General Assembly, prohibits camping overnight in any public area not designated for that purpose, including highway rest areas. 19 V.S.A. sec. 1504 (b). What actually constitutes camping is an open question: setting up a tent may be considered camping, while simply sleeping in the open or in a sleeping bag may not be.

(B) ASSAULT AND DISORDERLY CONDUCT. At its 1972 session, the Vermont General Assembly re-structured the criminal code with respect to "offenses against persons and property." The law now distinguishes between "simple assault," "aggravated assault" and reckless endangerment of another person.

(1) Simple assault: attempt to cause or causing bodily injury; negligently causing bodily injury with a deadly weapon; physical menacing. 13 V.S.A. sec. 1023 (as amended, Acts of 1971, No. 222 Sec. 2).

(2) Aggravated assault: attempting to cause or causing serious bodily injury "under circumstances manifesting extreme indifference to the value of human life"; attempting to cause or causing bodily injury with a deadly weapon; *drugging another person without his consent* (for other than medical purposes); causing physical injury with intent to prevent a L.E.O. from performing his duty. 13 V.S.A. sec. 1024 (as amended, Acts of 1971, No. 222 Sec. 3).

(3) Reckless endangerment is "conduct which places or may place another person in danger of death or serious bodily injury," and includes pointing a gun at someone whether or not it is loaded. 13 V.S.A. sec. 1025 (as amended, Acts. of 1971, No. 222 Sec. 4).

(4) Disorderly conduct consists of the following acts "with intent to cause public inconvenience, or annoyance, or recklessly creating a risk thereof":

    (a) engaging in fighting or in violent, tumultuous, or threatening behavior.

    (b) making unreasonable noise;

    (c) using abusive or obscene language in a public place;

    (d) disturbing a lawful assembly;

    (e) obstructing vehicles or pedestrian traffic. 13 V.S.A. sec. 1026 (as amended, Acts of 1971, No. 222 Sec. 5).

Under the *Coates* opinion, the entire disorderly conduct section may be unconstitutional. Certainly the "unreasonable noise" provision is extremely vague. In view of the recent United States Supreme Court decision of *Gooding v. Wilson*, ___U.S. ___(1972) (40 U.S.L.W. 4329, March 23, 1972), the obscenity provision may ultimately prove unconstitutional.

(5) Damaging property—whether real estate or personal property—is prohibited, 13 V.S.A. sec. 3701 (as amended, Acts of 1971, No. 222 Sec. 6).

(6) The old statue prohibiting firing guns, blowing horns or other "unnecessary or offensive noise" between sunset and sunrise was somehow preserved by the legislature. 13 V.S.A. sec. 1022. The standard of unnecessary or offensive noise may well be unconstitutionally vague.

VERMONT LAWS

(C) DRUGS. Unauthorized possession of drugs, including marijuana, depressants, stimulants, narcotics and hallucinogenics are crimes. Don't be misled by the rural nature of Vermont. Vermont has a narcotics squad which makes effective use of entrapment to make arrests. The long-haired stranger who gives you a ride or whom you meet at a party may turn out to be an agent. 18 V.S.A. sec. 4224 (as amended, Acts of 1971, No. 199, Sec. 16).

(D) HITCH-HIKING. As of this writing, there is no general state-wide law prohibiting hitch-hiking. However, a new statute which will become effective March 1, 1973 does state that "No person may stand *within the portion of the highway right of way* used for highway purposes for the purpose of soliciting a ride, . . ." (emphasis added). Acts of 1971, No. 258, Sec. 3, enacting 23 V.S.A. sec. 1056. In this writer's opinion, the statute prohibits soliciting a ride only if standing in the road; hitch-hiking while standing on the curb is permissible.

Presumably, towns still have the authority to regulate pedestrian traffic. 24 V.S.A. sec. 2291. Such power exists at present and town anti-hitch-hiking ordinances are in effect. There is no substitute for checking the ordinance of the town you are in. But in some towns—Burlington for example—hitch-hiking is prohibited only if standing in the roadway. Burlington Ordinances, Title 17, sec. 3557.

(E) TRESPASS. In legislating against use of snowmobiles on private land without the owner's consent, the General Assembly modified the criminal trespass law to prohibit *entry* on private land if notice is given either orally by the owner, agent, or an L.E.O., or by signs or placards. The statute does not apply to persons "entering on foot solely for the purpose of *lawfully* taking fish or game." 13 V.S.A. sec. 3705 (as amended, Acts of 1971, No. 229, Sec. 1). Presumably, merely walking across private property, without doing any damage to it, is no longer a criminal act.

(F) VAGRANCY. Though limited in its application, Vermont's anti-vagrancy statute may be employed to harass young visitors. Implicitly, a vagrant is defined as a "transient person, roving from place to place, and living without visible means of support." This status is by itself insufficient to charge a person with an offense. In addition, it must be coupled with one of the following forms of forbidden conduct:

(1) begging

(2) riding or attempting to ride on a freight train without permission

(3) entering or attempting to enter a dwelling house, barn, or building without permission of the owners or occupants. 13 V.S.A. sec. 3901.

Also:

(4) remaining in a building after being asked to leave, and

(5) kindling a fire on or near another person's land. 13 V.S.A. sec. 3905.

There are serious doubts as to the constitutionality of this statute. The overt activity is forbidden only to persons who are essentially homeless and without means of support. Presumably a person who is not a transient, who begs money, would not be subject to the penalties of the statute.

(G) WELFARE. Most single, young people will be eligible, if at all, for a state-funded aid program known as General Assistance (G.A.). 33 V.S.A. sec. 3001 et seq. Others who are disabled or who have children may be eligible for federally subsidized programs.

General Assistance is not munificent, but is better than nothing. Funds will be provided for food, shelter, and other basic necessities as required. Basic eligibility requirements are need and lack of any potential financial resources.

In theory, all residency eligibility requirements for the receipt of welfare have been declared unconstitutional by the United States Supreme Court. *Shapiro v. Thompson,* 394 U.S. 618 (1969). This means that a person cannot be denied assistance because of any statute or regulation which required him to be a resident of the state for any length of time. The Vermont general assistance statute permits the department to refuse aid to an individual when the commissioner "has reason to believe" that he came into the state for the purpose of receiving general assistance. This is simply a residency statute and should be unconstitutional, but in practical terms constitutional protection may be an illusion.

At least one state supreme court has held that programs which are totally funded by the state—as in General Assistance—are not subject to the *Shapiro v. Thompson* doctrine.

Although the statute requires that emergency assistance be granted regardless of other circumstances, bureaucratic stalling may create hardship. If an emergency exists, insist on your right to assistance. If denial persists, seek legal help. Unfortunately, however, emergency assistance may consist of a one-way bus ticket out of the state.

Finally, the Department of Social Welfare may require that an applicant be actively engaged in looking for employment, and deny assistance if this is not the case. In this event, there is no avoiding seeking legal help.

(H) ABORTION. Abortions performed by licensed physicians are no longer unlawful in Vermont. *Jacqueline R. v. Leahy,* 129 Vt. ___ (1972). The Vermont Supreme Court decision left somewhat vague the question as to the time limitation within which an abortion may be legally performed. The Attorney General has opined that the operation must be performed in the first twelve weeks of pregnancy. This seems to be a somewhat restrictive interpretation of the decision.

(I) MISCELLANEOUS. 1. In 1971 some Vermont towns passed ordinances under their authority to regulate public nuisances to limit, license, or prohibit assemblages of diverse sizes and sundry purposes. As an initial matter anyone wishing to hold a large gathering should make discreet inquiries as to whether a local ordinance exists, and, if so, what it requires.

Since the right to assemble is protected by the First Amendment of the United States Constitution and by the Vermont Constitution, a local ordinance may be unconstitutional, either on its face or in application. However, statutes requiring permits for meetings based on objective standards have generally been upheld by the courts.

2. Vermont has special laws protecting trees. 13 V.S.A. sec. 3606. Marking or damaging trees is prohibited. It is also forbidden to take certain rare plants. 13 V.S.A. sec. 3613, 3614.

VERMONT LAWS

3. The Vermont Constitution guarantees the right to fish in all "boatable" water and other waters not held privately. As a rule of thumb, this means that all good-sized rivers and lakes are open to the public, and public access ways exist if you take the trouble to look around for them. If you are 12 years old or older, fishing requires a license which can be obtained at any Town Clerk's office.

(J) RIGHT TO COUNSEL. Vermont law provides for assignment of counsel to "needy persons" who are charged with a "serious crime." 13 V.S.A. sec. 5234 (Acts of 1971, No. 161, Sec. 6). A needy person is one who is unable, without undue hardship, to provide for full payment of an attorney. A serious crime is one punishable by more than sixty (60) days in jail or a fine of more than one thousand dollars ($1,000). In addition, the United States Supreme Court has recently held that an individual facing *any* imprisonment must be assigned counsel if he cannot afford it. *James v. Strange,* ___ U.S. ___, 40 U.S.L.W. 4711 (June 12, 1972).

Experience has shown that some Vermont judges are reluctant to assign counsel to indigent persons. Their refusal has usually been premised on their assertion that the individual is not truly indigent, although some accused persons have reportedly been told that the crime was not serious enough. In view of this history, it is important to ascertain exactly what one is being charged with and the maximum possible penalty. *Ask*! Although the courts now have the express duty to make diligent inquiry, if you consider yourself indigent, state that fact and request assignment of counsel. If in doubt, make the request anyway. The law now expressly provides that release on bail does not necessarily disqualify a person from being needy.

Logically, if one cannot be imprisoned after trial without counsel being assigned, then one cannot be imprisoned before trial, in lieu of bail, without assignment of counsel. This has yet to be tested, however. The law is clear that one is entitled to assigned counsel at every stage of the proceeding at which there is a right to privately retained counsel.

If you believe you are unlawfully being denied counsel, contact the Vermont chapter of the American Civil Liberties Union, Craig Murray, Executive Director (802) 223-6304.

Michael Kupersmith

NOTES

SOME HUMAN RESOURCES IN VERMONT

UNITED COMMUNITY SERVICES
Burlington, Vermont 05401
"Directory of Human Resources for the Chittenden County Area"
- 1 – 25 copies 75 cents each
- 25 – 500 copies 50 cents each
- 500 – 1,000 copies 30 cents each

Checks should be made out to: Community Council of Greater Burlington, Inc.

This directory is essentially a list of most of the major human resource agencies of the state. It is an excellent listing.

COMMUNITY MENTAL HEALTH SERVICES
State Office Building
Montpelier, Vermont 05602 (802) 223-2311, Ext. 286

This program is responsible for the supervision of eleven mental health agencies throughout the state. These agencies are reimbursed for two-thirds of their net operating expenses by the Vermont Department of Mental Health.

PLANNED PARENTHOOD OF VERMONT, INC.
260 College Street (802) 863-6263
Burlington, Vermont 05401 (802) 863-5740

A. Educational services are free. The fee for clinical services is based on an individual's ability to pay.
B. Educational Outreach—Upon request speakers from Planned Parenthood will talk with groups about methods of contraception, will show contraceptive devices and perhaps use a movie. Planned Parenthood speakers are also able to answer questions about venereal disease.
C. Under 21 Club—A program of Planned Parenthood in Burlington.
D. Clinics—
   1. Personal interview to answer questions about contraceptive methods. An individual may choose not to accept any contraceptive devices.
   2. Pelvic examination by physician.
   3. Pap test.
   4. Optional test for gonorrhea.

VERMONT LEGAL AID SOCIETY, INC.
191 College Street
Burlington, Vermont 05401 (802) 863-2871

This office will handle civil cases for people who cannot afford their own attorneys. There are specific financial eligibility requirements.

CONSUMER INFORMATION CLEARINGHOUSE
University of Vermont Extension Service
Morrill Hall
Burlington, Vermont 05401 (802) 656-2990

Brings current information (by publication, press, TV, radio) to consumers in Vermont relative to products and services, buying schemes and frauds, pending and enacted legislation of interest to consumers, government agencies and other sources of help; publishes "Dollars and Decisions" newsletter bimonthly, free to Vermont consumers on request, and works cooperatively with the Vermont Consumer Protection Bureau. All services available to everyone free of charge.

VERMONT CONSUMER PROTECTION BUREAU
P.O. Box 981
94 Church Street
Burlington, Vermont 05401 (802) 864-0111

The Consumer Protection Bureau attempts to adjust complaints and eliminate unfair and deceptive trade practices in commerce within the state. There are no fees, as the office is a part of the State of Vermont Attorney General's Office. Jurisdiction is limited only by existence of other more appropriate agencies to handle particular concerns.

VERMONT DEPARTMENT OF HEALTH
115 Colchester Avenue
Burlington, Vermont 05401 (802) 862-5701, Ext. 58

Call the Office of Information at extension 58 or speak to a local public health nurse for information on free services in your area.

THE UNIVERSITY OF VERMONT EXTENSION SERVICE
Burlington, Vermont 05401

Services are free of charge. There is an extension service office in each county coordinating with state offices at the University of Vermont. County agents in agriculture, home economics, youth and 4-H, and area resource development are available to answer questions, or call upon various specialists available to them for assistance. A large variety of printed brieflets is available from the Extension Service. For example:

> "Understanding Vermont Soils"
> "The Home Vegetable Garden"
> "How To Do Batik"
> "Leaking Faucets"

SOME HUMAN RESOURCES IN VERMONT

VISITING NURSE ASSOCIATIONS located in areas of denser population may provide free well child clinics. Children receive physical examinations for normal growth and free immunizations are provided. Visiting nurses make home visits to the sick and fees are based on the type of service given and on the individual's ability to pay.

VERMONT DEPARTMENT OF SOCIAL WELFARE
Family Services Division
39 Pearl Street
Burlington, Vermont 05401   (802) 863-4587

Through its Family Services division, the department provides financial assistance, medical assistance, and social work services to the aged, blind, disabled, and needy families with dependent children.

Administers emergency food, housing, clothing and fuel and related programs and services, under a general assistance program, and also administers Medical and Food Stamp programs.

Hours are 8 to 4:30 weekdays. There is a 24-hour answering service.

NATIONAL WELFARE RIGHTS ORGANIZATION
c/o Office of Economic Opportunity
St. Albans, Vermont 05478   (802) 524-4446

The function of this national organization is to defend the rights of welfare recipients all over the country.

CIVIL DEFENSE
Vermont Department of Safety
Montpelier, Vermont 05602

Will provide first aid training and free informational materials to groups.

MEDICAL AND HEALTH CARE INFORMATION-CENTER
Mary Fletcher Unit—Medical Center Hospital
Burlington, Vermont 05401   (802) 864-0454

Sponsored by Medical Center Hospital of Vermont, the Chittenden County Medical Society and the University of Vermont Medical College, the Center provides 24-hour, comprehensive, health care information and state-wide referral services to the general public.

FREE VENEREAL DISEASE CLINIC
4th Floor Arnold Building
DeGoesbriand Unit
Medical Center Hospital
Burlington, Vermont 05401   (802) 864-0454

Open Tuesdays and Thursdays from 4:00—6:00 P.M. It provides diagnosis, testing and treatment—all absolutely free.

PEOPLE'S FREE CLINIC
165–167 Saint Paul Street
Burlington, Vermont 05401 (802) 864-6309

Open Monday, Tuesday, Wednesday and Thursday evenings. Provides general medical care, advice and treatment. There are physicians available each evening.

VERMONT WOMEN'S HEALTH CENTER
Colchester, Vermont 05446 (802) 655-1600

Open Monday–Saturday, 8–4. Offers pregnancy testing, pregnancy counseling, voluntary termination of pregnancy under 12 weeks, birth control counseling and devices, VD testing, and pap smears.

PEOPLE'S YELLOW PAGES
A directory of human resources of the area in the process of being put together; for information, write People's Yellow Pages, c/o Anita Landa, Plainfield, Vt. 05667.

AGENCIES PROVIDING SERVICES TO YOUNG PEOPLE IN CHITTENDEN COUNTY, VT.
This is a pamphlet compiled by Scott Lyman and Bruce Andrews. You can get a copy from the following address: Agency Pamphlet, c/o Scott Lyman, Howard Family Service Center, 260 College St., Burlington, Vermont 05401.

In other places around the country (especially in cities), a good place to contact for a community resources list is the Health and Welfare Council. Check the phone book for a local listing.

NOTES

APPENDIX I: A FEW THINGS YOU CAN DO AS A BEGINNING

(1) See what is happening in your area: Are there health groups? Is there a free clinic? If so, visit them and see what they are doing.

(2) Check to see how many people in your neighborhood or church group have parents in nursing homes or children in institutions. Would they be willing to share the caretaking responsibilities if you brought them home?

(3) Try to organize a health study group about medicine. Then check to see if there are local physicians who would be willing to meet with interested people and teach them about medicine.

(4) Find out if your local library has an adequate selection of health books. If not, does your local hospital?

(5) See if there are medic training courses being taught in your area. What are the requirements for taking them?

APPENDIX II

EMERGENCY CHILDBIRTH

A REFERENCE GUIDE FOR STUDENTS OF
THE MEDICAL SELF-HELP TRAINING COURSE
LESSON NO. 11

ACKNOWLEDGMENT

We wish to acknowledge with grateful appreciation the many services provided by the American Medical Association, through the Committee on Disaster Medical Care, Council on National Security, Board of Trustees and staff, in the preparation of this handbook.

From the inception of studies to determine emergency health techniques and procedures, the Association gave valuable assistance and support. The Committee on Disaster Medical Care of the Council on National Security, AMA, reviewed the material in its various stages of production, and made significant contributions to the content of the handbook.

EMERGENCY CHILDBIRTH

What To Do

1. Let nature be your best helper. Childbirth is a very natural act.
2. At first signs of labor assign the best qualified person to remain with mother.
3. Be calm; reassure mother.
4. Place mother and attendant in the most protected place in the shelter.
5. Keep children and others away.
6. Have hands as clean as possible.
7. Keep hands away from birth canal.
8. See that baby breathes well.
9. Place baby face down across mother's abdomen.
10. Keep baby warm.
11. Wrap afterbirth with baby.
12. Keep baby with mother constantly.
13. Make mother as comfortable as possible.
14. Identify baby.

What Not To Do

1. DO NOT hurry.
2. DO NOT pull on baby, let baby be born naturally.
3. DO NOT pull on cord, let the placenta (afterbirth) come naturally.
4. DO NOT cut and tie the cord until baby *AND* afterbirth have been delivered.
5. DO NOT give medication.

DO NOT HURRY—LET NATURE TAKE HER COURSE

If it becomes necessary for families to take refuge in fallout shelters there will undoubtedly be a number of babies born under difficult conditions and without medical assistance.

Every expectant mother and the members of her family should do all they can to prepare for emergency births. They will need to know what to do and what to have ready. (See "Expectant Mother's Emergency Childbirth Kit.")

SPECIAL SAFEGUARDS

A pregnant woman should be especially careful to protect herself from radiation exposure. She should have the most protected corner of the shelter and not be allowed to risk outside exposure.

She should not lift heavy objects or push heavy furniture. If food shortages exist, she should be given some preference.

Fear and possible exertion involved during an atomic attack will probably increase the number of premature births and of miscarriages.

PREPARATIONS

Usually there is plenty of time after the beginning of first labor pains to get ready for the delivery. Signs of labor are low-back ache, bloody-tinged mucous strings passing from the birth canal, or a gush of water from the birth canal.

The mother will need a clean surface to lie on. Her bed should be so arranged that the mattress is well protected by waterproof sheeting or pads made from several thicknesses of paper covered with cloth. Cover these protective materials with a regular bed sheet.

A warm bed should be made ready in advance for the baby. It may be a clothes basket, a box lined with a blanket, or a bureau drawer placed on firm chairs or on a table. If possible, warm the baby's blanket, shirt, and diapers with a hot water bottle. Warm bricks or a bag of table salt that has been heated can be used if a hot water bottle is not available.

A knife, a pair of scissors, or a razor should be thoroughly cleansed and sterilized in preparation for cutting the umbilical cord. If there is no way to boil water to sterilize them (the preferred method of sterilization), sterilize them by submersion in 70 percent isopropyl alcohol solution for at least 20 minutes or up to 3 hours, if possible. Sterile tapes for tying the umbilical cord will be needed. (Do not remove them from their sterile wrappings until you are ready to use them.) If no tapes are available, a clean shoestring or a strip of sheeting (folded into a narrow tie) can be boiled and used wet as a cord tie substitute.

STAGES OF LABOR

Labor is the term used to describe the process of childbirth. It consists of the contractions of the wall of the womb (uterus) which force the baby and, later, the afterbirth (placenta) into the outside world. Labor is divided into three stages. Its duration varies greatly in different persons and under different circumstances.

During the first and longest stage, the small opening at the lower end of the womb gradually stretches until it is large enough to let the baby pass through. The contractions (tightening) of the uterus, which bring about this stretching and move the baby along into the birth canal, cause pains known as labor pains.

These pains, usually beginning as an aching sensation in the small of the back, turn in a short time into regularly recurring cramplike pains in the lower abdomen. By placing your hand on the mother's abdomen just above the navel, you can feel each tightening of the uterus as an increasing firmness or hardness. It last for 30 to 60 seconds. The pains disappear each time the uterus relaxes.

At first these pains occur from 10 to 20 minutes apart and are not very severe. They may even stop completely for awhile and then start up again. The mother should rest when she is tired but need not be lying down continuously. She may sleep between tightenings if she can. She can take a little water or perhaps tea during the entire labor process. She should urinate frequently during labor so the bladder will be as empty as possible at the time of birth.

The skin in the vaginal area of the mother should be sponged occasionally with soapy water. Special attention should be given to cleaning the inner sides of the thighs and the rectal area with heavy lather. Soap or water should not be allowed to enter the vagina.

A slight, watery, bloodstained discharge from the vagina normally accompanies labor pains or occurs before the pains begin.

For first babies, this stage of labor may continue for as long as 18 hours or more. For women who have had a previous baby, it may last only 2 or 3 hours.

The end of this first stage is usually signalled by the sudden passing of a large gush of water (a pint or so), caused by the normal breaking of the bag of waters which surrounds the baby in the mother's womb. For some women, the bag of waters breaks before labor begins or perhaps as the first sign of its beginning. This should not cause the mother or those helping her any concern. It usually does not seriously affect the birth.

Through this first stage of labor, the mother does not have to work to help the baby be born. She should not try to push the baby down, but should try to relax her muscles. She can help do this by taking deep breaths with her mouth open during each tightening.

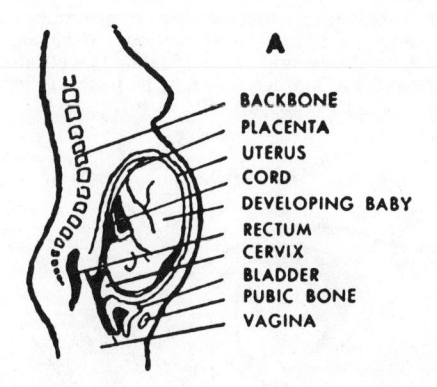

At full term, or after 40 weeks of pregnancy, the baby is ready to be born. The cervix through which baby must leave the uterus is shown clearly here, still closed. The contractions of the muscles of the uterus will open the cervix, and force the baby down through the vagina, or birth canal, to the outside.

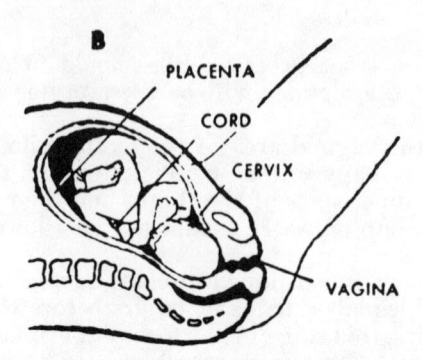

At the end of the first stage of labor the cervix is completely open and the baby's head is beginning to come down through the vagina. Contractions begin in the lower back and later are felt in the lower abdomen. At the time shown here contractions are probably coming every 2 minutes, lasting 40–60 seconds and very strong.

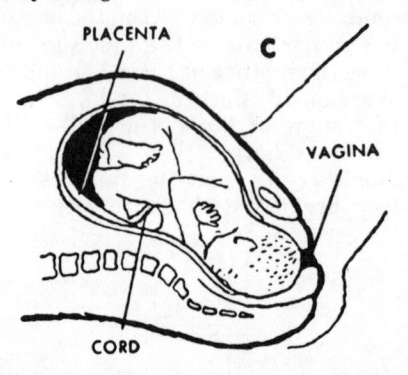

The first stage of labor usually lasts several hours and is hard work. The mother needs to relax, rest, and be reassured. Give her water and fruit juices. In this picture the second stage of labor is well along. It is shorter than the first stage and the mother will now be pushing down with each contraction, helping to force the baby into the world.

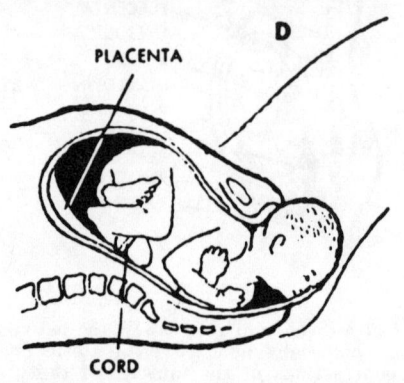

The head of the baby has been partially born. This shows the usual position with the face down and the back of the head up. The bag of waters in which the baby is enclosed throughout the pregnancy may have broken at the beginning of labor, before or during the first stage. It may break now, or have to be torn with the fingers.

APPENDIX II: EMERGENCY CHILDBIRTH 273

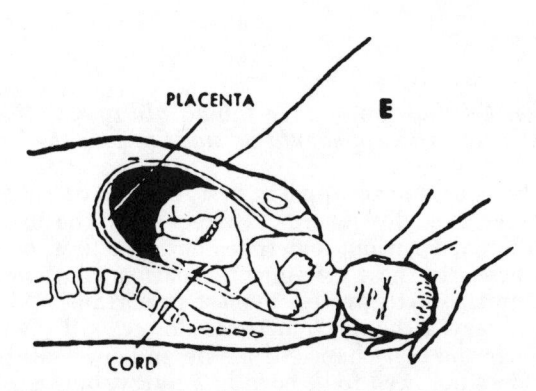

Here you see the baby's head turned to the right as is usual. The shoulders are about to be born. The head must turn so that the baby's body can fit into the birth canal and come through more easily. After the birth of the baby there will be further uterine contractions and the placenta will be separated from the uterine wall and expelled.

CHANGE OF FEELING

Gradually the time between the labor pains grows shorter and the pains increase in severity until they are coming every 2 to 3 minutes. It will not be long now before the baby is born.

At this stage the mother will notice a change. Instead of the tightness in the lower abdomen and pain across the back, she will feel a bearing down sensation almost as if she were having a bowel movement. This means the baby is moving down.

When this happens, she should lie down and get ready for the birth of the child. The tightening and bearing down feelings will come more frequently and be harder.

She will have an uncontrollable urge to push down, which she may do. But she should not work too hard at it because the baby will be brought down without her straining too hard. There will probably be more blood showing at this point.

The person attending the delivery should thoroughly scrub hands with soap and water. Never touch the vagina or put fingers inside for any reason. The mother also should keep her hands away from the vagina.

As soon as a bulge begins to appear in the vaginal area and part of the baby is visible, the mother should stop pushing down. She should try to breath like a panting dog with her mouth open in order not to push the baby out too rapidly with consequent tearing of her tissue.

She should keep her knees up and legs separated so that the person helping her can get at the baby more easily.

MOMENT OF BIRTH

The person helping the mother should always let the baby be born by itself. No attempt should be made to pull the baby out in any way.

Usually the baby's head appears first, the top of the head presenting and the face downward. Infrequently the baby will be born in a different position, sometimes buttocks first, occasionally foot or arm first. In these infrequent situations, patience without interference in the birth process is most important. The natural process of delivery, although sometimes slower, will give the child and the mother the best chance of a safe and successful birth.

The baby does not need to be born in a hurry, but usually about a minute after the head appears the mother will have another bearing down feeling and push the shoulders and the rest of the baby out.

As the baby is being expelled, the person helping the mother should support the baby on her hands and arms so that the baby will avoid contact with any blood or waste material on the bed.

If there is still a membrane from the water sac over the baby's head and face at delivery, it should immediately be taken between the fingers and torn so that the water inside will run out and the baby can breathe.

If, as sometimes happens, the cord, which attaches the child from its navel to the placenta in the mother's womb, should be wrapped around the baby's neck when his head and neck appear, try to slip it quickly over his head so that he will not strangle.

After the baby is born, wrap a fold of towel around his ankles to prevent slipping and hold him up by the heels with one hand, taking care that the cord is slack. To get a good safe grip, insert one finger between the baby's ankles. Do not swing or spank the baby. Hold him over the bed so that he cannot fall far if he should slip from your grasp. The baby's body will be very slippery. Place your other hand under the baby's forehead and bend its head back slightly so that the fluid and mucus can run out of its mouth. When the baby begins to cry, lay him on his side on the bed close enough to the mother to keep the cord slack.

The baby will usually cry within the first minute. If he does not cry or breathe within 2 or 3 minutes, use mouth-to-mouth artificial respiration.

Very little force should be used in blowing air into the baby's mouth. A short puff of breath about every 5 seconds is enough. As soon as the baby starts to breathe or cry, mouth-to-mouth breathing should be stopped.

CUTTING THE CORD

There should be no hurry to cut the cord. Take as much time as necessary to prepare the ties and sharp instruments.

You will need two pieces of sterile white cotton tape or two pieces of 1-inch wide sterile guaze bandage about 9 inches long to use to tie the cord. (If you do not have sterile material for tying the cord but do have facilities for boiling water, strips of sheeting—boiled for 15 to 20 minutes to make them sterile—can be used. Tie the umbilical cord with the sterile tape in two places, one about 4 inches from the baby and the other 2 inches farther along the cord toward the mother, making two or more simple knots at each place. Cut the cord between these two ties with a clean sharp instrument such as a knife, razor blade, or scissors.

A sterile dressing about 4 inches square should be placed over the cut end of the cord at the baby's navel and should be held in place by wrapping a "belly band" or folded diaper around the baby. If a sterile dressing is not available, no dressing or belly band should be used. Regardless of whether a dressing is applied or not, no powder, solution, or disinfectant of any kind should be put on the cord or navel.

If the afterbirth has not yet been expelled, cover the end of the umbilical cord attached to it (and now protruding from the vagina) with a sterile dressing and tie it in place.

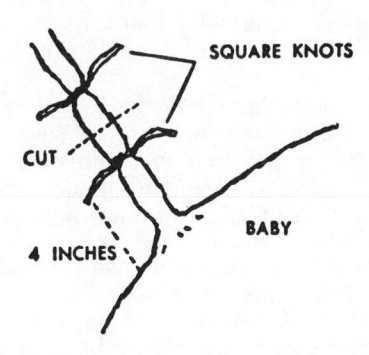

Cut between the square knots. Tie a square knot by bringing left tape over right tape for first loop and right tape over left for second loop. Tighten each loop firmly as tied. Use scissors or a razor blade to cut cord.

THIRD STAGE OF LABOR

Usually a few minutes after the baby is born (although sometimes an hour or more will elapse) the mother will feel a brief return of the labor pains which had ceased with the birth. These are due to contractions of the uterus as it seeks to expel the afterbirth. *Do not pull on the cord to hurry this process.*

Some bleeding is to be expected at this stage. If there is a lot of bleeding before the afterbirth is expelled, the attendant should gently massage the mother's abdomen, just above the navel. This will help the uterus to tighten, help the afterbirth come out, and reduce bleeding.

It may be desirable to put the baby almost immediately to the mother's breast for a minute or two on each side even though the mother will have no milk as yet. This helps the uterus contract and reduces the bleeding.

Someone should stand by the mother and occasionally massage her abdomen gently for about an hour after the afterbirth is expelled. After that, the mother should feel the rounded surface of the uterus through the abdomen and squeeze firmly but gently with her fingers.

The bedding should be changed and the mother sponged. Washing and wiping of the vaginal area should always be done from the front to the back in order to avoid contamination. A sanitary napkin should be applied.

Keep the mother warm with blankets. She may have a slight chill. Give her a warm (not hot) drink of sweetened tea, milk, or bouillon. Wipe her hands and face with a damp towel. She may drop off to sleep.

The mother's diet after delivery may include any available foods she wishes. She may eat or drink as soon as she wants to, and she should be encouraged to drink plenty of fluids, especially milk. Canned milk can be used and made more palatable by diluting with equal parts of water and adding sugar, eggs, chocolate, or other flavoring.

For the first 24 or 48 hours after delivery, the mother will continue to have some cramping pain in the lower abdomen which may cause a great deal of discomfort. Aspirin may help relieve these afterpains. She should empty her bladder every few hours for 2 days following the birth. If her bowels do not move within 3 days after delivery, she should be given an enema.

MISCARRIAGE

If a pregnant woman shows evidence of bleeding, she should restrict her activities and rest in bed in an effort to prevent possible loss of the baby. If a miscarriage does occur, keep the patient flat with the foot of the bed elevated from 12 to 18 inches to retard vaginal bleeding. Keep her warm and quiet, and give her fluids.

EXPECTANT MOTHER'S EMERGENCY CHILDBIRTH KIT

The public health and civil defense agencies of one State have planned a 1½-pound emergency childbirth kit made up of basic supplies that can be carried in a 1-yard square receiving blanket.

The kit consists of the following:

    One-yard square of outing flannel, hemmed (receiving blanket).
    Plastic (polyethylene flexible film) for outer wrapping of the kit if desired. (*Do not* wrap the baby in this plastic film.)
    One or two diapers.
    Four sanitary napkins (wrapped).
    Adhesive tape identification strips for mother and baby.
    Short pencil.
    Soap.

    Sterile package containing:
        Small pair of blunt-end scissors (cheapest scissors will do), or a safety razor blade with a guard on one side.
        Four pieces of white cotton tape, ½-inch wide and 9 inches long.[1]
        Four cotton balls.
        Roll of 3-inch gauze bandage.
        Six 4-inch squares of gauze.[1]
        Two or more safety pins.

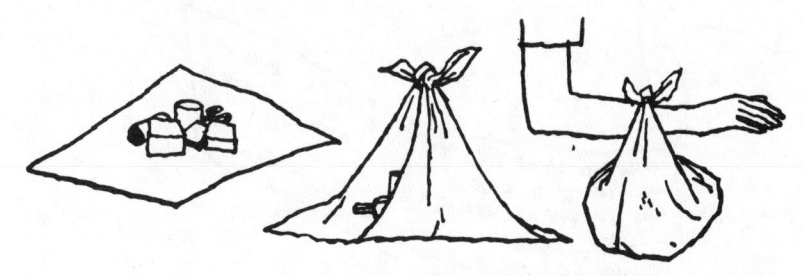

Instructions such as those contained in this chapter also should be considered a part of the emergency childbirth kit.

To make the kit ready to carry, lay the plastic (if used) out flat, and lay receiving blanket out flat on top of the plastic. Place the diapers, sterile package, soap, sanitary napkins, identification tapes, pencil, and instructions in the center. Pull two opposite corners of the receiving blanket and plastic together and tie. Do the same with the other opposite corners, pulling each side together well so that nothing will fall out. Then tightly knot the loose ends together in the same way, leaving an opening so that the kit can be slipped over the arm for carrying the kit while leaving the hands free.

---

[1] You will actually use only two tapes for tying the umbilical cord. The two extras are included as a safeguard in case one or two should be dropped or soiled. Extra 4-inch squares of gauze also are included.

Such an emergency delivery kit will weigh about 1½ pounds. The contents suggested are basic essentials only, for extreme emergency. Much more could be added, but the extra weight might mean leaving behind some other items needed for survival. Additional supplies could be stored in your home shelter to be ready in the event the birth takes place there. In case there is no need for an emergency delivery, either in the home shelter or in some evacuation situation, the supplies in the kit can be used in home care of the baby.

IDENTIFICATION TAPES

In emergency situations, identification will be particularly important, especially if the birth should take place in a group shelter rather than a family shelter, or in an evacuation situation.

Two wide strips of adhesive tape will be needed—one long enough to go around the mother's wrist, and the other long enough to go around the baby's ankle. Information should be written on these strips as shown below.

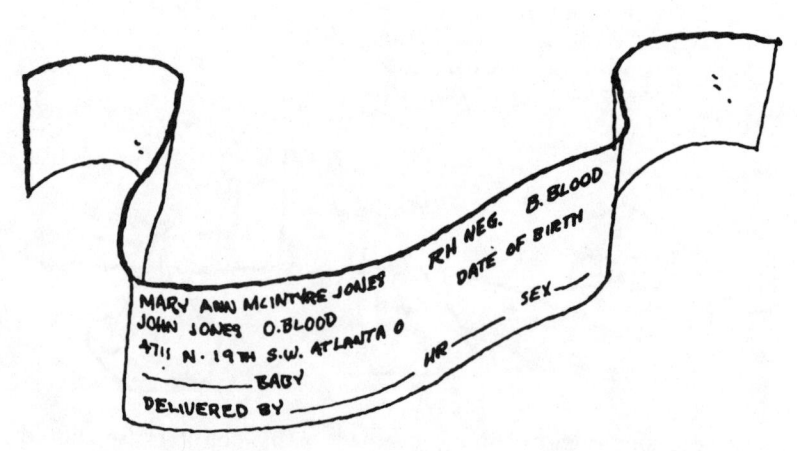

For Mother—Write parents' names, blood types, and mother's Rh factor, street address, and whether it is a first or later child.

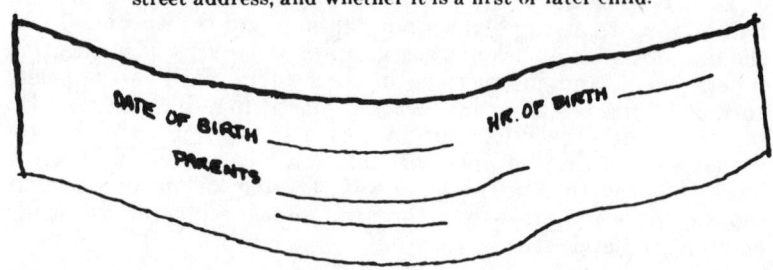

For Baby—Write date and hour of birth and parents' names and address.

APPENDIX III: UNIVERSAL DONOR CONTRACT

of _____
　　　　　　　　　　　　　　Print name of donor

In the hope that I may help others, I hereby make this anatomical gift, if medically acceptable, to take effect upon my death. The words and marks below indicate my desires.

I give:　　(a)　_____　any needed organs or parts
　　　　　　(b)　_____　only the following organs or parts

_____
　　　　　　　　　　　　(Specify the organ(s) or part(s)
for the purposes of transplantation, therapy, medical research or education;
　　　　　　(c)　_____　my body for anatomical study if needed.
　　Limitation or
　　special wishes, if any: _____

Signed by the donor and the following two witnesses in the presence of each other:

_____　　　　_____
　　　　Signature of Donor　　　　　　　　　　　Date of Birth of Donor

_____　　_____　_____
　　　Date Signed　　　　　　　　　　City　　　　　　　　　　State

_____　　　　_____
　　　　　　Witness　　　　　　　　　　　　　　　　Witness

This is a legal document under the Uniform Anatomical Gift Act or similar laws.

　　For further information consult your physician or

　　　National Kidney Foundation
　　　315 Park Avenue, South
　　　New York, New York 10010

BIBLIOGRAPHY

You can start to learn about health by reading about it. Any medical bookstore will have the standard textbooks. Some of the following might not be in a bookstore, but are worth ordering.

The Medicine Show, Editors of Consumer Reports, 1970, Revised Edition. Consumers Union, Mount Vernon, New York 10550. $2.00

The Medical Messiah, by James Harvey Young, Princeton University, Princeton, New Jersey, 1967. $2.00 (by Consumers Union)

Layman's Medical Dictionary, Frederick Ungau Publishing Co., 250 Park Avenue, New York, New York 10003. $1.75

Medical Corpsman and Medical Specialist. No. TM8-230. Available from: Superintendent of Documents, U.S. Government Printing Office, Washington, D.C. $1.75

Ship Captain's Medical Guide. Government Bookshop, P.O. Box 569, London S.E. 1, England. $3.60

Birth Control Handbook by McGill Students Society. From: Birth Control Handbook, 3480 McTavish Street, Montreal 112, Quebec, Canada. 25 cents for one, 10 cents for each additional copy

Composition of Foods. Bernice K. Watt, Annabel L. Merrill. From: Superintendent of Documents, U.S. Government Printing Office, Washington, D.C. $1.50

Emergency Medical Guide. John Henderson, M.D. McGraw Hill Book Company, Princeton, New Jersey. $3.95

Folk Medicine. D. C. Jarvis, M.D., Henry Holt & Company, New York, 1958. "I like Vermont medicine—I'm not sure there's much evidence for the clinical efficacy of apple cider vinegar and honey. But try it if you want."

Lange Medical Publications. P.O. Drawer "1", Los Altos, California 94022. "Have several inexpensive up-to-date paperback textbooks on pediatrics, obstetrics, internal medicine, diagnosis and treatment of poisoning, etc. available at reasonable prices."

Island. Aldous Huxley, Bantam Books, New York, 1963. "For a look at medicine the way it ought to be."

The Peckham Experiment. Innes H. Pearse and Lucy H. Crocker, George Allen and Unwin Ltd., 40 Museum Street, W.C., London, England. "A beautiful experiment in which medical care was seen to involve the life-style, home conditions, etc.—a model for a reasonable, non-sterile, socialized medical care system—ignored by the British politicians when they set up their present shoddy system."

Women and Their Bodies. Available from: Boston Women's Health Collective.

Commonsense Childbirth, by Lester D. Hazzell, Tower Publications, $5.95

Emergency Childbirth Manual, by Gregory J. White (available from the Police Training Foundation, 3412 Ruby Street, Franklin Park, Illinois 60131).

Husband-Coached Childbirth, by Robert Bradley, Harper and Row, $4.95.

Painless Childbirth, by Marjorie Karmel, Dolphin Books.

Textbook for Midwives, by Margaret F. Myles. 6th Edition, 1968, E. & M. Livingstone Ltd., Edinburgh, London. Printed by Darien Press, Great Britain.

Articles on Women's Health Problems including pamphlets on:
    A. Venereal Disease
    B. Common Infections of the Vaginal Area
    C. The Gynecological Examination
    D. Saline Abortions
    E. Vacuum Aspiration Abortions
        Available from: Women's Health and Abortion Project
                36 West 22nd Street
                New York, New York 10010

Remedies and Old Wives Tales, by W. W. Bauer, Doubleday & Company, Inc. Garden City, New York, 1969.

Syllabus of Laboratory Examinations in Clinical Science, by Tot. B. Page & Perry J. Culver, Harvard University Press, Cambridge, Mass. 1966—"You can do anything you want—with Page & Culver, a few chemicals, perhaps a microscope, and some anal compulsivity—" a clear and authoritative guide to laboratory examinations.

Handbook of Prescription Drugs by Richard Burack, Random House, New York, New York. "A guide to prescription drugs and their prices—buy two copies and give one to your physician."

* *Towards Earlier Diagnosis,* by Keith Hodgkin, E. & S. Livingstone Ltd., Edinburgh and London, 1966. $7.50. "A superb book—written by a family practitioner in England—tells you how to make diagnoses without hospitalization or expensive laboratory tests. Especially important in our age of mechanodiagnosis where physicians no longer talk to or touch their patients."

How to Raise a Human Being by Lee Salk & Rita Kramer, Random House, New York, New York. $5.95

INDEX

Abortion, 219-222
Abscess, 37
Agencies
    Abortion, 221-222
    Crisis centers, 146
    Human resource, in Vermont, 261-265
    Mental health, 157-159
Air temperature, effect of windspeed on, 55-56
Amphetamines, 137-138
Animal bite, 37
Animals, health of, 3-5
    diseases of, 5-6, 73-75, 80
Anxiety, 151-161
Artificial respiration, 31-32
Asthma, 37, 124-125
Athlete's foot, 229-230

Babies, home delivery of, 173-203, 267-278
Bad trips, 142-146
Bandaging, 33
Bang's Disease, 5
Bedbugs, 7, 9
Birth control, 209-218
    Mechanical means, 210-216
    Pills, 216-217
    Rhythm, 217-218
    Sterilization, 209-210
Birth of a baby, 173-203, 267-278
Bites, 37, 43
Bleeding, 31, 33
Blisters, 37
Bodies, women's. *See* Women's health
Boils, 37
Botulism, 83-85
Breast feeding, 204-207
Breast self-examination, 165-166
Breathing, artificial, 31-32
Burial, 248-250
Burns, 34-35, 51-54

Cancer, 165, 166, 168

Canning, 82-86
Cats, diseases of, 6
Chest wounds, 33
Chicken pox, 12
Chickens, diseases of, 5-6
Chiggers, 7
Childbirth, 173-203, 267-278
Child care, 223-226
Chills, 37
Choking, 38
Civil rights, 255-259
Cockroach, 8, 9
Colds, 37, 124
Communal diseases, 228-230
Communicable disease, 10-15, 71-75, 231-235, 236. *See also* Common Emergencies Guide, 31-48
Compost privy, 16-23, 78, 79
Constipation, 225
Convulsions, 39, 226
Cows, 5, 73-74, 80
Cremation, 250
Crisis centers, 146
Croup, 40
Cuts, 126

Death, 248-250
Dental health, 119-120
Diabetes, 40
Diarrhea, 40, 125, 223-224
Diet, 89-118
Dishwashing, 72
Dogs, diseases of, 6
Donor contract, 279
Drugs, 136-150
    Drug centers, 146
    Drug laws, 146-150
    Drugs, toxicity, 142-146
Dysentery, 13

Earache, 40
Emergency. *See* First aid
Epilepsy, 39
Exposure, 55-56

Eye irritation, 40

Family planning, 209-218
Farm equipment, 239-240
Fever, 41, 124, 225
Fire safety, 242-246
First aid
    Bleeding, 31, 33
    Breathing, 31, 32
    Burns, 34, 51-54
    Chest wound, 33
    Childbirth, 173-203, 267-278
    Choking, 38
    Convulsion, 39
    Drug toxicity, 142-146
    Fractures, 33-34
    Headache, 42
    Heart beat lost, 31
    Heatstroke, 42
    Insect bite, 8, 43
    Poisoning, 44, 58-62, 84
    Psychological, 151-161
    Shock, 35
    Snake bite, 45
    Stroke, 42, 46
    Supplies, 47-48, 51-54
    Toothache, 46, 120
    Unconsciousness, 46-47
    Wounds, 51-54
Fleas, 7, 9, 74-75
Flies, 8, 9, 72-73
Flu, 13, 124
Food hygiene and sanitation, 3-4, 71-73, 82-88
Fractures, 33-34
Freezing foods, 87
Freezing, skin, 41-42, 55-56
Frost bite, 41-42, 55-56

Gastroenteritis, 229
Gonorrhea, 13, 231-235
Gum sores, 120

Hallucinogens, 140-141
Headache, 42

Heart beat lost, 31
Heart emergency, 31, 42, 44
Heatstroke, 42
Helpful agencies. See Human resources.
Hepatitis, 13, 139, 236-238
Herbalism, 122-134
Hernia, 43
Home delivery of babies, 173-203, 267-278
Home nursing, 155-156
Hookworm disease, 12
Human resources, 261-264
Human waste, 16-23, 64-71, 76-79

Immunization, 4, 10-11, 223-226
Infections, 37
   Urinary, 231-235
   Vaginal, 167-168
Infectious diseases, 10-11, 12-15
   Athlete's foot, 229-230
   Chicken pox, 12
   Gastroenteritis, 229
   Gonorrhea, 13, 231-235
   Hepatitis, 13, 139, 236-238
   Influenza, 13, 124
   Meningitis, 43
   Mononucleosis, 228
   Mumps, 14
   Syphilis, 14, 168, 232-234
   Typhoid, 15
   Urinary tract infection, 228
Influenza, 13, 124
Insect bites, 43
Insect control, 6-10, 74-75, 228-229
Intestinal parasites, 74
I.U.D., 214-216

Latrines. See Toilets
Laws, Vermont, 146-150, 255-259
Legal help, 255-259
Lice, control of, 6-10, 74-75, 228-229
Liver, infection of, 236-238

Mastitis, 5, 73-74
Measles, 13, 14
Medic, role of, 1-29
Medical supplies, 47-48, 51-54

Meningitis, 43
Mental health, 151-161
Mites, 7, 9
Mononucleosis, 228
Mouth sores, 120
Mouth-to-mouth respiration, 32
Mumps, 14

Natural medicines, 122-134
Nausea, 43-44
Nosebleed, 44
Nutrition, 82-88, 89-118, 119

Organs, gift of, 279

Pain, 44
Parasites, intestinal, 74
Pasteurization, 64, 74, 80
Pediatric care, 223-226
Pigs, diseases of, 6
Pinworms, 229
Plants, poisonous, 127-129
Plants, as medicine, 122-134
Poisoning, 44, 58-62, 84-85, 127-129
Pregnancy, 173-203
Prenatal care, 173-193
Privy. See Toilets.
Protein, 90-91
Psychological problems, 151-161
Ptomaine poisoning, 82-85

Rash, skin, 44
Recipes, 95-97, 113-115
Reproductive organs, female, 163-202, 231-234
Rhythm. See Birth control.

Salmonellosis, 5-6
Sanitation, 64-80
   Food, 3-4
   Human waste, 16-23, 68-71
   Water, 24-29, 65-68
Seizure, 39, 226
Septic tank system, 22, 23, 79
Shit, 16-23, 64-71, 76-99
Shock, 35
Skin infections and rashes, 37, 44, 126

Snakebite, 45
Sore throat, 39, 226
Spiders, 8
Splinting, 33-34
Spoilage, in canning, 82-88
Sprains, 34, 126
Storage of food, 82-88
Stress, 151-156
Stroke, 42, 46
Suicide, 160-161
Syphilis, 14, 168, 232-234

Teeth, care of, 119-120
Tetanus, 10, 46
Ticks, 7, 9
Toilets, 16-23, 78, 79
Toothache, 46, 120
Tooth, extracted, 120
Transporting injured, 35-36
Trichinosis, 6
Tuberculosis, 5, 10, 15
Typhoid, 15

Unconsciousness, 46-47
Universal donor contract, 279
Urinary tract infection, 228
Urination, burning, 228, 231-235

Vaccines, 10-11
Vaginal infection, 167-168
Vegetarian diet, 89-118
Venereal disease, 13, 14, 168, 231-235
Vermont agencies, 146, 157-159, 221-222, 261-265
Vermont laws, 146-150, 255-259
Vitamins, 89-118
Vomiting, 43-44

Waste, human and animal, 64-80
Water, 64-68, 75-77, 79
Wells, 24-28, 79
Whooping cough, 14
Wind chill effect, 55-56
Withdrawal, 142-146
Women's health, 163-222
Wounds, 51-54, 124

Yogurt, 115

NOTES

NOTES